# Level 2

# Health and Social Care Diploma

# Level 2
# Health and Social Care Diploma

Val Michie
Caroline Morris
Layla Baker
Fiona Collier
Tina Marshall

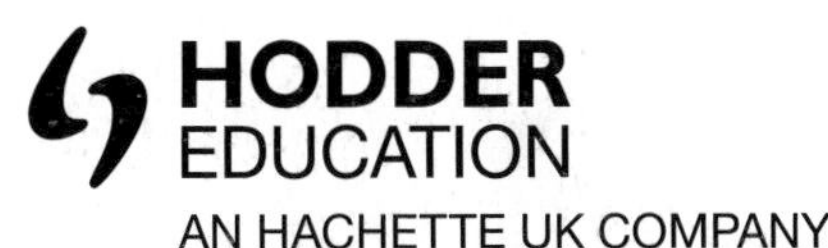

Orders: please contact Bookpoint Ltd, 130 Milton Park, Abingdon, Oxon OX14 4SB. Telephone: (44) 01235 827720. Fax: (44) 01235 400454. Lines are open from 9.00 to 5.00, Monday to Saturday, with a 24 hour message answering service. You can also order through our website www.hoddereducation.co.uk

If you have any comments to make about this, or any of our other titles, please send them to educationenquiries@hodder.co.uk

British Library Cataloguing in Publication Data
A catalogue record for this title is available from the British Library

ISBN: 978 1 444 135411

First Edition Published 2011
Impression number 10 9 8 7 6 5 4 3 2 1
Year 2015, 2014, 2013, 2012, 2011



Cover photo © Camille Tokerud / The Image Bank / Getty Images
Typeset by DC Graphic Design Limited, Swanley Village, Kent
Printed in Great Britain for Hodder Education, an Hachette UK Company, 338 Euston Road, London NW1 3BH.

# Contents

# Acknowledgements and Author biographies

**Acknowledgements and Author biographies**

Every effort has been made to trace and acknowledge ownership of copyright. The publishers will be glad to make suitable arrangements with any copyright holders whom it has not been possible to contact.

**Figure 4.3** Fall 2005 Judicial Database Systems Team Organisation; **P.75**. Statistics from NSPCC; **Chapter 10** References to Living with Dementia: A National Dementia Strategy DH 2009 Crown copyright; **Table 13.3** Responsibilities under the Manual Handling Operation taken from Getting to Grips with Manual Handling A Short Guide HSC 2006, contains public sector information published by the Health and Safety Executive and licensed under the Open Government Licence v1.0; **Page 177, 179, 181, 182** 'Living well with Dementia: A National Strategy' DH 2009 contains public sector information licensed under the Open Government Licence v1.0

The authors and publishers would like to thank the following for the use of images in this volume:

**Photo credits**

**1.1** © Monkey Business / Fotolia.com; **1.2** © Paula Solloway / Photofusion; **1.3** © Kelly Young / Fotolia.com; **2.1** © Tyler Olson / Fotolia.com; **2.4** © Susanne Güttler / Fotolia.com; **2.6** © Lisa F. Young / Fotolia.com; **2.7** © Arrow Studio / Fotolia.com; **3.1** © Marc Dietrich / Fotolia.com; **3.3** © PictureArt / Fotolia.com; **4.1** © Monkey Business / Fotolia.com; **4.4** © Monkey Business / Fotolia.com; **5.3** © Nikola Hristovski / Fotolia.com; **5.6** © Joanne Obrien / Photofusion; **5.8** © gwimages / Fotolia.com; **5.12** © Ocean/Corbis; **6.3** © Andy Dean / Fotolia.com; **6.4** © Radius Images/Corbis; **7.1** © 67photo / Alamy; **7.6** © mario beauregard / Fotolia.com; **7.9** © John Birdsall/John Birdsall/ Press Association Images; **7.13** © Paul Doyle / Photofusion; **8.4** © Bubbles Photolibrary / Alamy; **8.6** © Libby Welch / Alamy; **8.10** © MAMZ Images / Fotolia.com; **8.11** © Thomas Perkins / Fotolia.com; **9.1** © deanm1974 / Fotolia.com; **11.4** © Yannis Ntousiopoulos / Fotolia.com; **11.7** © Vladimir Mucibabic / Fotolia.com; **12.5** © Alexander Raths/ Fotolia.com; **12.9** © Terry J Alcorn / Getty Images; **12.11** © pressmaster / Fotolia.com.

**Author biographies**

**Val Michie** has an academic background in the biological sciences and in health and social welfare. Prior to becoming a Consultant in Education and Training for the Health and Care Sector in 2001, in which capacity she works with a wide range of training providers within the private, statutory and trades union sectors, she worked in medical research and then as a lecturer in FE, teaching health sciences, key skills and Health and Social Care. Her more recent role as a technical author has involved her in writing underpinning knowledge and assessment activities for a number of qualifications, including NVQs, Technical Certificates and BTECs in Health and Social Care. She is currently exploring issues related to dementia and elderly care in health and social care settings.

**Caroline Morris** has a background in the health service, having worked as a nurse, Registered Care Manager and, more recently, a teacher and lecturer, delivering in Health and Social Care since 1992. Caroline has provided services to OCR, Edexcel, OU and EDI as an external verifier in Public Services since 1997, and has been involved in writing materials and specifications for publishers and EDI and OCR awarding bodies. Caroline is carrying out post-graduate research in education to achieve PhD, and also undertakes inspections on behalf of BIIAB, EDI, OU and BAC.

**Layla Baker** is currently Subject Leader in Health and Social Care and Lead IV for BTEC courses, taught Health and Social Care for 14 years at Level 1, 2,3 and in Higher Education. She has worked in Further Education, Higher Education, 6th form college and is currently in a school teaching Key Stage 4 and 5. Layla has qualifications in BA Social Policy, Masters Health Service Studies, PGCE in Post 16 Education, QTS and is currently studying for a Masters in Teaching and Education. She has previously written textbooks and CD-roms for BTEC Firsts and BTEC Diplomas as well as learning materials for Age Concern.

**Fiona Collier** is a registered nurse with a varied experience within the field of Health and Social Care. In addition to her clinical skills Fiona has also worked as a teacher, trainer and internal moderator within Further Education providing work based training and education to health and social care workers. Fiona is presently working as a Consultant in Education and Training for the Health and Social Care Sector. This role involves designing, delivering and evaluating training as well as writing educational material for publishers and awarding bodies. Fiona has written the underpinning knowledge and assessments for a number of awards and qualifications including NVQs and VRQs.

**Tina Marshall** commenced her career in nursing as an auxiliary nurse in a large psychiatric institution in Surrey, and gained her Enrolled nurse qualification in May 1981. Tina then worked for several nursing agencies prior to her move to Somerset in 1986. In 1986 Tina worked for the NHS trust where she gained her D32 / 33 in assessing and verifying. She then completed her conversion course in 1986. Tina worked in a variety of settings including managing private nursing homes. In January 2007 she commenced work in City of Bristol College as Curriculum Manager for delivery of NVQs in Health and Social Care.

# Walkthrough

## We want you to succeed!

This book has been designed to support the new QCF Level 2 Diploma in Health and Social Care. This qualification has replaced the previous NVQ at Level 2. It has been written with the work-based learner in mind. Everything in it reflects the assessment criteria and evidence based approach that is applied to this vocational qualification.

We've included everything you will need for the mandatory units at this level. We've also included enough of the most popular optional units to see you through a full Diploma in Health and Social Care.

In the pages that follow you will find up-to-date resource material which will develop your knowledge, rehearse your skills and help you to gain your qualification. Each unit incorporates a step-by-step guide for you to follow allowing you to work your way through each unit with materials such as activities and real life case studies.

**Prepare for what you are going to cover in this unit, and prepare for assessment:**

The reading and activities in this chapter will help you to:

- Understand what is required for competence in your work role
- Be able to reflect on your work practice
- Be able to agree a personal development plan

**Reinforce concepts with hands-on learning and generate evidence for assignments**

Practice activity 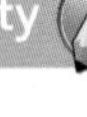

 Your own role in responding to complaints

This activity helps demonstrate your knowledge of your own role in responding to complaints.

Time to reflect 

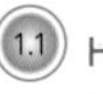 How does your job measure up?

Think about your duties and responsibilities.

1. Are they more or less what you expected them to be?
2. Do you sometimes find the job demanding and easier said than done or, on the other hand, insufficiently interesting or challenging?

Evidence activity 

 Describe the duties and responsibilities of own role

This activity enables you to demonstrate your knowledge of your own work role.

Research & investigate 

 Regulations

Look at the some of the regulations mentioned above.

1. What are the key principles?
2. Why would an effective care worker need to know these?

**Understand how your learning fits into real life and your working environment**

## Case Study

Charlotte

Charlotte Brown recently started working as a domestic at Tiny Tots Playgroup because, according to her mother, 'she absolutely loves children, is so good with them, she's always buying them presents, they love her to bits'.

1. Do you think Mrs Brown's assessment of her daughter's performance has any value?

**Check new words and what they mean**

## Key Term

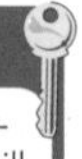

Sector Skills Councils (SSCs) are employer-led organisations that work to boost the skills of their sector workforces.

**You've just covered a whole unit so here's a guide to what assessors will be looking for and links to activities that can help impress them**

## Assessment summary

Your reading of this chapter and completion of the activities will have prepared you to demonstrate your learning and understanding of the principles of safeguarding and protection in health and social care. Assessment of Learning Outcomes 2,3,4,5 and 6 must be assessed in a real work environment. To achieve the unit, your assessor will require you to:

| Learning Outcomes | Assessment Criteria |
|---|---|
| Learning Outcome 1: Understand what is required for competence in your work role by: | 1.1 describing the duties and responsibilities of own role<br><br>See Evidence activity 1.1 on p. 20 |
| |  1.2 identifying standards that influence the way the role is carried out<br><br>See Evidence activity 1.2 on p. 23 |
| |  1.3 describing ways to ensure that personal attitudes or beliefs do not obstruct the quality of work.<br><br>See Evidence activity 1.3 on p. 24 |

**The internet's great for further research. There are pointers to some of the more useful information out there for assignments**

## Weblinks

| | |
|---|---|
| Care Quality Commission | www.cqc.org.u |
| Community Care Careers | www.communitycare.co.uk/jobs/search |
| General Medical Council | www.gmc-uk.org |
| General Social Care Council | ww.gscc.org.uk |
| General Teaching Council for England | www.gtce.org.uk |

# 1 Introduction to communication in health, social care or children's and young people's settings

## For Unit SHC21

### What are you finding out?

This chapter is about the importance of communication in such settings, and how we can overcome barriers to meet individual needs and preferences in communication.

You will need to be aware of the different ways of communicating, including verbal and non verbal. You will also need to be aware of the impact of confidentiality on your role.

The reading and activities in this chapter will help you to:

- Understand why communication is important in the work setting
- Be able to meet the communication and language needs, wishes and preferences of individuals
- Overcome barriers to communication
- Be able to respect equality and diversity when communicating
- Be able to apply principles and practices relating to confidentiality at work.

## LO1 Understand why communication is important in the work setting

### 1.1 The different reasons people communicate

As a worker you can provide a range of information to individuals who use services, to enable them to understand the support that is available to meet their needs. You could ask the individual for their opinions about the provision available and encourage them to make choices.

Exchanging information is important in order to develop your understanding of the needs of an individual, so that you can provide the support the client requires and improve the quality of service provision. If the information exchanged is inaccurate, mistakes can be made, for example, an individual could be prescribed the wrong medication if the GP did not know they were allergic to it. If information is not exchanged, individuals may not feel supported and workers will not be able to carry out their job roles as effectively as they could.

**Evidence activity**

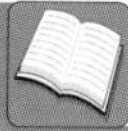

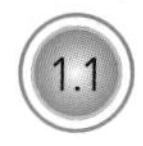 & 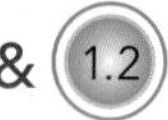

**1.1 & 1.2 Thinking about people you communicate with and why**

This activity will demonstrate your knowledge of the different reasons we communicate and how this affects all aspects of your work.

Think about all the people you communicate with. Why do you communicate with them? Make a list. You will be surprised!

### 1.2 How effective communication affects all aspects of the learner's work

You will establish many different relationships across the sector, some of which will be formal and others more informal. Two-way communication is required to form relationships and establish the boundaries. It will help to ensure that everyone concerned understands the purpose of the relationship and what they are aiming to achieve.

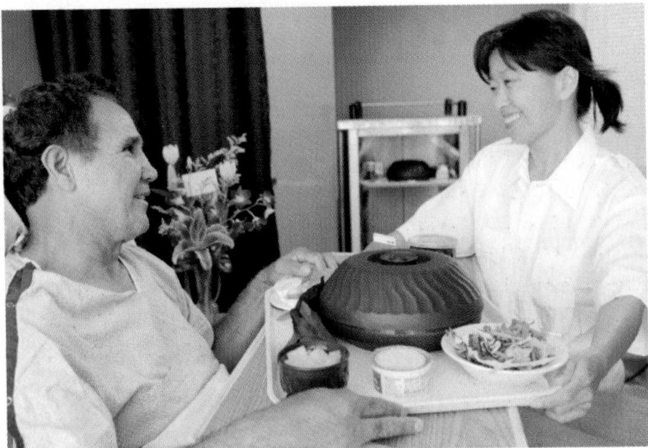

Figure 1.1 A multitude of job roles

The relationships between workers and service users, and also between colleagues, have a significant impact on the ability to provide effective care and support. Respect for each other can be developed through communication. Getting to know people by talking and listening to them will enable you to develop an understanding and awareness which will lead to stronger relationships in the longer term.

## 1.3 Why it is important to observe an individual's reactions when communicating with them

Conversations are such common, everyday events that people often think they do not require any specific or specialist skills. Some interactions will be informal, such as speaking with friends or family members. Other conversations will be more formal, for example, having a conversation with a health specialist, colleague or employer.

Communication in work settings may be complex. This means that it may have several purposes. As a practitioner, you will need to be aware that each individual has their own way of interpreting what is said, and observation can help you with this. How are they responding, does their body language match their spoken words? Effective communication means more than just passing on information, it means involving or engaging the other person or people with whom you are interacting.

Communicating has to be a two-way process where each person is attempting to understand and interpret, or make sense of, what the other person is saying. Often it is easier to understand people who are similar to us, for example, a person who has the same accent as us, or is in a similar situation. The decoding equipment in our brain tunes in, breaks down the message, analyses the message, understands it and interprets its meaning, and then creates a response or answer. When a practitioner is speaking with an individual they are forming a mental picture of what they are being told.

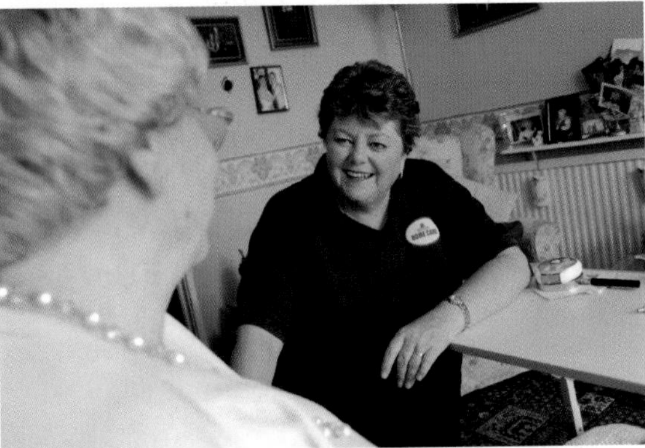

Figure 1.2 Interaction

### Evidence activity 

#### 1.3 Observing while communicating

This activity will help demonstrate that you understand why it is important to observe an individual's reactions when communicating with them.

What can observing an individual tell you about how they feel?

# LO2 Meet the communication and language needs, wishes and preferences of individuals

## 2.1 How to find out an individual's communication and language needs, wishes and preferences

As a practitioner, it is important that you become familiar with the needs of individuals to ensure you can communicate effectively with them. You can do this by:

- asking the person – they know best!
- looking in the care plan

- speaking to a family member, or a close friend
- asking other practitioners
- use reference books, if appropriate.

For example, in many cultures the use of touch or gestures and the use of personal space may differ. The ways in which people express themselves might also be different; or the way that men address women or the use of first names might be different. How people are addressed is important too. Some people prefer to be called by their first name while others may request to be called Mr or Mrs.

**Evidence activity** 

### 2.1 Finding out about someone's preferences

This activity helps demonstrate that you understand how to find out an individual's wishes and preferences.

How do you tell someone what you like to be called and how you like to be spoken to? Why is this important?

## 2.2 Communication methods that meet an individual's communication needs, wishes and preferences

Eye contact is a way of showing that the person who is listening is interested in the conversation. Eye contact will help the person you are communicating with realise that you are concentrating on what they are saying rather than on other conversations or activities that may be going on around you. Eye-to-eye contact can also help you to know how the other person is feeling. If either the individual or the practitioner is angry or upset, they might have a fixed stare that can send out that message; if they are excited or interested in someone, then their eyes will get wider. This means that when you are talking to an individual, the person can tell whether you like what you are hearing or not.

Good eye contact at appropriate times can encourage individuals to talk more openly. It conveys that you understand the individual's situation; you can put yourself in the person's position and can see things from their perspective, making it easier to provide support for them.

As a practitioner, you need to understand that eye contact conveys different meanings for people from different cultures. For example, direct eye contact is considered to be rude in some cultures and should be avoided. It is important to understand what is and what is not acceptable for the people with whom you are working. Also, some individuals may be unable or unwilling to make and/or maintain eye contact because of a disability.

### Listening attentively and responding

Active listening helps to maximise the effectiveness of communication. It is important to show not only that you are listening to the individual, but that you have actually heard and understood what has been said. By responding to what has been said, you will reassure the individual and encourage them to speak more openly. Responses can include nodding, smiling, or reflecting back what has been said. Making encouraging sounds can also indicate interest and can be used to gain further information. The person who is talking is encouraged by signals which show that the listener wants to know more.

### Looking interested

Using smiles and eye contact ensures that people know that you are interested in what is being said. You should display open body language, using gestures can also be helpful. Showing a person that you are interested in what is being said encourages them to communicate fully and can improve the level of detail they are prepared to give. Showing interest also helps to develop a trusting relationship which, over a period of time, can help improve communication.

**Research & investigate** 

### 2.2 Communication methods

Investigate the range of communication methods used in a specific setting, such as a nursery or learning disability provision, and list the benefits of each method.

## Time

Communication should never be rushed, as this may make an individual feel that they are not important, or that you lack respect for them. Also, taking too much time can be seen as dragging out the conversation and can make people feel uneasy. Timing should be appropriate for the purpose of the communication and take into account the needs of the individuals involved. It is important to give individuals time to say what they want to; this ensures that they feel respected and that their personal interests have been considered fully. Individuals should not be interrupted when they are speaking as this may make them feel that they are not being listened to properly.

## Use of technology, JAWS

JAWS is a computer program that reads information on the screen and speaks it aloud through a speech synthesiser. It works with any PC to provide access to software applications and the internet. It also outputs to refreshable **Braille** displays, providing Braille support for screen readers. Where the use of technology is appropriate to assist with communication, this should be encouraged so that everyone feels actively involved and no one is struggling to hear what others are saying or is unable to present their ideas or opinions.

### Key term

Braille is a system of writing and printing for blind or visually impaired people. Varied arrangements of raised dots representing letters and numerals are identified by touch.

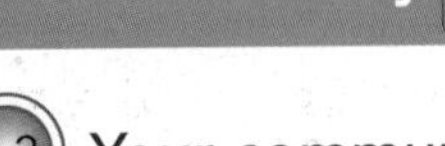

### Your communication experience and needs

This activity helps demonstrate your understanding of communication methods that meet needs.

Think about a time when you wanted to make a comment or complaint about a service you received. How did you do this? How did you feel? What was the outcome? Did you need someone to help you?

## Use of advocates or interpreters

An advocate is a person who tries to understand the needs and preferences of an individual and speaks on their behalf. Advocates are often needed when someone has a disability which makes it difficult for them to speak for themselves. An advocate should try and get to know the service user and develop an understanding of their culture and background, so that they can represent them accurately. The advocate should understand the person's needs and communicate these to practitioners or professionals involved with them. To ensure that they are unbiased, advocates are independent of the professional carers who work with the individual.

Interpreters can help people for whom English is not their preferred or first language. In the past interpreters may have been family members of the person in question, but this is now discouraged as far as is possible for reasons of confidentiality. For example, a mother whose daughter was interpreting for her may not want her daughter to know that she had cancer. Interpreters communicate meaning of one spoken language to another, while translators change written material from one language to another.

There are drawbacks to using translators and interpreters, as it may sometimes be difficult to grasp the exact meaning of a message or to express the meaning in the other language. Where an interpreter is used, it is important to remember to communicate with the service user rather than the interpreter, to ensure that the individual is empowered and feels valued.

In many services, leaflets concerning health topics or health facilities are produced in several other languages in addition to English, so that people from ethnic minorities can access the information. If information is not readily available in the relevant language it will need to be translated.

## Awareness of personal space and positioning

Seating arrangements and positioning should be considered carefully when communicating with others, and will depend on the circumstances and purpose of the communication. A person can convey confidence or lack of confidence through their body language, which can have an impact on the effectiveness of the communication. By developing an awareness of the signs and signals of body language, you will find it much easier to understand other people and to communicate more effectively with them.

Increasing understanding of body language can also help you to become more aware of the messages you are conveying to others.

## 2.3 How and when to seek advice about communication

Information and activities that cover this section can be found in section 3.4 below. Evidence Activity 2.3 can be found on page 10.

# LO3 Overcome barriers to communication

## 3.1 Barriers to effective communication

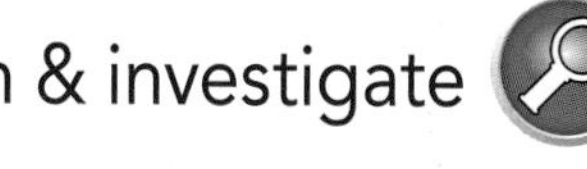

### Research & investigate

**3.1 Barriers to communication**

You are working in setting. There is a lot of noise going on, with new staff and new service users. What barriers do you think there are?

Research how you can overcome these barriers, and produce a simple plan outlining your solutions.

### Attitude of the worker

Your attitude can affect the way others communicate with you. When a worker is abrupt towards an individual, that person could feel intimidated and not want to communicate. They may feel that the worker is not interested in them and does not want to help. An insincere approach or lack of empathy may make an individual feel that they are wasting their time, and could make them reluctant to divulge personal information. A sincere and polite attitude is likely to promote more open communication from the service user.

### Limited use of technology

Some individuals need technological aids to support their communication. When there is limited availability of a technology, communication may be more difficult. For example, the absence of a **hearing loop** could be a barrier to an individual who uses a hearing aid. Workers who have limited experience of using technology (for example computers, fax machines or other technological devices), could find this interferes with their ability to communicate, for example they may not be able to communicate via email or use a fax machine. This could ultimately delay messages being received and responded to, and could undermine someone's authority if they need to ask for help.

### Key term

A **hearing loop** provides information on an induction loop system, to assist the hearing impaired by transmitting sound from a sound system, microphone, television or other source, directly to a hearing aid.

### Sitting too far away or invading personal space

Sitting too far away from a person may make them feel that they are not important or that the practitioner is not interested in what they have to say. It may also mean that they need to speak more loudly, which could compromise confidentiality or make them feel uncomfortable about communicating. Invasion of personal space (getting too close) can also make people feel uncomfortable. Most people prefer to get to know someone first and often only allow those who are close to them into their 'intimate zone'.

### Emotional distress

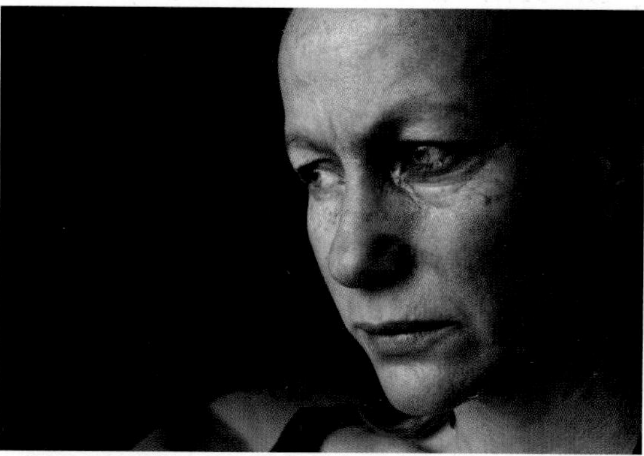

Figure 1.3 Confusion

Emotional issues, especially those that cause worry or distress, can make people behave erratically and unpredictably. When individuals have serious emotional needs they can be afraid or depressed because of the stresses they are experiencing. They may lack self-awareness or appear to be shy or aggressive, which has an impact on their ability to communicate. Listening involves learning about frightening and depressing situations, which can mean that practitioners sometimes avoid listening to avoid feeling unpleasant emotions. The practitioner can become emotionally distressed by the needs of the individual and can also make assumptions, or label or stereotype others.

Practitioners may have their own emotional issues that can create barriers. The practitioner may not be able to focus or may be tired due to worrying and lack of sleep. Listening and empathising takes mental energy, which may not be available if the practitioner has their own concerns. Practitioners who believe they do not have sufficient time to communicate properly can become stressed and so create a barrier.

When individuals are depressed, angry or upset, these emotions will influence their ability to understand what is being communicated to them, and their ability to communicate their own needs. Additionally, individuals who do not trust service providers or practitioners are less likely to share information with them.

## Poor or unwelcoming body language

A worker who displays negative body language in the form of crossed arms or legs, using inappropriate gestures, poor facial expressions, poor body positioning or constant fidgeting creates barriers to communication.

## Poor interpersonal skills

A worker who has poor **interpersonal skills** does not make an individual feel welcome. They may use inappropriate language or rely too heavily on technical terminology. Their manner and demeanour may be off-putting, which can create a barrier to successful communication. If the worker is not paying attention to the individual or is not listening properly they may miss important information. It is inappropriate to then ask for this to be repeated, as it will make the individual feel that they are not being valued.

### Key term

Interpersonal skills are the skills we use to interact with others.

## Lack of privacy

Conversations should not be held in a public place where others can overhear what is being said, as this lack of privacy can feel disrespectful. Interruptions by other people may make the individual feel intimidated and unimportant. A person is likely to communicate much more freely if they feel that what they are saying is being taken seriously and kept private.

## Lack of respect for individual

An individual is unlikely to communicate if they feel that they are not being respected. Addressing someone as 'dear' or 'lovey', or invading their personal space shows a lack of respect. Any action that is going to be taken should be clearly explained before it is actually carried out, and the opinions and choices of the individual should be respected. If someone feels that they are not being respected they may withhold information which could be vital.

## Stereotyping

Stereotyping means describing everyone in a particular category as being 'the same', or describing aspects of their behaviour or characteristics as 'the same'. It is an easy way of grouping people together. For example, it is stereotyping to believe that everyone over 70 years old is less mentally able or needs a walking aid, or that all children below the age of 4 are unable to make decisions for themselves. Sometimes individuals are stereotyped because of their language or the colour of their skin. Some people may assume that anyone who is not white cannot speak English, so they speak in 'broken English' to the individual without first finding out if they can speak English or if English is their preferred language.

Practitioners sometimes impose their own views and opinions on situations at work. These may be views and opinions they have learnt while growing up, or which they have assumed because they have friends who hold such opinions. A good practitioner will avoid stereotyping and labelling by making sure that they are informed and knowledgeable. They will also examine their own attitudes and values to make sure that they know themselves and are not unjustly judging others.

Evidence activity 

### 3.1 Barriers to effective communication

This activity demonstrates your understanding of the impact of barriers to effective communication.

How do you think a poor approach to communication can make an individual feel?

## 3.2 Ways to overcome barriers to effective communication

### Respecting cultural preferences and differences

Cultural differences can influence communication. Culture is much more than just the language that is spoken, it includes the way people live, think and how they relate to each other. In some cultures children are not allowed to speak if certain adults are present. Other cultures do not allow women to speak to men they do not know. Cultural differences can sometimes make relationships difficult; therefore workers across the sectors need to make sure they prepare well for this.

You must make sure that you acknowledge culture when communicating. For example, certain hand gestures are acceptable in this country but would not be in others. To show friendliness, in one culture you may say hello with a smile on your face; in another, you may make a silent formal bow; and in a third, you may even embrace the people warmly. Looking straight into the eyes of the person you are speaking to is desirable in most conversations in this country, but would be considered rude in others. These cultures believe that looking down shows proper respect for another individual. A practitioner who feels that eye contact is important must learn to accept and respect this cultural difference.

These examples show that people of different cultures communicate differently even when they have the same motive to communicate.

It is important across the sectors for information to be made available in a person's chosen language. It may also be appropriate to employ interpreters to support individuals so that they can be actively involved in any communication and understand the support available or the procedures being carried out.

When communicating it is important to remember the following points:

- Do not make assumptions when meeting a person – they could appear to be demanding simply because they feel insecure or because they are not familiar with their surroundings.
- Treat a person with a same-sex partner accompanying them in the same manner as everyone else.
- Show respect for the values of individuals.
- Do not invade personal space – often people feel uncomfortable with this until they develop trust.
- Acknowledge the beliefs and differences of individuals from other cultures.
- Develop knowledge and understanding of different cultures in order to avoid making mistakes or causing offence.

### Asking questions to clarify points, aiding understanding of communication

- Ask an individual to summarise their understanding of the situation so that further explanation can be given if necessary.
- Always ask if there is anything that is not understood – this can prevent mistakes being made or something being interpreted in the wrong way.
- Ask questions relating to timing, place and procedures to enhance understanding.

Evidence activity 

### 3.2 Overcoming barriers to effective communication

This activity demonstrates your understanding of how to overcome barriers to effective communication.

Hamid is a new service user. He speaks little English but is keen to get to know people. How can the service, and you, help Hamid integrate?

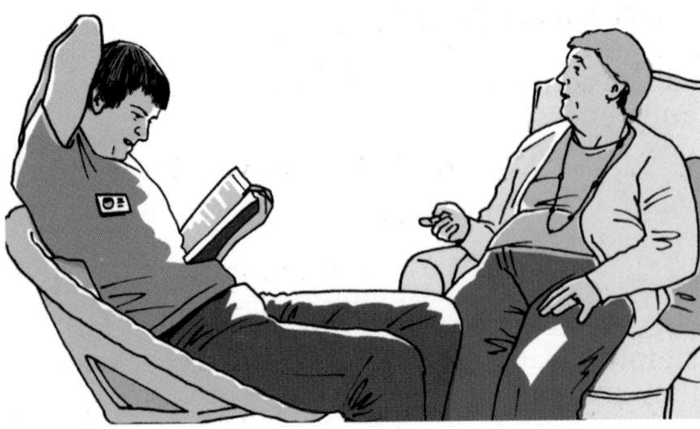

Figure 1.4 Listening

## 3.3 Ways to ensure that communication has been understood

### Asking questions to clarify points, aiding understanding

Asking the right questions without being too intrusive is an important skill to develop. It will help you to clarify the important points and understand the communication. Questions should be short and to the point. Using language and vocabulary that is easy to understand will help to avoid confusion. You should avoid asking multiple questions, as these may be difficult for the individual to answer.

Closed questions (with 'yes' and 'no' answers) should be used to gather factual information when you need to know about specific points, such as date of birth, allergies, medication being taken.

Open questions should be used where more detailed information is required, as these give the individual the opportunity to give longer answers. These questions give more of an insight into how the individual is feeling or about their views and opinions.

### Using language appropriate to the individual's understanding

It is important to avoid using language that individuals do not understand, for example using adult language when working with a child would be inappropriate. Likewise, using sophisticated language when communicating with an adult with learning difficulties is not suitable either. If acronyms or technical terminology are used these should always be explained, to ensure that the person understands what has been said. You should always assess the individual you are communicating with before progressing with your communication, so that the interaction is as effective as possible

### Environmental barriers

A health and social care environment can be noisy, distracting and confusing at times. It is important that the member of staff recognises this and reduces any background noise to a minimum, for example how often have you seen individuals placed next to a noisy television that no one is watching. What effect do you think this will have on their ability to concentrate or converse with others? It is also important that you ensure that the environment is freely accessible, and that the placement of furniture encourages individuals to interact with each other. The placement of notices in freely accessible locations will also inform individuals of activities and events. This will not only encourage conversation between carers and individuals, but will also encourage individuals to plan for the event, and to participate and socialise with other individuals and their families.

### Language barriers

Successful communication hinges on how well you listen and respond to others. Here are some language behaviours that may hinder the communication process:

- Dominance: If someone dominates the communication process, communicating becomes a one-way process and responses from individuals are hindered.
- Inappropriate self-disclosure: If someone talks too much about themselves, then the topic or focus of the communication changes.
- Self-protection: Individuals often protect themselves from meaningful contact by talking exclusively about safe topics; avoiding uncomfortable issues; emotionally detaching themselves from the topic of conversation.
- Swearing: Such language may be powerful, but it usually turns others off.
- Using jargon: People often use words that belong exclusively to their area of expertise.
- Judging others: As a health and social care worker it is important that you do not impose your own value judgements on others. Avoid telling others that their ideas or opinions are bad or wrong. Simply say, 'I disagree.'
- Patronising: Condescending words, tone or behaviour, will make individuals and their families feel angry and defensive.

- Pressurising: Using threats – implied or explicit – to persuade someone of your point of view.
- Being insensitive: Being callous or unaware of your own feelings and the feelings of others.

## Sensory loss

Some older people may have difficulty communicating because of poor eyesight or hearing. You can assist individuals who have visual impairment by making sure that their eyesight is tested regularly, that their spectacles are clean and worn properly, and that their possessions are kept in the same, familiar place. You could also learn the correct way to guide and assist a partially sighted person while they are walking, and find out what visual aids are available in your nursing home, for example large print books and newspapers or talking books. When communicating with visually impaired individuals, it is important that you:

- Let them know you are nearby in a quiet and unhurried manner.
- Introduce yourself by name.
- Use appropriate forms of touch to initiate and then sustain the conversation.
- Ask the individual what form of communication best suits them.
- Allow the individual to take your arm before you lead them around.
- Treat the person as an individual, and never assume that all visually impaired people have the same communication needs.

You can support individuals with hearing impairment by making sure that their hearing aid is tested regularly, that it is clean and worn properly, and that the battery is not flat. You can also learn the correct way to replace a hearing aid battery, or talk to colleagues about how the hearing impaired use sign language. You can also find out what aids are available, for example flashing lights instead of telephone bells or door bells. When communicating with hearing impaired individuals, it is important that you:

- Speak clearly, listen carefully and respond to what is said to you.
- Minimise any distractions, for example a noisy television.
- Make sure any aids to hearing are working.
- Use written forms of communication that are appropriate.
- Use signing, where appropriate, by involving a properly trained interpreter.

**Evidence activity** 

### 3.3 Ensuring communication is understood

This activity will demonstrate you understand how to ensure communication is understood.

Describe two examples of how ineffective communication can occur and explain how these may affect individuals.

## 3.4 Sources of information and support or services to enable more effective communication

If there are problems identified with communication there are a range of services which can be accessed. Never presume that you or anyone else can be heard, understood and responded to, without first thinking about the person involved. Check first to ensure you are supporting someone to communicate as effectively as possible by working with them to overcome as many challenges and barriers as possible. It may be necessary to access additional support or services to help make communication better or clearer. People may have problems in communicating with others due to:

- Intellectual impairment leading to problems comprehending and processing information.
- Sensory difficulties (hearing, vision).
- Problems in understanding social interaction (for example autism).
- Speech problems (for example articulation problems).
- Others not listening and valuing what they are trying to communicate.

Many different professionals may be involved in this, but a person's motivation and efforts are equally important. Key experts likely to be encountered include speech and language therapists to help with communication problems, advocates, interpreters and clinical psychologists to help with problems affecting mental processes and emotions.

Health professionals need to:

- Take time and have patience.
- Value what is being communicated.
- Recognise non-verbal cues.
- Find out about the person's alternative communication strategies if verbal communication is difficult (for example their typical non-verbal cues, use symbols, sign language).
- Explain things clearly in an appropriate way (verbally and with pictures etc).
- Be prepared to meet the person several times to build up rapport and trust.
- Use the knowledge and support of people's carers.

**Evidence activity** 

 2.3 &  3.4 **How, when and where to seek support to enable more effective communication**

This activity will help demonstrate that you understand how, when and where to seek support to enable more effective communication.

Who can offer advice and guidance in your setting to ensure communication needs are met?

## LO4 Be able to respect equality and diversity when communicating

### 4.1 How people from different backgrounds may use and/or interpret communication methods in different ways

It is important to respect the fact that people have different cultural preferences and values, and therefore different priorities. You will need to recognise the diverse attitudes of those with whom you come into contact, and must not condemn or treat people differently if their values are different from yours.

Body language can be interpreted differently by different cultures. Certain cultures use gestures or touch much more than others, and gestures can mean different things in different cultures. In some cultures, touching someone shows understanding and empathy, but in British culture it might be considered unacceptable in a work situation. Making direct eye contact when communicating may be considered acceptable and even desirable in one culture (for example British), but rude and totally unacceptable in another (for example Greek). In order to avoid causing any offence or misunderstanding, it is worth taking time to find out about an individual's cultural background.

It is important to develop your knowledge and understanding of different cultures. For example, you should know that in some cultures, young women can only receive medical attention if they are accompanied by an older family member. Also, decisions about whether to have treatment or care are often made collectively by the senior members of the family rather than by the individual. These considerations may not at first seem to be directly linked to communicating with services users, but they do have an impact on the way people communicate and with whom.

**Evidence activity** 

 4.1 **Communicating with people from different backgrounds**

This activity will demonstrate your understanding of how people from different backgrounds may use and/or interpret communication methods in different ways.

List the main points you think you may need to consider when communicating with people from different backgrounds.

### 4.2 Communication that respects equality and diversity

Tips for communicating with people from different cultures include:

1. Understand the individual's values: Understand that people from other cultures

might have entirely different value systems from yours. It is useful to check the person's records for information, or speak to a member of their family or a friend if appropriate or possible. Ask someone else from the same culture, either another worker or an advocate. Use reference books and/or the internet if necessary.

2. Give the appropriate amount of personal space: Different cultures have different norms regarding a person's public space (in which others can stand and converse with you) and their private space (reserved only for people who are close to you). For example, people from Arab countries do not share the British concept of 'personal space' – for them it is considered offensive to step or lean away while talking to some. Make sure you leave the correct amount of space between yourself and others when you talk to them. If you are unsure, you can always ask what the other person prefers.
3. Do not belittle their religion: Remember, most people believe passionately in their religion, and they may have different beliefs from yours. If you have trouble dealing with this, you may wish to avoid discussing the topic of religion altogether.
4. Learn to recognise physical cues: Physical gestures that are acceptable when communicating vary widely between different cultures. When people visit other countries they often miss subtle cultural cues, which lead them to misinterpret others. For example, the use of irony or the implication of a laugh may be shown only in a squinting of the eyes or a shaking of the hand, which a cultural outsider might miss.
5. Know relationship differences: Many foreigners think British relationships are superficial (with a brief, 'Hi, Jim', and never a backward glance). British people might think relationships in other cultures are too sentimental. So, know that if a person strikes you as too outspoken or withdrawn, it may be considered normal in their culture.
6. Learn about their culture: Learn about greetings, goodbye rituals, before-meal ceremonies, food and clothes. This will help you understand people from other cultures and improve your communication with them.
7. Accept that there may be lapses in communication: Even the best communicators fall short when jumping across the large gap that exists between different cultures. Humour and non-defensiveness are the best way of dealing with these situations.
8. Ask: There is no better tool for effective communication than asking a question. If something strikes you as funny or inappropriate, if you feel the other person is neglecting you or is offended, simply ask them what you can do to change the situation. Misunderstandings can create big problems unless they are discussed openly.

**Evidence activity** 

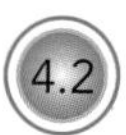


**Communication that overcomes language barriers**

This activity will help demonstrate that you can communicate in a way that respects equality and diversity. Think about a time when you were on holiday or speaking to a person whose first language was not English. How did you feel? What changes did you make to your method of communication?

## Needs and preferences

Individuals should always be given the opportunity to express their needs and preferences. Practitioners should not make assumptions and definitely should not make decisions on behalf of the service user unless they have been given permission to do so or are acting as an advocate for the person.

## Respecting individuals' rights to confidentiality within legal and organisational procedures

Individuals have a right by law, under the Data Protection Act 1998, to have confidentiality maintained and their personal information kept private. When an individual knows and understands that their information will not be shared with others, unless it is absolutely necessary, they will feel that they can trust the person they are communicating with and will feel more at ease with them. They are likely to share more detailed information, which could result in them ultimately receiving more effective levels of care.

A142252



# LO5 Apply principles and practices relating to confidentiality at work

## 5.1 Explain the term 'confidentiality'

### What is confidentiality?

Confidentiality means that personal and private information obtained from or about an individual must only be shared with others on a 'need-to-know' basis. Information given to a worker should not be disclosed without the person's informed permission. Confidentiality is an important principle in health and social care because it provides guidance on the amount of personal information and data that can be disclosed without consent. A person disclosing personal information in a relationship of trust reasonably expects his or her privacy to be protected, i.e. they expect the information to remain confidential. The relationship between health and social care professionals and their patients/clients centres on trust, and trust is dependent on the patient/client being confident that personal information they disclose is treated confidentially.

However, confidentiality can be countered when there is a public interest in others being protected from harm.

**Case Study**

**5.1 Confidentiality**

Ms X lives with her two children in a small market town. She is to have a minor operation and arrangements need to be made for the care of her children while she is in hospital and convalescing.

Arrangements for the care of the children are being discussed at a case conference by Ms X and the family's GP, social worker and health visitor. The elder child's school will be informed of the final arrangements.

Various pieces of information are known to the four people at the case conference, although not each piece of information is known by each individual. The privacy interests of Ms X, her children and their absent father may be different.

Here are some criteria that can influence whether or not information is disclosed or shared:

- confidence that the recipient of the data will handle it responsibly
- the need for consent to disclosure and respect for refusals to consent
- the accuracy, relevance, and pertinence of the data.

1. Can you think of any other considerations?

   It is not always easy to decide which pieces of information should be shared. Consider the following:

   The GP knows that the absent father is HIV positive. To the best of the GP's knowledge, neither the social worker nor the health visitor are aware of this. It is also possible that Ms X is unaware.

contd.

## Case Study *contd.*

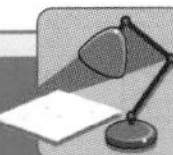

2. In these particular circumstances, should the GP share this information with the following people, and why?
   (a) Ms X
   (b) the health visitor
   (c) the social worker
3. As a health or social care professional it is vital that you apply the principles of confidentiality. Inappropriate disclosure of information can have a significant negative impact on people's lives. What could be the impact of disclosure in this situation?

# 5.2 Confidentiality in day-to-day communication

## Maintaining confidentiality

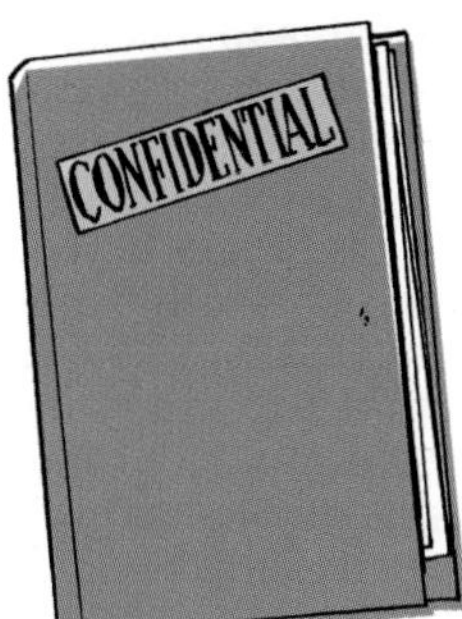


Figure 1.5 Safe and secure

Maintaining confidentiality is a very important aspect of building trust between a client and a worker. Without trust, communication is less likely to progress between two or more people. Building trust involves honouring commitments and declaring conflicts of interest. It also means making sure that the policy which relates to ways of communicating with people is followed.

The right to confidentiality means that a person's notes must not be left lying around or stored insecurely (for example, left in a car). Computerised information relating to the person should only be accessed by those who have the authority to do so, so it should be password protected and the password given only to authorised staff. Conversations with clients should not be so loud that others can hear and, if the content of the conversation is personal, the interaction should be in a room where others are not present and the door is closed. People have the right not to be spoken about in such a way that they can be identified.

There are occasions when a worker may have to break confidentiality. Such situations arise when:

- a person is likely to harm themselves
- a person is likely to harm others
- a child or vulnerable adult has suffered, or is at risk of suffering, significant harm
- a person has been, or is likely to be, involved in a serious crime.

It must also be remembered that other professional workers will need to have specific information on a need-to-know basis and, in these circumstances, information may have to be passed to others.

## Evidence activity

### 5.2 Confidentiality in day-to-day work

This activity demonstrates that you understand the need for confidentiality in day-to-day work.

A client's cousin has telephoned from Australia asking for an update on their family member's health. They say that due to the distance, they will not be able to get over to visit for a long time so they should be given the information.

What action do you take and why?

## Legal requirements

The approach of courts of law to record keeping tends to be that 'if it is not recorded, it has not been done'. Workers across the sectors have both a professional and a legal duty of care to their clients, so their record keeping should be able to demonstrate:

- a full account of their assessment and the care that has been planned and provided
- relevant information about the condition of the patient/client at any given time
- the measures taken by the worker to respond to their needs
- evidence that the worker has understood and honoured their duty of care, that all reasonable steps have been taken to care for the patient/client and that any actions or omissions on the part of the worker have not compromised their safety in any way
- a record of any arrangements that have been made for the continuing care of a patient/client.

## Organisational policies

### 5.3 Situations where information normally considered to be confidential might need to be passed on

Confidential information is personal details from our lives which we may not want to share with others. It can include our address, phone number, birth date, employment history or other personal information. It may also include information about our past or present health and development. Individuals have the right to keep information of this type private. While the rights and desires of families to keep their personal details private are important, there are also some circumstances under which identifying information should be shared.

This is called 'need to know'. To ensure the health and safety of individuals with special needs, carers and staff who interact with them should be informed of any specific dietary needs, intolerances or allergies. For example, staff who prepare and serve food should be fully aware of who has food allergies and what each person is allergic to. It is also necessary to pass on information if a person, or other people, may be at risk. For example if a person discloses information about the poor treatment, or neglect, of another person. You must tell the person you are passing this information on and report it to your manager.

**Research & investigate**

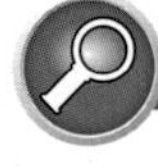

**5.3 Confidentiality procedures**

Select a service user group and find out the confidentiality procedures that apply.

### 5.4 How and when to seek advice about confidentiality

All organisations have their own policies and procedures regarding recording and reporting of information to make sure that all practitioners observe the regulations that apply to them. Confidentiality is an essential component of an accessible service. Some users of services bring issues with them and provide personal details in order for practitioners to help them. By being assured that their information is going to be recorded, stored and shared appropriately, individuals feel more able to disclose information that they may not have been previously happy to discuss. Some people feel intimidated by, or reluctant to talk about, their issues. Young people, refugees and offenders, for example, may feel especially vulnerable. Users of services need reassurance that they will not be judged, and that anything they tell workers will not be shared with others without the client's knowledge and consent. The few exceptions to this are usually outlined in the policies the organisation follows. In order for policies to operate successfully, there needs to be commitment from all the staff.

Many different organisational policies refer to responsibility in relation to recording and reporting of information, including:

- Confidentiality policies.
- Health and well-being policies.
- Information governance policies.
- Health and safety policies.
- Child protection policies.
- Assessment, recording and reporting policies.
- Codes of Conduct and National Standards Frameworks relating to practitioners across the sectors, which also apply within organisations.

## Meet the needs of individuals

Only information required to meet the individual's specific needs should be recorded and reported. Information that is not relevant should not be recorded at all. For example, financial information would not be relevant to a patient who has been admitted to hospital for an operation; however, it may be needed to determine an individual's ability to pay for adult social care services. Information describing personal characteristics such as age, gender, disability, ethnicity, religion and sexual orientation should only be used to support the provision of high-quality care to meet individual needs. This information can be used to meet the requirements of legislation, regulations and policies and to demonstrate good practice.

The Caldicott Principles were developed for the NHS in relation to the recording and sharing of personal information. These principles can easily be applied to any organisation or setting. The Caldicott Standards are based on the Data Protection Act 1998 principles.

## The Caldicott Principles

1. *Justify the purpose(s) of using confidential information*

   Every proposed use or transfer of patient-identifiable information within or from an organisation should be clearly defined and scrutinised, with continuing uses regularly reviewed by an appropriate guardian.

2. *Do not use patient-identifiable information unless it is absolutely necessary*

   Patient-identifiable information items should not be included unless it is essential for the specified purpose(s) of that flow. The need for patients to be identified should be considered at each stage of satisfying the purpose(s).

3. *Use the minimum necessary patient-identifiable information that is required*

   Where use of the patient-identifiable information is considered to be essential, the inclusion of each individual item of information should be considered and justified so that the minimum amount of identifiable information is transferred or accessible as is necessary for a given function to be carried out.

4. *Access to patient-identifiable information should be on a strict need-to-know basis*

   Only those individuals who need access to patient-identifiable information should have access to it, and they should only have access to the information items that they need to see. This may mean introducing access controls or splitting information flows where one information flow is used for several purposes.

5. *Everyone with access to patient-identifiable information should be aware of their responsibilities*

   Action should be taken to ensure that those handling patient-identifiable information – both clinical and non-clinical staff – are made fully aware of their responsibilities and obligations to respect patient confidentiality.

6. *Understand and comply with the law*

   Every use of patient-identifiable information must be lawful. Someone in each organisation handling patient information should be responsible for ensuring that the organisation complies with the legal requirements.

Caldicott Guardians are senior staff in the NHS and social services appointed to protect patient information to ensure that it is used for the purposes intended, meeting the individual needs of the patients in their care.

### Evidence activity 

 **5.4 How and when to seek advice about confidentiality**

This activity demonstrates your understanding of how and when to seek advice about confidentiality.

What is the impact of the Caldicott Principles on service delivery?

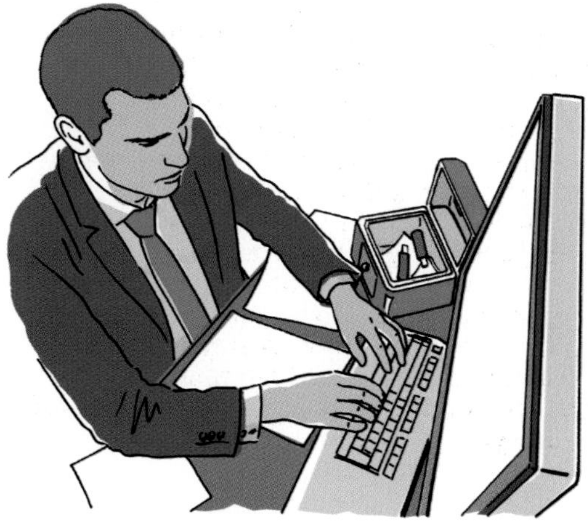

Figure 1.6 Confidentiality

## Assessment summary

Your reading of this chapter and completion of the activities will have prepared you to be able to engage in communication in health, social care or children's and young people's settings

To achieve the unit, your assessor will require you to:

| Learning outcomes | Assessment criteria |
|---|---|
| Learning outcome 1: Understand why communication is important in the work setting by: | 1.1 identifying the different reasons people communicate<br><br>See Evidence activity 1.1, p. 1 |
| | 1.2 explaining how effective communication affects all aspects of the learner's work<br><br>See Evidence activity 1.2, p. 1 |
| | 1.3 explaining why it is important to observe an individual's reactions when communicating with them.<br><br>See Evidence activity 1.3, p. 2 |
| Learning outcome 2: Be able to meet the communication and language needs, wishes and preferences of individuals by: | 2.1 showing how to find out an individual's communication and language needs, wishes and preferences<br><br>See Evidence activity 2.1, p. 3 |
| | 2.2 demonstrating communication methods that meet an individual's communication needs, wishes and preferences<br><br>See Evidence activity 2.2, p. 4 |
| | 2.3 showing how and when to seek advice about communication.<br><br>See Evidence activity 2.3, p. 10 |
| Learning outcome 3: Be able to overcome barriers to communication by: | 3.1 identifying barriers to effective communication<br><br>See Evidence activity 3.1 p. 7 |
| | 3.2 demonstrating ways to overcome barriers to effective communication<br><br>See Evidence activity 3.2, p. 7 |

| Learning outcomes | Assessment criteria |
|---|---|
| Learning outcome **3**: Be able to overcome barriers to communication by: | 3.3 demonstrating ways to ensure that communication has been understood<br>See Evidence activity 3.3, p. 9 |
| | 3.4 identifying sources of information and support or services to enable more effective communication<br>See Evidence activity 3.4, p. 10 |
| Learning outcome **4**: Be able to respect equality and diversity when communicating by: | 4.1 describing how people from different backgrounds may use and/or interpret communication methods in different ways<br>See Evidence activity 4.1, p. 10 |
| | 4.2 showing communication that respects equality and diversity<br>See Evidence activity 4.2, p. 11 |
| Learning outcome **5**: Be able to apply principles and practices relating to confidentiality at work by: | 5.1 explaining the term confidentiality<br>See Case study 5.1, pp. 12–13 |
| | 5.2 demonstrating confidentiality in day-to-day communication<br>See Evidence activity 5.2, p. 13 |
| | 5.3 describing situations where information normally considered to be confidential might need to be passed on<br>See Research and investigate 5.3, pp. 14 |
| | 5.4 explaining how and when to seek advice about confidentiality.<br>See Evidence activity 5.4, p. 15 |

Good luck!

## Weblinks

| | |
|---|---|
| Community Care | www.community-care.co.uk |
| Royal National Institute for the Deaf | www.rnid.org.uk |
| Royal National Institute of the Blind | www.rnib.org.uk |
| Social Care Sector Skills Council | www.skillsforcare.org.uk |
| Health Care Sector Skills Council | www.skillsforhealth.org.uk |
| Skills for Justice Sector Skills Council | www.skillsforjustice.com |

# 2 Introduction to personal development in health, social care or children's and young people's settings

## For Unit SHC22

### What are you finding out?

Personal development is not just to do with education or training and the development of skills and interests. It is also about developing a better understanding of yourself, your values, beliefs and experiences, and how they impact on your behaviour. It is about appreciating what motivates you to learn so that you can achieve your full potential.

Personal development is important because life without change may lead to a duller existence. The thought of change can be unwelcome – 'I am quite comfortable as I am, thank you.' But in order to handle new challenges, achieve a better quality of life or become accomplished in our work, we need to move out of our comfort zone, reflect on our experiences and ... change, even if it's just a minor adjustment.

As Mark Twain said, 'Twenty years from now you will be more disappointed by the things you didn't do than by the ones you did do. So throw off the bowlines. Sail away from the safe harbour. Catch the trade winds in your sails. Explore. Dream. Discover.'

Personal development is stimulating and energising. It opens doors, in our personal lives and at work. Learning does not end when we finish school.

The reading and activities in this chapter will help you to:

- Understand what is required for competence in your work role
- Be able to reflect on your work practice
- Be able to agree a personal development plan
- Be able to develop knowledge, skills and understanding.

## LO1 Understand what is required for competence in own work role

### 1.1 Describe the duties and responsibilities of own role

Work in the health and social care sector covers many job roles. Loosely, these can be categorised into three areas:

1. **Ancillary** – domestics, electricians, porters, etc.
2. **Administration and managerial** – office staff, receptionists, senior management, (such as chief executives and owners or managers of private care providers), etc.
3. **Providers of care** – nurses, teachers, care workers, midwives, social workers, nursery workers, etc.

**Key Term**

Ancillary workers in health and social care are staff who do not provide hands-on care.

There are many organisations, internet sites, professional journals, newspapers and so on, which describe job roles within health, social care, children's and young people's settings. Descriptions will include:

- entrance requirements for each role
- qualifications
- skills
- personal qualities
- professional development and career pathways associated with job roles
- hours of work
- rates of pay.

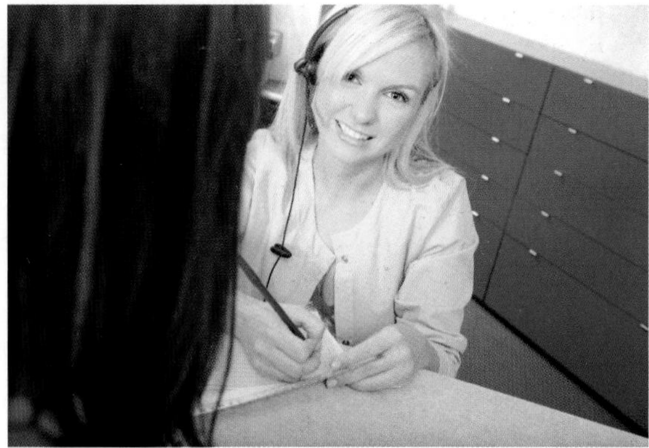

Figure 2.1 A multitude of job roles

The internet is a good starting point for exploring roles within the health and social care sectors. Websites you may find interesting include:

1 Healthcare careers www.connexions-direct.com/jobs4u
2 Social care and counselling www.connexions-direct.com/jobs4u
3 Community care www.communitycare.co.uk/jobs/search
4 Skills for Health www.skillsforhealth.org.uk
5 Skills for Care and Development www.skillsforcareanddevelopment.org.uk
6 Directgov www.direct.gov.uk

## Research & investigate

### 1.1 Fancy a change?

Think about a couple of jobs in a health or care setting that you'd like to be in now, instead of your current role. Research as much information as you need in order to decide whether either of the jobs would be appropriate for you, for example, you could search the internet or visit your local connexions office or Jobcentre.

1. What do you think the key roles of each job are?
2. Are you suited for each or either role?
3. Would you enjoy either or each of them?

Possibly, you applied for your current job role because the job description caught your eye and you thought you would enjoy the duties and responsibilities involved.

1 Duties are the tasks or activities that you are paid to carry out. They are listed in your job description and contract of employment.

2 Responsibilities are to do with the qualities that underpin the way you work, for example that you are reliable, dependable, conscientious and trustworthy; that you conduct yourself as required and demonstrate respect, consideration and maturity; that you comply with policies and procedures and Codes of Practice as relevant to the care setting. Being responsible means being accountable for your actions and being prepared to improve.

## Time to reflect

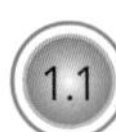

### 1.1 How does your job measure up?

Think about your duties and responsibilities.

1. Are they more or less what you expected them to be?
2. Do you sometimes find the job demanding and easier said than done or, on the other hand, insufficiently interesting or challenging?

## Evidence activity

### 1.1 Describe the duties and responsibilities of own role

This activity enables you to demonstrate your knowledge of your own work role.

Write a job description for your work role that outlines your duties and responsibilities.

## Time to reflect

### 1.1 How do you measure up?

1. Compare the job description that you wrote for Evidence Activity 1.1 with the official description for your job role. How do they compare?
2. Are you carrying out your duties as required, and do you conduct yourself in a responsible manner?

## 1.2 Identify standards that influence the way the role is carried out

Standards are a required level of quality, and care has to meet certain standards. Standards include:

- Codes of Practice
- regulations
- minimum standards
- national occupational standards.

### Codes of Practice

Codes of Practice set out the criteria against which providers are assessed by. They also describe the standards of conduct and practice with which workers must carry out their activities and ensure that what they do is competent and consistent with the values of their employer. These standards are how registrants' 'fitness to practice' is determined. For a care worker to work in a certain profession, they have to register with their particular Professional Council and then work to the Codes of Practice which they deem fit. Not following their Code of Practice could result in them being taken of the register and no longer allowed to work in that role.

Codes of Practice are specific to work roles:

- Codes of Practice for Social Care Workers and Employers: General Social Care Council (GSCC)
- Codes or Standards of conduct, performance and ethics for nurses & midwives: Nursing and Midwifery Council (NMC)
- Code of Conduct and Practice for Registered Teachers: General Teaching Council (GTC)
- Standards of Conduct Performance & Ethics: Health Professionals Council (HPC)
- Code of Practice for Doctors: General Medical Council (GMC)

## Research & investigate

### 1.2 Codes of Practice

Look at the websites for the above groups (www.gscc.org.uk; www.nmc-uk.org; www.gtce.org.uk, www.hpc-uk.org, www.gmc-uk.org).

1. Examine their Codes of Practice.
2. Are there any similarities between the codes?

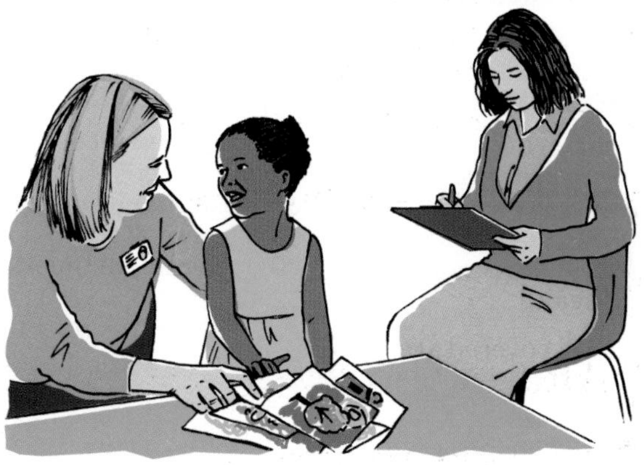

Figure 2.2 Inspection

### Regulations

Regulations are the rules which organisations and care workers must follow.

The Care Standards Act requires providers of health and care services to ensure that care provision is fit for purpose and meets the assessed needs of people using the services. The NHS & Community Care Act requires that all individuals are appropriately assessed and care plans are put into place. Care workers need to ensure they understand the regulations regarding provision and standards.

Health and safety laws, such as the Health and Safety at Work Act, Management of Health and Safety at Work Act, Food Safety Act, Food

Safety (General Food Hygiene) Regulations, COSSH, RIDDOR and so on, need to be followed to ensure individuals receiving care are safe and free from harm. Care workers need to ensure they understand health and safety regulations.

Confidentiality laws such as the Data Protection Act, Freedom of Information Act, Access to Medical Records and so on, regulate how information is collated, stored, accessed and deleted. Care workers need to ensure they understand confidentiality regulations.

### Research & investigate

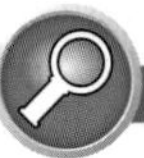

1.2 Regulations

Look at the some of the regulations mentioned above.

1. What are the key principles?
2. Why would an effective care worker need to know these?

## National Minimum Standards

The Care Standards Act 2000 requires providers to ensure care provision is fit for purpose and meets the assessed needs of individuals. These requirements are written into National Minimum Standards (NMS) by the Department of Health.

Areas covered are:

- children's homes
- fostering services
- boarding schools
- care homes for adults
- domiciliary care
- residential special schools
- care homes for older people
- independent healthcare.

But whilst NMS are specific to individual health and care settings, all describe how a worker is expected to demonstrate competence in their work role. As they are 'national' they ensure that individuals receive the same level of care regardless of where they live.

## National Occupational Standards

National Occupational Standards (NOS) are benchmarks of performance and provide a way to assess how well someone can do a job. They are work-related statements of the ability, knowledge, understanding and experience that an individual should have in order to carry out key tasks competently and effectively. The Health and Social Care (HSC) NOS and the Children's Care Learning and Development (CCLD) NOS have been compiled by the **Sector Skills Councils:** Skills for Care, Skills for Health and the Children's Workforce Development Council.

### Key Term

Sector Skills Councils (SSCs) are employer-led organisations that work to boost the skills of their sector workforces.

### Research & investigate

1.2 Standards and best practice

Look at:

2. The Codes of Practice for your work role. Sum up how they impact on your work role.
3. The key regulations which you have to follow in your role. Summarise the main regulations of your role.
4. The NMS for your work setting. Sum up how they impact on your work role.
5. The NOS for one of your key areas of work. What abilities, knowledge, understanding and experiences do they say you need to be able to carry out your work competently and effectively?

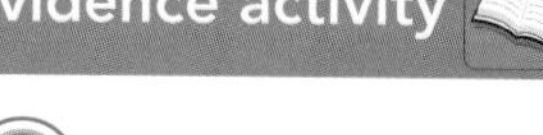

Evidence activity

### 1.2 Identify standards that influence the way the role is carried out

This activity enables you to demonstrate your understanding of the expectations about your own work role as expressed in relevant standards.

Identify your key duties and responsibilities referring to Codes of Practice, Regulations, Minimum Standards and National Occupational Standards.

## 1.3 Describe ways to ensure that personal attitudes or beliefs do not obstruct the quality of work

We all have attitudes; how we think, behave or what we value. Attitudes are very personal and different individuals have different attitudes.

A belief system is a set of ideas and principles about what is right and wrong, true or false. Like attitudes, beliefs are very personal. One individual's religious and political beliefs will be different from another's. Their ideas about, for example, how to dress, what to eat, how to behave, what is right and wrong, just and decent, will also differ.

### Time to reflect

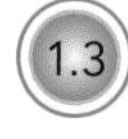

#### 1.3 Who do you think you are?

Think about a time when you felt that you had been unfairly judged, perhaps ridiculed for your attitudes or beliefs.

1. How did this treatment make you feel?

Now think about whether, in your personal life, you ever judge people unfairly because of their values, beliefs and experiences.

2. Why do you treat them unfairly?
3. Do you think you have any right to judge people like this?
4. How do you think you would have made them feel?

You are unlikely to agree with the attitudes and belief systems of all the individuals you work with, nor will you share many of their experiences. However, best practice involves putting your own personal attitudes and beliefs to one side and respecting, promoting and responding positively to those of the people you work with.

Allowing your own personal attitudes and beliefs to influence the way you work with people will prevent you seeing them as individuals and taking their individual needs into account. A lack of respect for others' values, beliefs and experiences threatens their right to fair treatment, and regard for their individual needs is neglected.

Tips to ensure personal attitudes or beliefs do not obstruct the quality of work.

- Find out about individuals – their history. Understanding the individual may challenge your own attitudes and values.
- Find out about their attitudes and beliefs – ignorance can often be a barrier. Understanding may promote tolerance.
- Be professional at work. Even if you fundamentally disagree with another individual's attitudes and beliefs, they have the right to hold them, the same right as you have. Respect this.
- Promote **empathy**. Considering life from their perspective may help you to appreciate their attitudes and beliefs.

### Key term

Empathy means identifying with that person's position, in order to understand from their perspective.

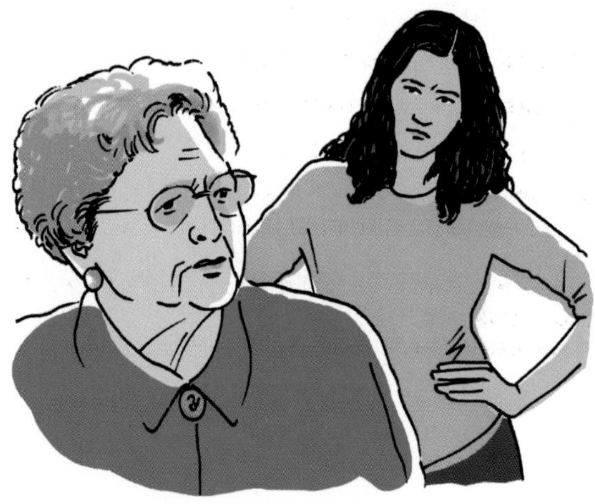

Figure 2.3 Respect? What's that?

## Case Study

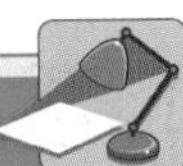

###  1.3 Dorothy and Jessica

Dorothy is an elderly resident at the care home where Jessica works. She has a wealth of life experiences – she served as a nurse during World War II and not only had the opportunity to nurse a number of very interesting people, she also got to travel through Europe. She has been a committed Christian since her early childhood, which she spent in South East Asia where her mother and father were missionaries. Her husband was killed in action during the war and as a consequence and much to her disappointment she has no children. She is also a staunch Conservative.

Jessica is 23 years old. She worked in a supermarket when she first left school, but the proximity of the care home to where she lives and the opportunity to swap shifts suits her better as it allows her, as a single parent, to play a more active role in bringing up her little boy. She is divorced from her husband because of the pressure he put on her to conform to his cultural background, including embracing his religion and social customs. She has no religious beliefs but, because of her father's influence, is a loyal trade unionist.

Jessica doesn't enjoy working with Dorothy. She has no time for her 'happy clappy God talk' and stories about what she got up to in the war, and makes unkind jibes at her politics and the reasons she doesn't have any children. As a result, Dorothy feels lonely and neglected; she has no confidence in Jessica as a care worker and is frustrated and angered by her lack of respect.

1. What do you think lies behind Jessica's unkind treatment of Dorothy?
2. How might the tensions between the two ladies be resolved?

## Evidence activity

###  1.3 Describe ways to ensure that your personal attitudes or beliefs do not obstruct the quality of your work

This activity gives you an opportunity to demonstrate that your personal attitudes and beliefs do not obstruct the quality of your work.

1. Identify some individuals with whom you work whose personal attitudes and beliefs are different from your own.
2. In what ways are their values, beliefs and experiences different from yours?
3. Describe how you should deal with this so that the quality of your work isn't affected.

# LO2 Be able to reflect on own work activities

## 2.1 Explain why reflecting on practice is an important way to develop knowledge, skills and practice

Being able to reflect on our actions and experiences, learn from them and adapt our behaviour accordingly are some of the most important personal development skills we can acquire. They are of equal importance in a professional development scenario.

We need to consider our:

- Knowledge – what we know or do not know.
- Skills – how able we are at doing something or not.
- Practices – how we behave or perform a task.

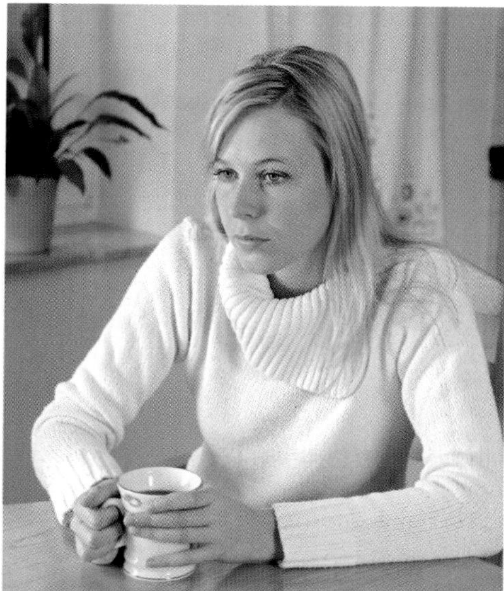

Figure 2.4 Reflection

Reflective practice is the process that enables us to achieve a better understanding of ourselves, our knowledge and understanding, our skills and competencies, and workplace practices in general. It involves:

- Considering what we do.
- Considering why we do it like that.
- Considering whether it is successful.
- Considering whether it could be done better.
- Planning for any changes to what we do.

## Research & investigate

### 2.1 The voice of experience

Talk to some of your supervisors about reflective practice.

What does reflective practice mean for them?

How has it helped them both professionally and in their personal lives?

What could reflective practice mean for you?

Engaging in **critical** reflective practice can be difficult. It challenges our comfortable assumptions about ourselves. However, it is very important for improving quality of service.

## Key term

Critical means examining thoroughly, both the positives and the negatives.

Through being reflective:

1. We become more self-aware. Being self-aware allows us to have raised awareness of others and an increased sensitivity to their needs and how we care for them.
2. We are able to identify weaker work practices, monitor standards and consider alternative approaches and activities in the pursuit of best practice.
3. We have the opportunity to consider our own and others' learning and development needs, thereby ensuring competent practice and improved quality of service.
4. We are able to explore and deal with any negative feelings or anxieties associated with our work, and as a result develop a more positive attitude and improved relationships.

## Evidence activity

### 2.1 Explain why reflecting on practice is an important way to develop knowledge, skills and practice

This activity enables you to demonstrate your understanding of the importance of reflective practice in continuously improving the quality of service provided.

Explain why engaging in critical reflective practice is so important in your ability to continuously improve the quality of service you give to the people you work with.

## 2.2 Assess how well own knowledge, skills and understanding meet standards

'We cannot move forward, if we don't know where we are now.'

Quite simply, this stage is assessing where we stand currently with our knowledge skills and understanding of how to meet standards. Doing this will allow care workers to move forward on the right path to fully recognising and understanding standards which are appropriate for them.

As you read in the introduction, personal development is not just to do with education, or training and the development of skills, although development in these areas is very important to become a knowledgeable, competent and insightful worker and help progress up the career ladder.

How would you assess your knowledge, performance and understanding at the moment? Obviously you feel it is in need of developing or you wouldn't be reading this! But to someone who doesn't work in the health and care sector or use its services, you might already appear to be rather clever! Complimentary though that may be, it is not a valid measure of your abilities. In order to show that you are indeed knowledgeable, competent and insightful, you need to meet the standards set by the various organisations that have an interest in boosting the skills of the health and care sector workforces.

Whatever setting you work in, be it health, social care or with children and young people, there are Codes of Practice, Regulations, National Minimum Standards and National Occupational Standards setting out the standards that are required and expected of you at work and, indeed, by which you can measure yourself.

It's important that you do measure or monitor your knowledge, understanding, conduct and competence, for your own personal and professional development and also for the health, safety and well-being of the people you work with. To do this, you need to regularly reflect and evaluate how you compare with standards.

## Case Study

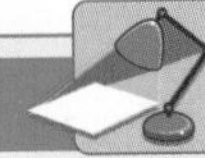

### 2.2 Charlotte

Charlotte Brown recently started working as a domestic at Tiny Tots Playgroup because, according to her mother, 'she absolutely loves children, is so good with them, she's always buying them presents, they love her to bits'.

1. Do you think Mrs Brown's assessment of her daughter's performance has any value?
2. Explain your answer.
3. How would you suggest that Charlotte evaluate her performance?

## Evidence activity

### 2.2 Assess yourself

Using the template below, and the research you did in 1.2 on standards which are relevant to you, complete the following table.

| Standards | Strengths of knowledge, skills and understanding | Areas of knowledge, skills and understanding to develop |
|---|---|---|
| Codes of Practice | | |
| Regulations | | |
| Minimum Standards | | |
| National Occupational Standards | | |

## 2.3 Demonstrate the ability to reflect on work activities

There are two main types of reflection:

1. Reflection *on* action, which is reflecting on an activity after it has happened. Reflecting *on* action allows you to learn from what has happened – learning from experience. For reflection *on* action to make any difference to your practice, you have to make a commitment to *take action* as a result. In other words, you have to be prepared to move out of your comfort zone!
2. Reflection *in* action, which is reflecting on an activity whilst it is happening. Reflecting *in* action allows you to make changes to an activity whilst it is happening, usually because something unexpected or unwanted happens. Reflection *in* action requires you to think on your feet, quickly – learning on the job.

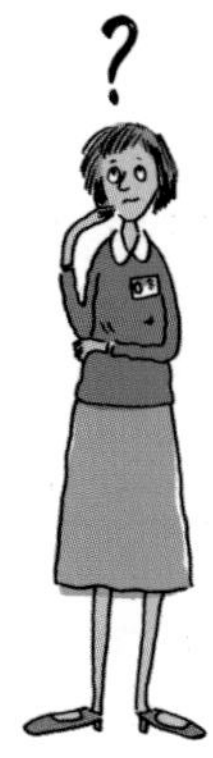
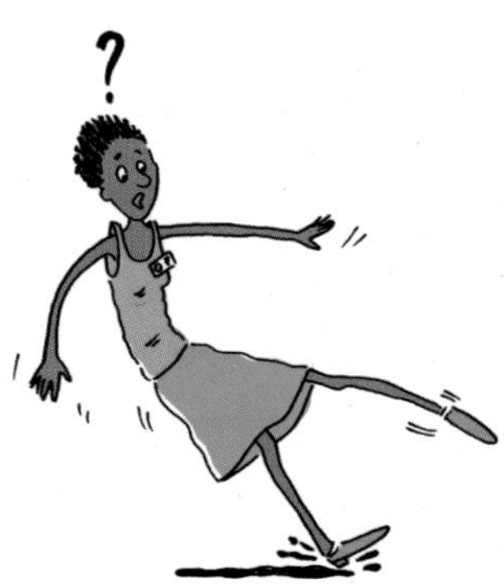

Figure 2.5 Reflection on action and reflection in action

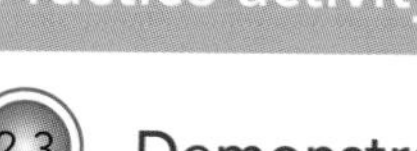

### Practice activity

### 2.3 Demonstrate the ability to reflect on work activities

This activity gives you an opportunity to practise demonstrating your ability to reflect on your work practice.

Identify an activity that you carried out recently. Complete the table below to show that you are developing the skills of reflective practice.

1. Think critically about your behaviour whilst carrying out the activity, for example:
   - What were you doing?
   - What were you trying to achieve?
   - How were you feeling when you started the activity?
   - What were you thinking about at the time?
   - What influenced the way you did the activity?
   - Where were you?
   - Why were you in that place?
   - Who else was there? What were they doing?
2. Assess the impact of your behaviour, for example:
   - How did the activity make you feel?
   - How did the activity make you behave?
   - Why did you behave as you did?
   - What were the consequences of your behaviour for yourself?
   - What were the consequences of your behaviour for others?
   - How did others feel?
   - How do you know this?

*contd.*

## Practice activity *contd.*

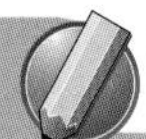

3. Evaluate the impact that the activity had, for example:
   - Did the activity achieve what it was meant to achieve?
   - What went well?
   - What did you do well?
   - What did others do well?
   - What went wrong or did not turn out as it should have done?
   - In what way did you or others contribute to this?
   - Whose interests seem to be served by the way the activity was carried out?
4. Review how the activity could be changed, for example:
   - Could you have done things in a different way?
   - Could others have done things in a different way?
   - How else could the activity be carried out?
   - What would be the consequences of making these changes?
5. Plan for change, for example:
   - How will you carry out the activity next time?

# LO3 Be able to agree a personal development plan

## 3.1 Identify sources of support for own learning and development

Reflection can come from your own considerations. However, there are other sources which can help evaluate learning and development. Feedback from others is useful because it can offer a viewpoint on your work which you may not see for yourself.

Sources of support may include:

- Support within the organisation:
  - formal support
  - supervision
  - appraisal
  - informal support.
- Support beyond the organisation:
  - colleagues from other care organisations
  - friends and family.

### Within the organisation

#### Formal support

In any job role there is a range of support available to support care workers.

- Induction. Induction is a process of introducing an individual to their new role and their responsibilities. This could help an individual to identify their strengths and weaknesses at the outset and may establish areas they need to develop.
- Training. Organisations will all have systems in place for training and CPD (**Continuing Professional Development**). These could be run in-house (internally within the organisation) or with another training provider (externally). It may be that advertised training courses prompt thoughts such as 'I need help with that!'.
- Training days/inset days/development times. Organisations will often have specific periods for care workers to develop their skills and knowledge; this could also prompt discussion about ways to improve.

#### Key term

Continuing Professional Development is the process by which a workforce can maintain, improve and broaden their knowledge and skills and develop the personal qualities required in their work lives.

### Supervision

Your line manager or supervisor is a very important source of feedback as they are ultimately responsible for your work and conduct. Feedback from a line manager or supervisor should happen during appraisal and should be constructive, that is, positive and helpful. Negative feedback is destructive and doesn't promote personal development and change. Supervision feedback could be formal, in set meetings or reviews. However, supervision is also beneficial in a more informal manner: regular catch ups, meetings, chats over coffee, bumping into each other at the photocopier and discussions as simple as 'how's it going?' can also be important.

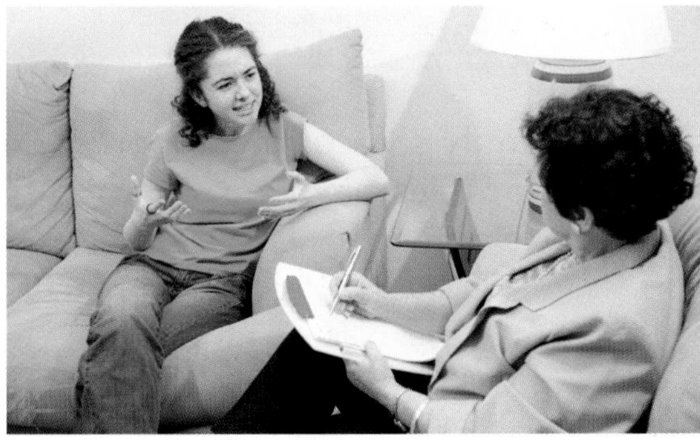

Figure 2.6 Seek feedback from the people you work with

### Appraisals

Appraisals are an opportunity for you to reflect on your work practice and behaviour, talk about your strengths and plan for change in areas that are weak and need developing. Appraisals and performance reviews are another example of formal supervision in that they are planned, carried out according to official workplace policy and conducted in private.

They are an opportunity for you and your line manager or supervisor to get together to:

1. Assess your performance against relevant standards and agreed **performance indicators**, for example attendance on courses, a specific skill, a specific target.
2. Discuss your knowledge, understanding and achievements, including what you have learnt and achieved since your last appraisal/review; your personal attitudes and conduct; and your learning and personal development needs.
3. Exchange views about your work practices – your strengths and how you can improve; your concerns and how they might be dealt with; how you would like your career to develop and what you need to do to further your development.
4. Agree a date for a further meeting, to ensure that your development is continuously reviewed.

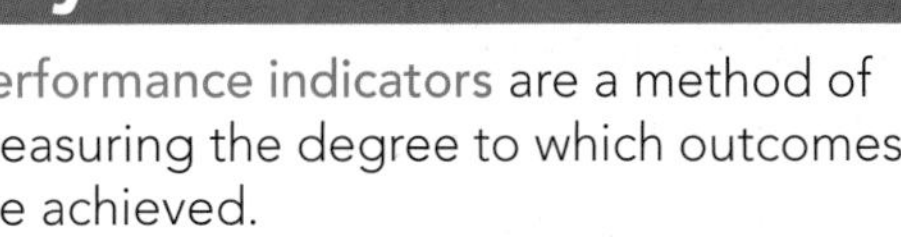

**Key term**

Performance indicators are a method of measuring the degree to which outcomes are achieved.

To be successful, appraisals and performance reviews should be used as the basis for making and reviewing your personal development plan. You will read about personal development plans shortly.

### Informal support

Informal supervision, whilst not quite as structured as appraisals and performance reviews, is a very useful source of support. Informal supervision takes place on the job, by someone who is trained and who has the relevant experience.

Sources of support for personal development within your workplace include the individuals and colleagues you work with on a day-to-day basis. They will be very much aware of your skills and developmental needs and happy to help you develop your care and team working skills if they know you will accept their support with a positive attitude and act on their advice. If, however, you are hostile to criticism and ignore it, they will think twice before giving any advice, however thoughtful their intentions.

Feedback from the people you work with is probably the most important advice to take on board – they may see you in practice daily. Your relationship with them is a partnership, and partnership working demands a mutual show of respect, and so you must value other people's opinions, choices and suggestions about the way you support and care for them.

## Beyond the organisation

### Colleagues from other care organisations

You may work with people from other services. Speaking to them and receiving input and support from them could provide a perspective from outside the confines of your own organisation. Sometimes, we only see what we already see. Seeing a different person's point of view from a different organisation could challenge your existing perspective.

### Friends and family

Although non-specialist, the people who know you could help with identifying your needs (remember confidentiality must be paramount at all times here). They may suggest courses, training or different ways of working as they know you best and may already be aware of areas you need development in.

## But remember ... finish the job! Take action!

As with reflective practice, for feedback to make any difference to your practice, you have to be prepared to act on it and make changes. Think about the feedback you're given. You may not agree with the changes you're asked to make, for example you may be asked to do something in a way that you feel is inappropriate, is not within your level of responsibility or would compromise health and safety. In situations like this, talk with your supervisor or line manager. However, most feedback will be positive and changes you're asked to make will be well within your capability.

Welcome feedback; ask for it and accept any criticism with a positive attitude to show that you are intent on doing your best and learning from your mistakes. Having a positive attitude and being willing to learn will encourage you to reflect on what you've been told. It will also help you deal with any negative comments and complaints and keep them in perspective.

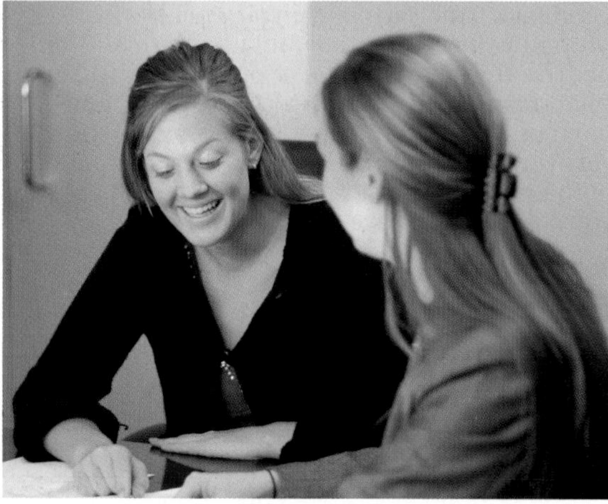

Figure 2.7 Formal supervision

### Research & investigate

#### 3.1 Formal supervision in your workplace

Check out how often formal supervision (appraisal or performance review) should take place at your workplace, when and where your next appraisal or performance review will take place, and who will carry it out with you.

### Practice activity

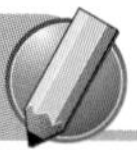

#### 3.1 Identify sources of support for own learning and development

This activity enables you to practise identifying sources of feedback to evaluate your performance and inform your development.

1. Consider your work placement. Make a list of all the various sources of support available to you.
2. Show this list to your supervisor to see if there are any more you could add to it.
3. Ask each source of support for some feedback on your progress and development.

## 3.2 Describe the process for agreeing a personal development plan and who should be involved

A personal development plan may have different names but is a record of information such as agreed objectives for development, proposed activities to meet objectives, timescales for review and so on.

Personal development planning is a process that involves reflecting on your knowledge, understanding, attitudes, behaviour, work practice and achievements, and planning for your personal and career development. It aims to help you understand what and how you are learning, and to review, plan and take responsibility for your own development.

Personal development planning will help you:

1 Become a more effective, independent and confident learner.

2 Understand how you learn and apply your learning to different situations, thereby developing in your job role, both as a person and a practitioner.

3 Set personal goals and evaluate and review your progress towards achieving them.

4 Develop a positive attitude to learning and self-development throughout your life.

Personal development planning is a structured and supported process. It is a good idea to seek support from others when you are planning and reviewing your development. This may include support from:

- carers
- advocates
- supervisor, line manager or employer
- other professionals

Your organisation may employ a Staff Development Officer, who can map your development needs with appropriate training courses and opportunities for **mentoring** and **coaching**.

## Key terms

Mentoring refers to a developmental relationship in which a more experienced person helps someone who has less experience.

Coaching is a method of directing, instructing and training a person or group of people, in order that they achieve some goal or develop specific skills.

Your organisation may employ a training officer or an NVQ assessor, each of whom have a responsibility to help you assess your learning and development needs and support you in meeting them.

You may also have a colleague who is a Trade Union Learning Representative. Their function is to refer you to appropriate learning opportunities.

And of course, staying knowledgeable about your duties and responsibilities and the Standards and Codes of Practice that relate to your job role will ensure that you constantly assess and review your performance and think about ways to develop.

Sources of support for planning and reviewing your development outside of your workplace include organisations such as:

- Connexions (www.connexions-direct.com) which supports young people living in England who want advice on getting to where they want to be in life.
- Your local College of Further Education, which will assess your current skills and abilities and refer you to a learning programme that will meet both your personal and career development needs.
- Websites such as the Careers Advice Service (www.careersadvice.direct.gov.uk), many of which can help you self-assess your current circumstances.

There is no excuse for sitting there and letting the world pass you by! Don't be disappointed in 20 years by the things you don't do now!

## Practice activity

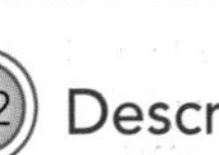

### 3.2 Describe the process for agreeing a personal development plan and who should be involved

This activity enables you to describe the process for agreeing a personal development plan and who should be involved.

1. Make a list of all the information you would need for developing a personal development plan.
2. Make a list of all who should be involved.

## 3.3 Contribute to drawing up own personal development plan

Once you have collated all your information, the next stage is to actually complete your Personal development plan. Clearly, different organisations will have different development plans based on their own systems and requirements.

Below is an example of a personal development plan.

| Focus Area | Area to develop | Action to take | Target to achieve | Target date for completion | Resources needed | Staff | Achievement |
|---|---|---|---|---|---|---|---|
| | | | | | | | |
| | | | | | | | |
| | | | | | | | |
| | | | | | | | |
| | | | | | | | |
| | | | | | | | |
| | | | | | | | |
| | | | | | | | |

Figure 2.8 Example of a personal development plan

## Key

- Focus area – this is the general area a concern falls into, for example communication skills, practical skills, attendance and punctuality, report writing/record keeping skills, organisation, health and safety and so on.
- Area to develop – this is the specific area which needs to be developed. Not to be written critically, but factually and objectively.
- Action to take – what action needs to be taken to redress the area to be developed. This could be attendance on a course, shadowing another member of staff, improved outcomes or just more focus and attention.
- Target to achieve – all targets should be SMART.

S – Specific
M – Measurable
A – Achievable
R – Realistic
T – Time-based

This makes them more likely to be successful as it is clear what is expected and by when.

- Target date for completion – this could be one overall date, or could be broken down in to frequent target dates to check progress at regular intervals.
- Resources needed – this could be financially to pay for training or books, or it could be human resources such as staff who could support you with your targets, or it could be time for you to work on your areas to improve.
- Staff – the member of staff responsible for your target should clearly be defined so that they and you know who is responsible. It may be that different staff are responsible for different targets based on their skills and experience.
- Achievement – here is where the review of your progress can be recorded. If the target has been met, then it may be signed off and new targets for the next time period can be set. If the target has not been met, then productive, non-critical discussions should follow as to why not to help to rectify and remove any problems to development.

### Practice activity

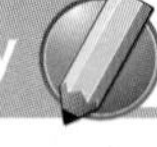

### Contribute to drawing up your own personal development plan

This activity enables you to practise drawing up your own personal development plan.

1. Ask for a blank copy of your work placement's personal development plan.
2. Based on the feedback from the sources of support you requested in previous sections, complete the plan as fully as you can.

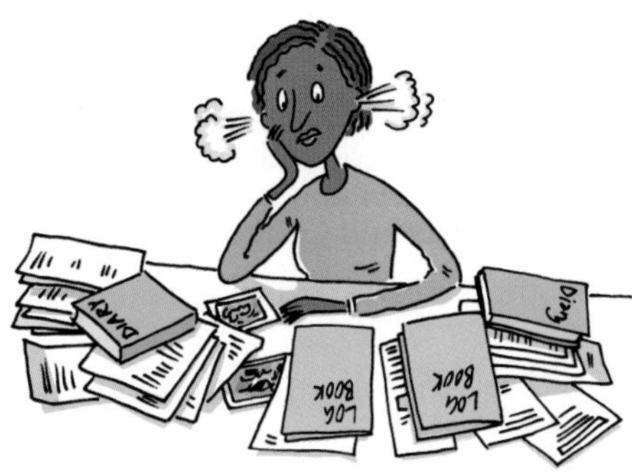

Figure 2.9 Preparing to agree your PDP!

## LO4 Be able to develop knowledge, skills and understanding

### 4.1 Show how a learning activity has improved your own knowledge, skills and understanding

If a learning activity has been completed, we need to evaluate whether it has improved our knowledge, skills and understanding.

It is important to evaluate the outcomes:

1. So that the individual can reflect on how their abilities have improved.
2. So that supervisors and managers can see evidence of improvements.
3. So that the people who organise learning activities can see whether they have been useful or not.

As mentioned in section 2.1, development could have been in:

- Knowledge – what we now know which we didn't know before.
- Skills – what we are able to do which we weren't able to before.
- Practices – how we now perform a task in an improved way to before.

We each need to take responsibility for our own development. Hence it is best to seek out learning activities that are enjoyable and that will most benefit the way we work.

Learning is most effective if you use your preferred learning style. Learning styles are simply different ways of learning and include visual, auditory and kinaesthetic.

Visual learners learn best through seeing, for example:

- they may need to see somebody's body language and facial expression to fully understand an interaction
- they may learn best from visual displays such as diagrams, illustrated text books, DVDs, flipcharts and hand-outs
- they may take notes during a class or training session, to help them absorb the information.

Auditory learners learn best through listening, for example:

- they may enjoy discussions, talking things through and listening to what others have to say
- they may be good at 'reading between the lines', for example they are alert to tone of voice, pitch, speed and other nuances of speech
- it may be that written information does not inspire them to learn.

Kinaesthetic learners learn through doing, for example:

- they may prefer a hands-on approach
- they may need activity to learn
- they may find it hard to sit still for long periods.

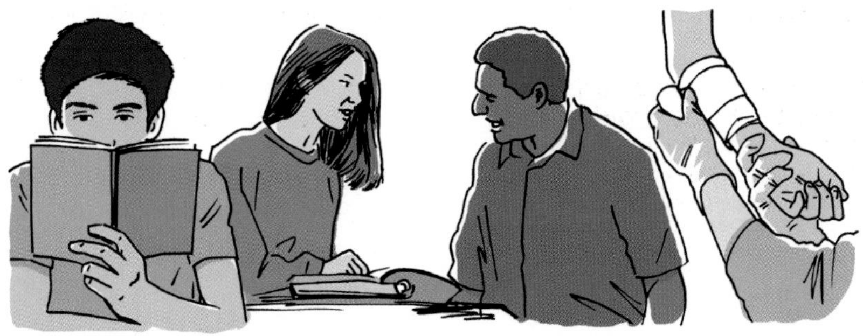

Figure 2.10 Different learning styles

**Evidence activity** 

 4.1 **Evaluate how learning activities have affected practice**

This activity enables you to demonstrate how learning activities have affected your practice.

Think about five learning activities you have participated in that were intended to develop your work practice, and complete the table below to show how your practice has been affected as a result.

| Learning activity and learning style | Effect on your practice? |
|---|---|
| 1. | |
| 2. | |
| 3. | |
| 4. | |
| 5. | |

1. What do you conclude about your learning activities, which have had the greatest impact on your work?
2. How can you apply this conclusion to your future learning and development?

## 4.2 Show how reflecting on a situation has improved own knowledge, skills and understanding

You looked at reflective practice earlier in this chapter and were given an opportunity to explain its importance in improving the service you provide as well as demonstrating your ability to reflect on your work practices. This section asks you to identify how your work has improved as a result of reflective practice.

The reflection process requires you to think critically about areas such as the following and how each affects your work:

1 Your personal beliefs, values and experiences.

2 Your awareness of, attitude to and relationships with the people with whom you work.

3 Your skills, competences and work practices and whether they meet and maintain expected standards and Codes of Practice.

4 Yours and others' training and development needs.

5 Any negative feelings or anxieties you have about your work.

**Case Study** 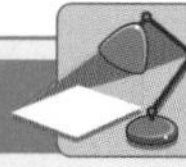

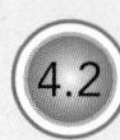 4.2 **Adele**

Adele recently considered her performance at work. She realised that she was really good at what she called 'customer service', she spoke on the phone really well and listened to what individuals had to say. She also realised though that sometimes she spoke in slang, and although not meaning to, she thought she might sound unprofessional.

She also considered how, when she received emails from colleagues she didn't really get on with, she usually deleted them without reading. Days later, they would come and find her to speak to her, making her dislike them even more. She reflected that if she read the email initially and responded, then they wouldn't need to challenge her about it, and maybe this was a **self-fulfilling prophecy** she had created.

Lastly, she reflected on her organisation skills. She felt that although she was excellent on a computer, her written skills were poor and her report writing at work at times illegible.

Adele resolved to tackle all three areas of concern.

1. How has this reflection been beneficial to Adele?
2. What suggestions would you make for Adele?
3. Why would her care worker be pleased with Adele's reflection?

## Key term

Self-fulfilling prophecy means a prediction that directly or indirectly causes itself to become true.

Reflction enables you to identify learning and development needs in order that skills, competences and work practices continuously improve.

## Time to reflect

### How are you getting on?

Most of the activities in this chapter have asked you to think about the effect of your behaviour and work practices on other people. This one looks at how you are affected.

1. Are there any aspects of your job role or other people's work practices or behaviours that you don't enjoy or can't cope with?
2. How do you think things could be improved such that work became more enjoyable and manageable for you?
3. Who can you talk to about your concerns and suggestions for improvement?

## Practice activity

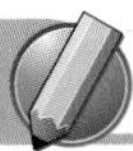

### Show how reflecting on a situation has improved own knowledge, skills and understanding

This activity enables you to practise reflecting on a situation that has improved own knowledge, skills and understanding.

1. Identify three work practices that are carried out at your workplace which you can reflect on.
2. Identify the strengths and areas to develop in each practice.
3. Describe how you think each could be improved.
4. Discuss your ideas for improvement with your line manager or supervisor.
5. If agreed, put your ideas for improvement into practice.

## 4.3 Show how feedback from others has developed own knowledge, skills and understanding

Section 3.1 considered the different sources of support which could be used to assist development. In this section, consideration will be given to how to use this feedback to develop your own knowledge, skills and understanding.

## Case Study

### Yosef

Yosef is a good natured member of the workforce. He has lots of good intentions but never gets around to sorting anything out; he can sometimes be a bit 'haphazard'. He has done what his course has required, and has asked for feedback from varied sources of support. He has 'stored' this information at the bottom of his bag, which is screwed up and not organised. He has not looked at it since, as he thinks he is 'doing great at work, it's brilliant!'.

If Yosef was actually to look at his feedback there are some positives, but there are also some significant concerns and areas where he needs to develop.

1. Explain why ignoring this could be a problem for Yosef.
2. Explain why Yosef not developing or recognising his 'concerns' is a problem for his care setting.
3. In the longer term, what may happen to Yosef?

There is little point gaining feedback if one does little with it.

- If written, it needs to be read fully.
- If spoken, it needs to be listened to (and notes taken if needed).
- It needs to be stored appropriately.
- The feedback needs to be summarised into strengths (positives) and areas to develop (weaknesses).
- The feedback needs to be analysed maturely and critically. Although at times it can be difficult to confront one's own failings, little progress will be made if it is taken personally.
- If it is felt that feedback is too critical or harsh, it is perfectly acceptable to challenge it and present your opinions and perspectives. Just because someone else has said it, it doesn't ALWAYS mean it is right!
- Discuss the feedback with your supervisor.
- Act on the feedback!
- List actions you could take and changes you could make to present in your PDP.

## Practice activity

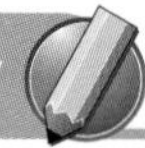

### Show how feedback from others has developed own knowledge, skills and understanding

This activity enables you to show how feedback from others has developed your own knowledge, skills and understanding.

1. Review the feedback you gained in Practice activity 3.1.
2. Summarise the strengths that the feedback suggests.
3. Summarise the areas you need to develop that the feedback suggests.
4. How has this feedback developed your own thoughts of your development?
5. What action do you plan to take from this feedback to develop your own knowledge, skills and understanding?

## 4.4 Show how to record progress in relation to personal development

Your personal development plan is an ongoing record of your strengths, goals and objectives, learning and development needs, and achievements. In other words, it is a record of your progress in relation to your personal and professional development.

Why record personal and professional development? Especially when time is at a premium and doing the learning can seem more important than noting down what we've learned?

Recording is important for a number of reasons:

- it helps us reflect and review
- it reminds us of what we've learnt

- it helps us build our CV and provides information for potential employers
- it provides the framework for appraisals and promotion boards
- it's a regulatory requirement for some professions
- it provides evidence when we need to prove competence, for example when applying for **professional registration.**

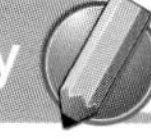

## Key term

Professional registration demonstrates that you have met standards of competence and is a requirement for employment of a number of professionals.

Records of personal development should include information such as:

- What you've learnt and when, how you learnt it and any evidence that verifies your learning.
- Evidence to show how your learning has developed your practice, for example, statements from your line manager, colleagues and the people you work with.
- How you've used support and in what ways you found it useful.
- How well you feel that you are progressing towards your long-term goals.
- How your learning needs are developing.

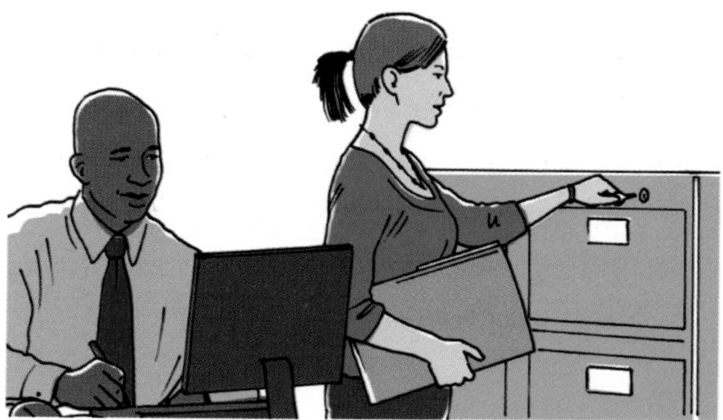

Figure 2.11 Completing and storing your PDP

Records can take the form of a simple learning journal or log-book, on paper or in a computer file; and a ring-binder can be used for storing evidential statements, course notes, certificates, reading lists and lists of books, articles and so on that you've read and that have helped you.

More formal personal development action plans and portfolios of evidence record learning in a more organised way, for example they might include summaries of evidence, personal references and cross-referencing of learning. Alternatively, you could use an on-line system, which will provide a set format guiding you in what to record and when to update your record. However you choose to record your development, make it fit with your circumstances, the expectations of your employer and any regulatory requirements you have to comply with.

When thinking about how to record your personal development plan, bear in mind issues of confidentiality. If you refer by name to the people you work with, you must ensure confidentiality as per your organisation's legal requirements. You might also want to bear in mind the location of your record and its accessibility. You need to update your record regularly, but you also need to be able to take it with you if you change jobs.

## Practice activity

### 4.4 Show how to record your progress in relation to personal development

This activity enables you to practise showing how to record your progress in relation to your personal development.

Create your own personal development plan, find an on-line pro-forma or get hold of one that is produced by your workplace. Start using it to keep a record of your personal development, updating it as regularly as you think appropriate or your workplace policy requires.

## Assessment summary

Your reading of this chapter and completion of the activities will have prepared you to demonstrate your learning and understanding of the principles of safeguarding and protection in health and social care. Assessment of Learning Outcomes 2,3,4,5 and 6 must be assessed in a real work environment. To achieve the unit, your assessor will require you to:

| Learning Outcomes | Assessment Criteria |
|---|---|
| Learning Outcome 1: Understand what is required for competence in your work role by: | 1.1 describing the duties and responsibilities of own role<br><br>See Evidence activity 1.1 on p. 20 |
| | 1.2 identifying standards that influence the way the role is carried out<br><br>See Evidence activity 1.2 on p. 23 |
| | 1.3 describing ways to ensure that personal attitudes or beliefs do not obstruct the quality of work.<br><br>See Evidence activity 1.3 on p. 24 |
| Learning Outcome 2: Be able to reflect on own work activities by: | 2.1 explaining why reflecting of practice is an important way to develop knowledge, skills and practice<br><br>See Evidence activity 2.1 on p. 25 |
| | 2.2 assessing how well own knowledge, skills and understanding meet standards<br><br>See Evidence activity 2.2 on p. 26 |
| | 2.3 demonstrating the ability to reflect on work activities.<br><br>See Practice activity 2.3 on p. 27 |
| Learning Outcome 3: Be able to agree a personal development plan by: | 3.1 identifying sources of support for own learning and development<br><br>See Practice activity 3.1 on p. 30 |
| | 3.2 describing the process for agreeing a personal development plan and who should be involved<br><br>See Practice activity 3.2 on p. 31 |

| Learning Outcomes | Assessment Criteria |
| --- | --- |
| Learning Outcome 3: Be able to agree a personal development plan by: | 3.3 contributing to drawing up own personal development plan. See Practice activity 3.3 on p. 32 |
| Learning Outcome 4: Be able to develop knowledge, skills and understanding by: | 4.1 showing how a learning activity has improved on knowledge, skills and understanding See Evidence activity 4.1 on p. 34 |
| | 4.2 showing how reflecting on a situation has improved own knowledge, skills and understanding See Practice activity 4.2 on p. 35 |
| | 4.3 showing how feedback from others has developed own knowledge, skills and understanding See Practice activity 4.3 on p. 36 |
| | 4.4 showing how to record progress in relation to personal development. See Practice activity 4.4 on p. 37 |

Good luck!

## Weblinks

| | |
| --- | --- |
| Care Quality Commission | www.cqc.org.u |
| Community Care Careers | www.communitycare.co.uk/jobs/search |
| General Medical Council | www.gmc-uk.org |
| General Social Care Council | ww.gscc.org.uk |
| General Teaching Council for England | www.gtce.org.uk |
| Government Careers Advice website | www.careersadvice.direct.gov.uk |
| Healthcare Careers | www.connexions-direct.com/jobs4u |
| Health Professionals Council | www.hpc-uk.org |
| Ofsted | www.ofsted.gov.uk |
| Nursing and Midwifery Council | www.nmc-uk.org |
| Social Care & Counselling careers | www.connexions-direct.com/jobs4u |
| Skills for Health | www.skillsforhealth.org.uk |
| Skills for Care and Development | www.skillsforcareanddevelopment.org.uk |
| Government website (public services) | www.direct.gov.uk |

# 3 Introduction to equality and inclusion in health, social care or children's and young person's settings

## For Unit SHC23

### What are you finding out?

In our society we live with a variety of different **cultures** and have grown up in this multicultural environment. We are all aware of racial tensions that can occur and the origins of this behaviour, a prime example would be the slave trade, importing overseas persons, and the treatment they incurred when arriving in Britain. On arriving in Britain they were seen as slaves, inferior people with no rights, and no expectations were placed on them to integrate within British society. Within this chapter we are going to explore equal rights in health and social care and children's and young person's settings. We are going to identify the terms, 'equality' and 'inclusion' and what they mean to the people we are caring for. Equality identifies that all persons are treated fairly and equally. An example of equality would be the idea that a person who is unable to walk has the same rights as a person who can walk. A good example of this is the paraplegic Olympics, which give disabled persons the right to compete in the Olympics.

The United Kingdom is one of the most diverse countries in Europe. Of its 61 million residents, almost 8 per cent – about 4.6 million people – are from ethnic minority groups, and in London over 300 languages are spoken. There are slightly more women than men in the UK, and an estimated 6 per cent of people are lesbian, gay or bisexual. There is also religious diversity: while 45 per cent of people in the UK identify themselves as having no religious belief, 47.5 per cent of people say they are Christian, 3.3 per cent are Muslim, and there is also a strong representation of Hindu, Jewish, Sikh and Buddhist faiths. There are also around 11 million disabled people in Great Britain, representing around 18 per cent of the population.

http://www.cqc.org.uk

Within this chapter we will identify where you may come across inequality and exclusion within settings and the resources available to you to promote equality and inclusion.

The reading and activities in this chapter will help you to:

- Understand the importance of equality and inclusion
- Be able to work in an inclusive way
- Know how to access information, advice and support about diversity, equality and inclusion.

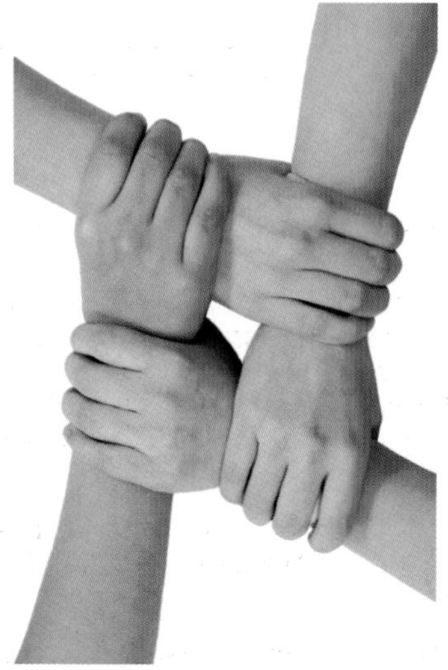

Figure 3.1 Equality and diversity

### Key term

Culture is the behaviours and beliefs characteristic of a particular social, ethnic or age group: for example youth culture or drug culture.

# LO1 Understand the importance of equality and inclusion

## 1.1 Explain what is meant by diversity, equality, inclusion and discrimination

### Diversity

**Diversity** is defined as being when many different types of things or people are included in something. Within the health and social care setting, diversity is always prominent in care homes for the elderly. This is due to different age groups, different cultures and different beliefs. The easiest way to look at diversity is to go back to your childhood days and school. Think how diverse your school was: did you have people from different cultures; were there thin and larger children at school? Did you know someone who was vegetarian, homosexual, was someone taller then you? The questions of diversity can continue into many areas in the school setting. As we have grown up and explored the wider world in our workplace, on our way to work, shopping and so on we have found many differences. The term 'Diversity' has become well known as the name of a dance group who clearly illustrate diversity through different age groups, different cultures and height differences. Using this model we can identify different or diverse groups in everyday living.

**Key term**

Diversity is when many different types of things or people are included in something.

In care practices we have many different abilities, sexual preferences, ages and backgrounds. Within childcare settings we can identify children from diverse backgrounds.

**The General Medical Council** defines diversity as 'the differences in the values, attitudes, cultural perspectives, beliefs, ethnic backgrounds, and sexuality, skills, knowledge and life experiences of each individual in any group of people'. This definition refers to differences between people and is used to highlight individual needs. The government addresses diversity for children in the publication 'Every Child Matters'.

The need to address diversity has certain **legislation** attached to it: the **Human Rights Act 1998** and the **Equality Act 2010** identify the need to address differences and embrace them.

**Key terms**

The Equality Act 2010 is a legislation framework to protect the rights of individuals and advance equality of opportunity for all.
The Human Rights Act 1998 is key legislation for the protection of individual's fundamental rights.
Legislation is statutory law.
The General Medical Council are the regulators of doctors and ensure good medical practice.

**Evidence activity** 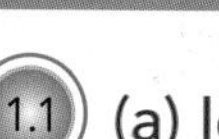

**1.1 (a) Identifying types of diversity**

This activity will show you can identify different types of diversity.

List the different diversities within your workplace within these three areas

| Staff | Clients | Visitors | Explain why they are diverse |
|---|---|---|---|
| | | | |

### Equality

The definition of equality is that everyone be equal. The Equality Act of 2010 identifies the need to ensure that everyone is treated fairly and equally. A good example of equality is equal rights for women and men. In the U.K. the suffragettes won the right for women to vote in 1918 and this was a huge advance for women's rights and equality.

The Equality Act identifies the areas in which we can all expect to be treated as an equal, these include:

- basic human needs, housing, warmth
- education and employment

- transport
- health and social care
- sufficient money to live
- childcare.

This legislation ensures that we all have the right to housing that is warm and safe; we are all able to access education and employment on the same equal basis. We are all entitled to use of public transport and no one should live in poverty, as the legislation identifies financial support for those who need it. We are all entitled to childcare provision.

The legislation is there to ensure we all have equal access to services and the same choices in life. No one will be discriminated against as we will all be seen on an equal basis. To ensure that we all have the same rights and opportunities, we need to embrace individual differences.

An example of equality in the healthcare setting might be by employing different sexes to do the same role. Men and women can do the same job. In care homes we often check with the female clients if they mind a male attending to their personal hygiene, how often do we check with the male clients if they mind a female attending to their personal hygiene needs?

When we are applying for employment we would be shocked to see a vacancy with two salaries advertised suggesting males will be paid at a higher rate.

In a childcare setting we do not allow only the girls to play with dolls and the boys only to play with cars. This would not be equal.

We address equality in everyday life, we expect to be treated the same as everyone else within our family, within our communities and within the wider environment. On buying this book you know you are receiving the same information as everyone else who has bought the book as this is equal and fair.

## Inclusion

We have identified the meanings of diversity and equality; we are now going to look at **inclusion** (the action of being included in to a group). It is fine to say that everyone has equal access but we also need to ensure that no one is prevented from joining in an activity due to any differences: this is the main topic for inclusion.

### Key term

**Inclusion** means to include all.

### Evidence activity

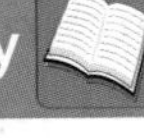

**1.1 (b) Explain your understanding of equality**

This activity will demonstrate that you can explain your understanding of equality.

Mr Jones is to be admitted to the home in the afternoon; Mr Singh is also being admitted in the afternoon. The care assistant is preparing the information documents and care plan paperwork. Mr Jones is blind and has a niece looking after him, and Mr Singh has no one looking after him. The information packs are all written in English. What preparation can you do prior to their arrival to ensure equality?

An example of inclusion would be that at school, no matter what your academic abilities you are included in the learning. Within a healthcare setting an example of inclusion would be that all the residents join in a group activity, regardless of their differences.

When we look at inclusion, because some people may have difficulties in being included due to their differences, we need to ensure that we make suitable adaptations so that the individual can be included. A good example of this would be the Paralympics.

Within the work setting it is part of our role to ensure we include everyone and make sufficient adjustments for those with differences. The importance of involving everyone is to ensure that isolation does not occur. Can you recall a situation when you were excluded, and how this felt? It is not a comfortable feeling and tends to make the individuals feel not wanted, not part of the community and disadvantaged.

## Discrimination

The definition of discrimination in the *Oxford Dictionary* is the unjust or prejudicial treatment of different categories of people, especially on the grounds of race, age or sex.

It is frequently forgotten in residential homes that persons of any age can enjoy sex and are able to have an active life even if they are possibly unable to function in other daily living skills.

We face discrimination frequently: people in wheelchairs have limited access to venues, how many times have you been past a person in a wheelchair and not greeted them in the way you

Evidence activity 

### 1.1 (c) Demonstrate your knowledge of inclusion

This activity will allow you to demonstrate your knowledge of inclusion.

Write down an example of a situation in the workplace when you have taken some of the residents out. Write about how it went: were there any residents that could have been included but were left out due to disabilities? How could you have included them? What will you do next time?

would a person standing up? If you have ever broken a leg and needed a wheelchair you will appreciate how difficult this is, being unable to reach things and relying on others to assist you. Although supermarkets have access and hire wheelchairs for those who need them, customers in shops are not very supportive and are unaware of how difficult it can be for these people, they just continue with their trolleys, rushing around. The main complaint from people in wheelchairs is the lack of eye contact or people speaking above them. Have a look when you next go shopping.

With young people there is a general prejudicial belief that they are up to trouble, for example if they wear a hooded top this is confirmation they are into drugs. This was highlighted when a law was proposed that would mean hoods were not allowed to be worn by youngsters in shopping malls. This is discrimination as it classifies all young people as the same because of their age.

Our role is to be aware of these discriminations and prevent them. We can do this by reinforcing a positive attitude and embracing differences.

Evidence activity 

### 1.1 (d) Demonstrate your knowledge of discrimination

This activity will allow you to demonstrate your knowledge of discrimination.

In the table below, fill in different types of discrimination that you can identify.

| General discrimination | Against you | Against others |
|---|---|---|
| | | |
| | | |
| | | |

## 1.2 Describe ways in which discrimination may deliberately or inadvertently occur in the work setting

In a care setting you have many residents/clients who have a variety of knowledge and experience. Sometimes these experiences can lead to prejudicial beliefs. Someone who fought in the war against the Argentines may be prejudiced against anyone from that country. We may inadvertently deal in prejudice with televisions in a communal lounge; believing men want to watch football whilst not taking account of the wishes of all the men. Some men do not like football and some of the women may not like sport. This type of prejudice can become quite difficult to handle. Think of a situation you have been involved in and ways to pacify the situation. Generally we would identify the majority who wish to watch the programme and arrange another area for the others to watch their preferences.

When someone enters care for the first time we should identify their individual likes and dislikes. By doing this we ensure that we are able to cope with their individual needs. This includes dietary preferences. Sometimes we may come across different religions and beliefs that we are unaware of. We need to identify their preferences to maintain their religion, this is our role. Therefore we need to explore these preferences and identify how we can help the individual to become part of the community and not feel isolated.

In childcare settings we need to identify the child's and parent's culture, on first meeting them, and then we can ensure we maintain their culture. It would be very easy just to make sure all children wash their hands before meals. But the Islamic religion, for example, does not believe in washing in still water. For these children we can then ensure that they are washing their hands without the plug in the sink.

Inadvertent discrimination in this instance would presume that everyone from an Indian religion is Muslim and that all the children must therefore wash in free flowing water. This highlights the importance of finding out individual needs and preferences at the beginning before starting to provide care.

Another example of inadvertent discrimination would be preparing a Sunday roast for all your residents and pouring gravy over every meal without checking first that everyone wanted gravy.

**Evidence activity** 

### 1.2 Describe the ways discrimination may deliberately or inadvertently occur in the work setting

This activity demonstrates that you can describe ways in which discrimination may deliberately or inadvertently occur in the work setting.

Think of your workplace and identify two types of discrimination and two types of inadvertent discrimination that could occur. Write a brief outline of what you could do to prevent these types of discrimination.

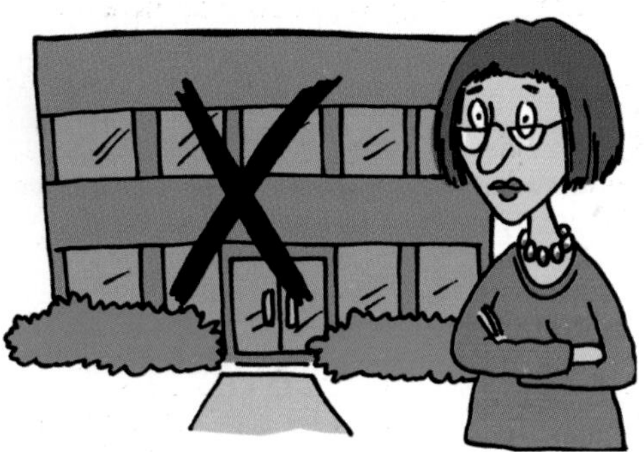

Figure 3.2 Age discrimination

## 1.3 Explain how practice that supports equality and inclusion reduces the likelihood of discrimination

Recall a time when your friends have asked you for a night out, and think about how you come to the decision of where you were going. This was an agreed view of the majority of the group. When people are living in a shared environment they may not be able to vocalise their choices and wishes, therefore we need to ensure we understand all their choices and needs. Then we are able to include everyone.

By understanding the diversity of needs we can establish likes and dislikes within a community and enhance the living conditions. Sometimes we have different cultures living in the same environment, instead of identifying these as special circumstances, for example vegetarians, by giving them a label, we could embrace this culture and have a theme night of vegetarian foods. By doing this we explore differences and enable others to learn and maybe enjoy the food.

An example we often come into contact with within care homes of older persons, is their misunderstanding of overseas staff. Communication and prejudices are most prominent. Initially we need to understand how these prejudices have come about, a classic one may be an individual brought up in India, where the locals were their servants. Communication from the resident/client may be abrupt and rude, this may be the way the resident/client would have spoken to the servants and this would have been the correct manner in those times.

The need to educate the resident/client about the role of the carer is paramount as the resident/client needs the care that the carer is trying to deliver. By enabling this education we will enable a better service for the individual and increase her/his knowledge. We need to support the carer, our work colleague, during this time.

I am sure all of us can think of a time when a resident/client has been sharp in their manner towards us; this can make us less enthusiastic to attend to their needs and we rely on the support of our colleagues to manage this behaviour.

**Evidence activity** 

### 1.3 Explain how your practices support equality and inclusion and reduce the likelihood of discrimination

This activity demonstrates that you can explain how your practices support equality and inclusion and reduce the likelihood of discrimination.

List the resources available to you to enable choices and support individuals to have choices.

Reflect on the advantages of giving choices; identify what could happen if individual choices were not allowed.

The use of supervision in the setting enables us to support and encourage inclusion from all.

## LO2 Be able to work in an inclusive way

### 2.1 Identify which legislation and codes of practice relating to equality, diversity and discrimination apply to own role

Within any work setting, health, social care or children's and young person's settings, we have guidelines and protocols on acceptable behaviour. Every work setting has policies and procedures; these give the outlines of our roles.

When starting employment in these settings you are introduced to the policies and procedures and are asked to keep up to date with changes in these.

The General Social Care Council (GSCC) provides codes of practice for social care workers and employers. Within these codes are directives of good practice for treatment of individuals. These codes include their right to be respected, promotion of individual rights and preferences, the right to be given support to control their lives and the right to make informed choices.

Policies and procedures are formed via legislation and good practices guidelines. Legislation for NHS employers can be found at www.nhsemployers.org/EmploymentPolicyAndPractice, within this you can find the Equality Act 2010. For children you can find the relevant information at www.dcsf.gov.uk/everychildmatters/earlyyears/equalityanddiversity, this is where you need to look for relevant legislation.

Good practice guidelines can be found at www.nmc-uk.org/About-us/Equality-and-diversity/Equality-and-diversity-about-us, this is the organisation that regulates qualified nurses. Another place where the information is freely available is at www.cqc.org.uk.

Where you are working there will also be policies (a principle or rule of what should occur in certain situations) and procedures (a series of actions or operations on how to do a task).

**Evidence activity** 

**2.1 Identify which legislation and codes of practice apply to your own role**

This activity demonstrates your ability to identify which legislation and codes of practice relating to equality, diversity and discrimination apply to your own role.

List the relevant legislation and good practice guidelines that are in effect in your workplace.

### 2.2 Show interaction with individuals that respects their beliefs, culture, values and preferences

In a care home setting weekends can be a busy time. Residents/clients of Christian faith may wish to visit the local church or a church service may be present in the home, but how do we manage the spiritual needs of residents/clients of the Jewish faith? In the Jewish religion Saturday is their day of worship, is this recognised in your setting?

In a care environment it is important to identify individual choices and values. The need to ensure preferences prior to admission is paramount. The Care Quality Commission will be looking for evidence of equality and diversity within the home whilst on their inspections.

There is a need to ensure that everyone can understand the rights and choices available to them. Individuals are able to request an advocate to voice their needs. Female residents are able to ask for female carers only.

On admission it is important to identify how a person would like to be addressed, for example Mr Smith, Harry or Sir. This should be noted in their care plans so everyone will be aware of what their preferred name is.

**Evidence activity** 

### 2.2 Show interaction with individuals that respects their beliefs, culture, values and preferences

This activity demonstrates that you understand how to show interaction with individuals that respects their beliefs, culture, values and preferences.

Mr X is physically disabled and has a wheelchair. He wishes to visit his neighbour every Saturday. Mr X is sometimes confused and may get lost. The distance from the home to his neighbour is one mile. Mr X has strong arm muscles and is able to move in his wheelchair independently. On the way to his neighbours is a steep hill that has a main road running down the side.

What are the risks?

Should Mr X be allowed to go?

What can be done to reduce the risks?

## 2.3 Describe how to challenge discrimination in a way that encourages change

We have identified what is classed as discrimination, now we need to look at ways of dealing with discrimination in a positive manner that will encourage a change in behaviour. We have discussed that discrimination is generally due to misunderstanding and limited knowledge. Sometimes this is due to fear of the unknown.

Therefore it is important that we challenge every discrimination that we identify and, even more importantly, challenge inadvertent discrimination as the persons are likely to be unaware of this occurring.

Imagine you have walked into a nursery and the children are put into two groups, boys and girls. The group activity is very feminine for the girls and very masculine for the boys. What can you do? The main way to educate and enable choice is to identify a time to switch the activities, informing the organisers of the session that this will enable a more accurate reporting of abilities.

In the home care setting we may come across people who have taken a dislike to another resident/client for no obvious reason. A way we can challenge this is to engage both in an activity or discussion on something they both have in common. We can only address this if we know what both people like and dislike. This again comes from the initial assessment on arrival.

Training courses can challenge the way we think and encourage positive discussions to look at our actions and modify our behaviours. The most effective way of challenging behaviour is to model good behaviour; this is used frequently in childcare settings.

If we examine our own behaviour, analyse our own prejudices and perceptions, we feel confident to discuss them freely and listen to alternative views. The reception from others will be more positive. Behaviour is copied: a test of this is to sit in a room with your colleagues and start quietly yawning; you will be amazed how many of your colleagues start doing the same thing (if you are not comfortable with yawning try scratching your arm discreetly).

**Evidence activity** 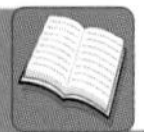

### 2.3 Challenge discrimination in a way that encourages change

This activity demonstrates your ability to describe how to challenge discrimination in a way that encourages change.

A gentleman has been admitted to a home and has shown an interest in a female resident within the home. The family of the woman are accepting of the relationship but the gentleman's relatives are against the relationship. They say that their father was in love with their mother and although she has died they feel he would not want another relationship. The gentleman is insistent that he wants this relationship and becomes angry if not allowed to mix with his female friend.

What rights do the family have?

What support can you get for the gentleman?

What would you do?

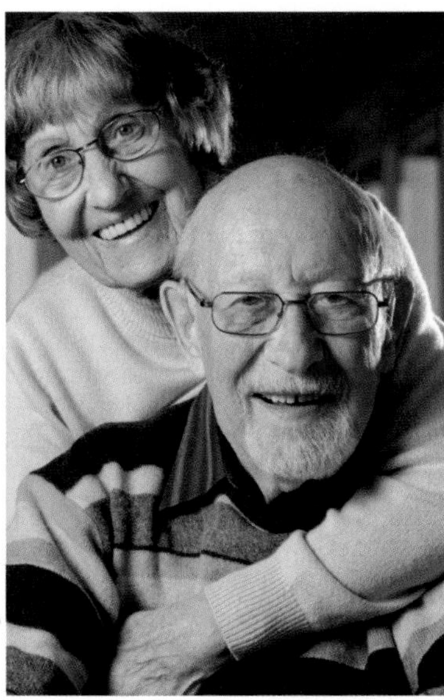

Figure 3.3 Relationships between older people

## LO3 Know how to access information, advice and support about diversity, equality and inclusion

### 3.1 Identify a range of sources of information, advice and support about diversity, equality and inclusion

When working in a setting we have already identified the need to find out about client's individual choices, values and beliefs. Finding these out may initially be difficult if the person is not able to verbalise these issues clearly, we can rely on their relatives if the individual agrees. We can also find out some factual information regarding their religion, for example, from medical records. Sometimes we need to spend extra time with the individual to establish their likes and dislikes. Occasionally we may need to identify who they feel more comfortable with when speaking about their personal preferences. With children we need to let them explore by doing things, an example of this would be letting them play with sand to gauge their enjoyment of this activity; they may prefer to play with water instead. Children may have limited experience from which to form a judgement of their likes and dislikes.

As carers we need to ensure that a client's preferences will not exclude them from the group, either in a residential premises or a childcare group. Our role is to maximise their involvement within the community they are in.

You may come across a person who does not enjoy socialising, and this needs to be respected as their choice. Ways of including them would be to always offer them the opportunity to attend a function, even if they say no it is important to show them they are part of a group and entitled to attend if they wish. Sometimes it is easy to assume that someone will always say no and so never invite them, this is not inclusion and does not make the person feel valued.

With equality and diversity you may sometimes require some advice on how to enable individuals in your care. Because people are so individual and diverse it is impossible to find a book containing all the situations you may come across with answers for every situation. The Equality Act 2010 has the legislation relating to the legal requirements of the act. Policies and procedures will give you some ideas, but sometimes you will still come across a situation where you are unsure.

There are many places to find answers to any situation. In a care setting you have a variety of skilled people working with you that you can ask, the nurse in charge, doctor, relative or colleague. Within the care setting you have a handover time, care plans and so on; these are prime times to address any concerns you have regarding equality and diversity. The first person to discuss any issues with, however, would be the person you think is being treated unfairly. A more indirect questioning of how they feel will generally bring up words of 'lonely, not part of the group, not important' and so on. If this is the information you are getting from the individual you know inequality of care has occurred either directly or indirectly.

When a client/resident is being seen by the doctor or another professional who may not be so informed of the person's choices it is your role to ensure their preferences are heard and acted upon.

Just because someone needs a care environment it does not follow that they have lost their rights, and as a care worker your role is to support that person in the ways that are their preferred choices.

In childcare settings the values are the same, you may be the voice for the child if they are unable to express their preferences. The parent may state they have difficulties in getting their child to have a nap in the afternoon; you may, through your observations, have identified the child falls to sleep to the sound of a certain type of music. By informing the parents they can try this and the child gets their choice.

## Evidence activity 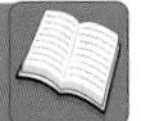

### 3.1 Identify a range of sources of information, advice and support about diversity, equality and inclusion

This activity demonstrates your ability to identify a range of sources of information, advice and support about diversity, equality and inclusion.

List all the relevant legislation relating to diversity, inclusion and equality. Here is some relevant legislation to help you start your research:

- Human Rights Act 1998
- Disability Discrimination Act 1995
- Disability Discrimination Act 2005
- Special Educational Needs and Disability Act 2001
- Race Relations (Amendment) Act 2000
- Equality and Human Rights Commission

## 3.2 Describe how and when to access information, advice and support about diversity, equality and inclusion

There are many situations when we should question and challenge behaviour. Sometimes we will need support to promote diversity, equality and inclusion.

We need to assess situations very carefully to identify clearly what the problems are. As we have discovered, discrimination may come from our previous learning of situations; an example of this would be if our parents had told us that people with ginger hair are all very intelligent. We would have the understanding that all red headed people are clever and are not in need of any educational help. This would be a prejudice and may cause isolation for the individuals. Therefore we need to examine and challenge our own beliefs. One way that we can challenge our beliefs is to ask colleagues about their understanding of red headed people. Another way we challenge our beliefs is through coming into contact with a red headed person; their reaction is sometimes different to what we believe it will be. Reflective practice allows us to explore our attitudes.

Sometimes in the care setting we can find that different people react differently to alternative approaches, an example of this would be a male resident having a shave from a female compared to having a shave at the barbers. As previously stated, sometimes we do not initially know someone's personal preferences and so have to explore these over a period of time. Information we obtain on admission may not initially identify preferences, or may be taken from a relative who has not been involved in their care for many years.

It is important to also note that preferences may change, and moving into a home environment and seeing how others enjoy or do things differently may be a factor itself in changing preferences.

When someone new needs our care there are some things we are able to do to ensure we promote equality and diversity. An example of this is to identify the religion of the person and ensure that all staff are aware of their cultural needs. The easiest way of finding detailed information is by using the internet. There are other resources: colleagues, libraries and information in the local communities.

Another time that you may need to seek advice or information is if someone you are caring for needs information on their medical diagnosis. You could again ask a colleague or, in a care home setting, ask the doctor to inform the person.

In any organisation part of the policies and procedures are the complaints guidelines. Everyone has the right to complain. Complaints should be seen as a positive outcome. Complaints highlight any inequalities or discrimination. Some people may be reserved about complaining and will require help and support to do this; there may also be a need for advocacy.

With young people, especially the much younger child, support will include their parents and possibly social services or other agencies involved in their care. To gain support in childcare go to the website below:

**http://www.dcsf.gov.uk/everychildmatters/strategy/improvingquality/qualificationsandtraining/childrensworkforce**

Part of anyone's job who works in the health, social care or children's and young person's setting, is the duty to maintain their knowledge of up-to-date legislation and practices. Within your employment, regular supervision meetings with your line manager should identify training needs and offer support to deal with any diversity, equality or inclusion problems.

Remember though that any problems should not just be kept for supervision meetings, as they can escalate quickly and therefore should be sorted out promptly.

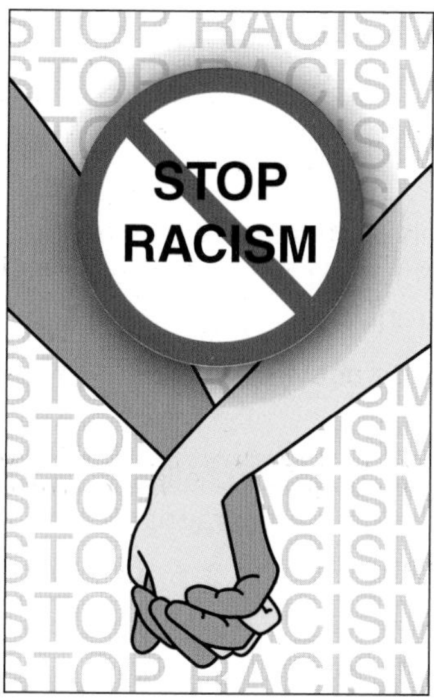


Figure 3.4 Sources of information

## Evidence activity 

 3.2 **Identify how and when to access information, advice and support for diversity, equality and inclusion**

This activity enables you to demonstrate that you can identify how and when to access information advice and support for diversity, equality and inclusion.

Think of a situation where you might have to access support for someone due to discrimination. Where would you go for support? Write an action plan of what help and support you would get and where you would access this help.

Prepare a leaflet of the information for anyone new into the services.

## Assessment summary

Your reading of this chapter and completion of the activities will have prepared you to demonstrate your learning, understanding and competence in equality and inclusion in health, social care or children's and young person's settings. Assessment criteria 2.2 and 3.2 must be observed in the workplace by your assessor. To achieve this Level 2 Introduction to equality and inclusion in health, social care or children's and young person's settings, your assessor will require you to:

| Learning Outcomes | Assessment Criteria |
|---|---|
| Learning objective 1: Understand the importance of equality and inclusion by: | 1.1 explaining what is meant by:<br>diversity (Evidence activity 1.1a, p. 41)<br>equality (Evidence activity 1.1b, p. 42)<br>inclusion (Evidence activity 1.1c, p. 43)<br>discrimination (Evidence activity 1.1d, p. 43) |
| | 1.2 describing ways in which discrimination may deliberately or inadvertently occur in the work setting<br><br>Evidence activity 1.2, p. 44 |
| | 1.3 explaining how practices that support equality and inclusion reduce the likelihood of discrimination<br><br>Evidence activity 1.3, p. 44 |

| Learning Outcomes | Assessment Criteria |
|---|---|
| Learning objective 2: Be able to work in an inclusive way by: | 2.1 identifying which legislation and codes of practice relating to equality, diversity and discrimination apply to own role<br>Evidence activity 2.1, p. 45 |
| | 2.2 showing interaction with individuals that respects their beliefs, culture, values and preferences<br>Evidence activity 2.2, p. 46 |
| | 2.3 describing how to challenge discrimination in a way that encourages change<br>Evidence activity 2.3, p. 46 |
| Learning objective 3: Know how to access information, advice and support for diversity, equality and inclusion by: | 3.1 identifying a range of sources of information, advice and support about diversity, equality and inclusion<br>Evidence activity 3.1, p. 48 |
| | 3.2 Describing how and when to access information support about diversity, equality and inclusion<br>Evidence activity 3.2, p. 49<br>Reflective accounts require an explanation of a situation, what happened, what you did, what you could have done differently and what you have learned. Reflective accounts are seen as good evidence as this will show your learning and development. This can also be assessed through oral or written questions.<br>Professional discussion is a discussion on an agreed topic of the unit with your assessor. Professional discussion should be planned with sufficient time for you to read up on the topic and then discuss with the assessor. Witness or expert testimony is where someone in your workplace writes a statement saying that you have demonstrated the competence or knowledge for this unit. If you have evidence of prior learning in the subject, possibly a training day you have been on, this is classed as recognition of prior learning.<br>Direct observation is required for most units; this is where your assessor will observe you in the workplace. |

Good luck!

## Weblinks

| | |
|---|---|
| Department of Health for Social Care | www.dh.gov.uk/en/SocialCare |
| The General Social Care Council | http://www.gscc.org.uk |
| Skills for Care | www.skillsforcareanddevelopment.org.uk |
| Care Quality Commission | www.cqc.org.uk |
| Human Rights Act 1998 | www.direct.gov.uk |
| Equality Act 2010 | www.equalities.gov.uk |
| The Equality Act 2010 (in chapters) | www.legislation.gov.uk |
| Government website for children | www.education.gov.uk/schools/careers/workforceremodelling/supportstaff |
| The Children's Workforce Development Council | www.cwdcouncil.org.uk |

# 4 Introduction to duty of care in health, social care or children's and young person's settings

## For Unit SHC24

### What are you finding out?

This chapter introduces the concept of duty of care and also covers ensuring that any complaints made are responded to appropriately. The ability to change things is important, and ensuring that individuals have an awareness of and access to a robust complaints system is crucial and will be explored in this chapter.

The reading and activities in this chapter will help you to:

- Understand the meaning of duty of care
- Be aware of the dilemmas that may arise about duty of care and the support available for addressing them
- Know how to respond to complaints.

## LO1 Understand the meaning of duty of care

### 1.1 The term 'duty of care'

### What is duty of care?

Duty of care is the requirement to exercise a level of care towards an individual to avoid injury to that individual or their property. It is based on the relationship of the different parties, the negligent act or omission and the reasonable likelihood of loss to that individual.

A negligent act is an unintentional but careless act which results in loss. Only a negligent act will be regarded as having breached a duty of care. Whether an act is negligent can only be considered in the context in which it happened.

In Scotland this area of the law is called **delict**, while in England, Wales and Northern Ireland it is called the law of **tort**. Delict and tort differ from the law of contract. Contracts generally specify the duties of each of the parties and the remedy if these duties are breached. When the parties enter into a contract, they obtain specific rights and certain duties. In delict or tort these duties operate through the nature of the parties' relationship regardless of the contractual obligations.

### Key terms

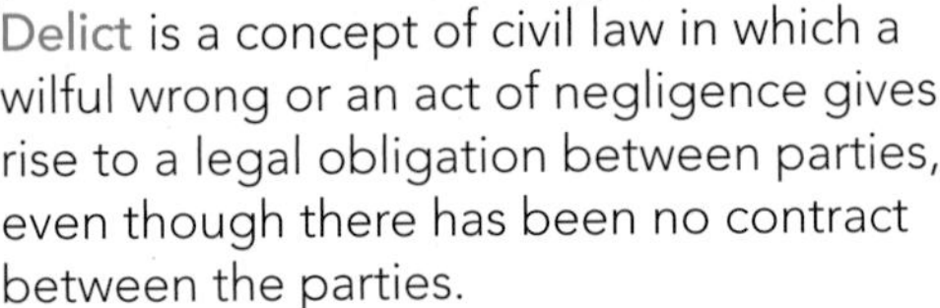

Delict is a concept of civil law in which a wilful wrong or an act of negligence gives rise to a legal obligation between parties, even though there has been no contract between the parties.

Tort is any wrongdoing for which an action for damages may be brought.

Although much of the law of delict and tort has been developed by the courts, there are also now a number of statutory rules which apply, for example to employment, disability discrimination, health and safety, data protection and occupier's liability.

### Research & investigate

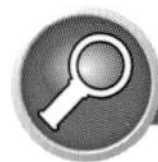

#### 1.1 Duty of care

Ask your manager or senior in charge what they understand by 'duty of care'. How do they ensure they are meeting these requirements? Have they experienced any breaches of this duty?

## Does a duty of care exist?

This depends on the relationship between the parties. A duty of care is not owed to everyone, only to those who have a suitably close relationship. There is no **liability** if the relationship between the parties is too remote. Closeness in this context, of course, also implies a professional relationship or responsibility.

### Key term

Liability is the state of being legally obliged and responsible.

## Is there a breach of that duty?

Liability only arises if the action breaches the duty of care and causes a loss or harm to the individual which would have been reasonably foreseeable in all the facts and circumstances of the case.

In a social care context, a duty of care will usually exist where the social care worker has some professional or work responsibility for delivering a service to an individual. A breach would arise where a negligent act or omission to act resulted in harm to that individual and the harm was foreseeable.

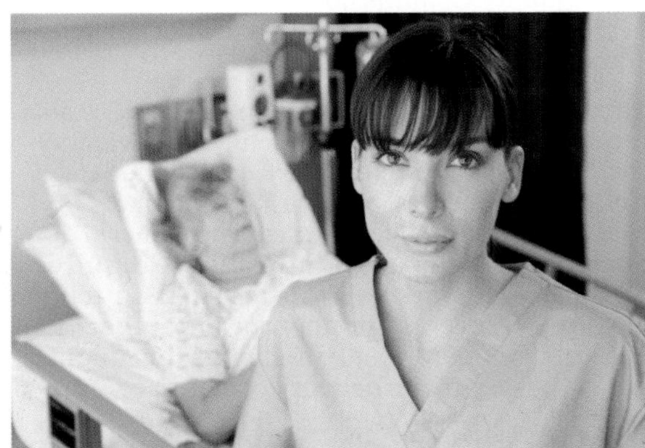

Figure 4.1 Duty of care

# 1.2 How the duty of care affects own work role

## Your duty of care

As a care worker, you have a duty:

- to take reasonable care for your own health and safety, and for the health and safety of others, while at work
- to follow reasonable directions given by, or on behalf of, the employer on issues related to health or safety
- to use relevant safety equipment provided for your use
- to report a workplace accident to the employer as soon as practicable after it occurs.

As a care worker you must not:

- intentionally or recklessly interfere with or misuse safety equipment provided by your employer
- intentionally create a risk to the health or safety of another at your workplace.

### Time to reflect

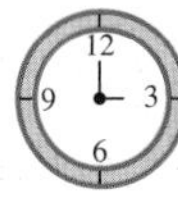

**Duty to individuals**

What do you think your duty to individuals is?

Does it match up with the expected duty of care?

In 1932 a court was asked to consider a case involving snails that had found their way into a glass of ginger beer! The woman who consumed the ginger beer suffered from nervous shock as a result of seeing the snails in the bottom of her glass and, in a landmark case, she brought an action against the publican who had served her the drink. She was able to establish that the publican owed her a duty of care and that he had breached that duty of care by unwittingly allowing the snails to get into her glass. After great deliberation, the court upheld the unfortunate woman's claim and the doctrine of duty of care was born. Since 1932 the courts have been full of people claiming that a duty of care was owed to them by someone, that the person has been negligent in observing that duty of care and has, as a result, breached it. That 1932 case has led to a society in which there is a huge amount of litigation, where, for example, councils are being sued for failing to put up signs that warn of pending dangers, publicans sued for allowing intoxicated people to drive off from their premises, and homeowners sued when a trespasser trips over an object left in an awkward place in their own home.

## Case Study

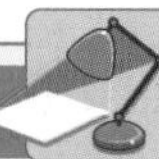

### 1.2 Did Heidi follow the duty of care?

On a ward there has been one staff nurse and one Health Care Assistant (HCA) short on the day shift for two weeks. For the last three days there has been a further Health Care Assistant missing due to sickness. The one remaining day shift HCA, Heidi, tries her best but by the end of the first day is aware that even with help from the nurses, it is impossible to carry out even the minimum of necessary duties to a basic standard. She speaks to the ward sister about her concerns and is assured by her they are trying to get cover, but is told that with support from the nurses, it should be possible to keep going for a couple more days.

On the third day Heidi makes a mistake. She gives a drink to a patient who was designated 'Nil by Mouth' as they were to be operated on later in the day. Heidi is warned that she faces a serious investigation. She is very upset.

It is clear that the sister should have acknowledged her responsibilities under the NMC Code of Professional Conduct and have made greater efforts to get immediate cover. Heidi should have been able to raise her concerns formally if nothing happened when they were raised informally. However, Heidi cannot be blamed if others failed in their duty of care. Clinical governance should mean the focus of any investigation is at least as much on the staffing shortages and why they weren't tackled as one mistake by the HCA.

Health and social care professionals have a duty of care to ensure the safety and well-being of service users. Most professions have set out good practice guidelines. Not following these guidelines may amount to abuse or neglect. All health and social care professions have identified certain principles and ways of working as 'good practice'. Being aware of what 'good practice' means can help you to identify abuse or neglect.

## Research & investigate

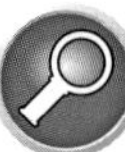

### 1.2 Good practice

Find out what is meant by 'good practice' in your workplace. How do people ensure they work to this at all times?

Health authorities, including primary care trusts and mental health trusts, and local authority social services are legally responsible for all the staff they employ. This includes making sure that appointed staff have the necessary qualifications and skills to carry out their roles, and that there is no reason to believe that staff could pose a risk to others. This involves following up references and checking with the Criminal Records Bureau that prospective staff have no criminal convictions which may affect their work. Health authorities and social services departments should ensure that staff receive the ongoing supervision, training and support needed to carry out their work. A health authority or local authority is liable if a member of their staff is found guilty of professional misconduct.

Health and social care services as a whole are regulated by a national regulatory agency, the Care Quality Commission. This agency inspects health and social care services to check that standards are being met.

Most health and social care professions are also regulated by independent agencies relevant to their profession, such as the General Medical Council for doctors, and the Nursing and Midwifery Council for nurses. The General Social Care Council's code of practice requires all social care workers to '(bring) to the attention of your employer or the appropriate authority resource or operational difficulties that might get in the way of the delivery of safe care.'

www.gscc.org.uk

In order to be allowed to do their jobs, workers in these professions have to be registered with their regulatory agency. An individual who is found guilty of professional misconduct, whether through abuse or neglect, will be disciplined by their specific professional agency or regulator.

Over the past two decades the idea of choice has become important to the health and social care professions, and to the government departments that make policies impacting on these sectors. It is now widely accepted that individuals should be able to make informed choices about the most suitable treatments for themselves. However, a patient does not have a legal right to demand a particular treatment, and complete choice does not always happen in practice, for example, the preferred treatment may not be available within an individual's local area.

## Empowerment and duty of care

A crucial aspect of relationship building in your job role is making sure that people are able to make choices and take control over as much of their lives as possible. This is known as empowerment.

One of the difficulties in trying to work out when a duty of care exists is that courts always have the benefit of hindsight. Whether a duty of care is owed or not very much depends on the facts of the matter, including the positions of the people involved. For example, an expert giving advice to a non-expert can be expected to have a duty of care to the non-expert. The expert is considered to have superior knowledge and the non-expert rightfully expects to be able to rely on that superior knowledge. The expert thus assumes a duty of care in giving the advice and, if that advice is given negligently and without care, then he or she can expect a court to find that the duty of care has been breached.

Many people who receive care services are not able to make choices about what happens in their lives. This might be due to many factors, for example their physical ability, where they live, who provides care and the way services are provided.

Individuals who are unable to make choices and exercise control may also suffer from low self-esteem and lose confidence in their own abilities. There are other factors which may impact on self-esteem, including the degree of encouragement and praise a person is given from important people in their lives, the amount of satisfaction people get from their jobs and whether they have positive and happy relationships with friends and family.

Self-esteem has a major effect on people's health and well-being. Individuals who have a positive and more confident outlook are far more likely to be active and interested in the world around them than those lacking confidence and belief in their own abilities. Therefore it is easy to see how this can affect an individual's quality of life and their overall health, safety and well-being.

Often individuals are told the level of support they will be given and when it will be given. Services have limited budgets and resources which have to be managed in order to deliver services efficiently and effectively. They obviously try to consider and take account of the needs of the individuals, but here lies a tension,

### Evidence activity 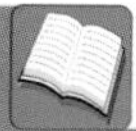

**1.2 How duty of care offers choice**

This activity helps demonstrate your understanding of how your duty of care affects your job role and the choices offered to others.

Explain how you think duty of care offers choice to individuals.

How would you feel if there was not a choice in the services you were receiving?

How do you think others will feel?

as resource and budget constraints must be adhered to. It is your role to try and ensure that your practice empowers individuals as far as possible.

# LO2 Be aware of dilemmas that may arise around duty of care and the support available for addressing them

## 2.1 Dilemmas that may arise between the duty of care and an individual's rights

### Consequences of breaching a duty of care

Historically, a breach of a duty of care, once it has been proved, generally leads to damages being awarded to the injured party. In the United Kingdom, damages tend to be awarded only to **compensate** the injured party for their actual financial loss. In the United States, however, the level of damages awarded is often much greater. In courts in the United States juries are able to penalise defendants in cases where a duty of care has been breached by awarding what is called exemplary damages. The reasoning behind such awards is that they will discourage others from breaching their duty of care and set examples of the outcomes of poor practice.

## Key term

Compensate means to give something, such as money, as payment or reparation for a service or loss.

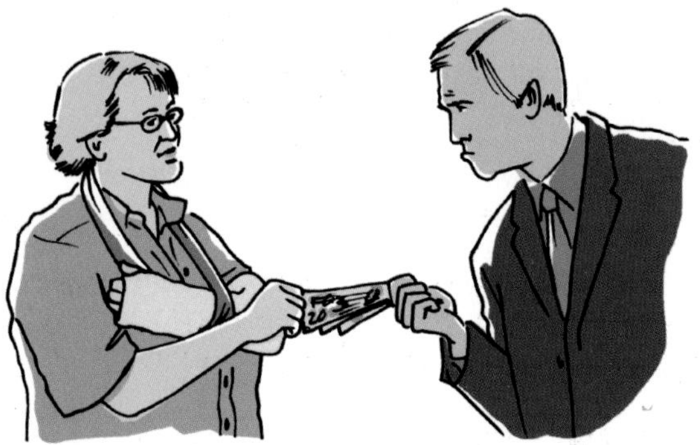

Figure 4.2 When it all goes wrong

It is important that rights are supported by:

- making sure that all staff understand the organisation's policies and guidelines relating to the rights of individuals
- ensuring that individuals are made fully aware of the organisation's complaints procedures
- discussing choices and preferences with individuals
- ensuring that professional colleagues are made aware of an individual's choices and preferences
- supporting individuals to maintain their rights and independence
- refusing to participate in discriminatory or prejudicial behaviour.

The duty of care in childcare may involve conflicts in some situations. Issues related to the duty of confidentiality about children and their parents are an example. A dilemma may arise which would normally require complete confidentiality, but which if not disclosed to parents of other children may put those children at risk. This would then be a breach of the duty of care to the other children. A decision to observe one duty could result in a breach of the other, and it is not always the case that one duty automatically has priority over the other. These situations require discussion, and advice and direction should be sought either from the employer or the sponsoring service or from a legal advisor.

There is no doubt that people working in health and social care are at risk of claims for breaches of duty of care. Employers and self-employed carers must ensure that they carry adequate insurance and comply with its terms. In addition, it is critical that carers comply with all obligations under any sponsored scheme or employment contract, a contract with a carer or with any licensing body.

## Research & investigate

### 2.1 Dilemmas

Find out what dilemmas you may encounter in your workplace, how are these worked through and a resolution agreed.

## 2.2 Where to get additional support and advice about how to resolve such dilemmas

Health and social care services usually involve the individual having contact with a number of staff. This could include frontline staff, a manager, volunteers, the local authority complaints manager, and inspectors and regulators as well as contract monitors. This creates a complex interaction of roles which can be confusing for the individual. It is therefore important to try to reduce duplication, but it is also important that staff are not confined to rigid roles that detract from a holistic approach to services. For example, in domiciliary services, even though the service might be monitored by both inspectors and a contract monitor, good practice might entail domiciliary staff being trained to spot possible abuse or changes in the well-being of an individual that might trigger the need for a care plan review. If domiciliary staff are not trained to do this it increases risk to the individual and wastes a resource that might reduce that risk. The same argument could be seen to apply to contract monitoring staff.

There is a legal underpinning to this argument in that if a local authority becomes aware – or ought to be aware – of risks to an individual they are likely to have a duty of care and obligations under the Human Rights Act 1998, and potentially under *No Secrets* guidance, to take action, whether or not a breach of contract is involved.

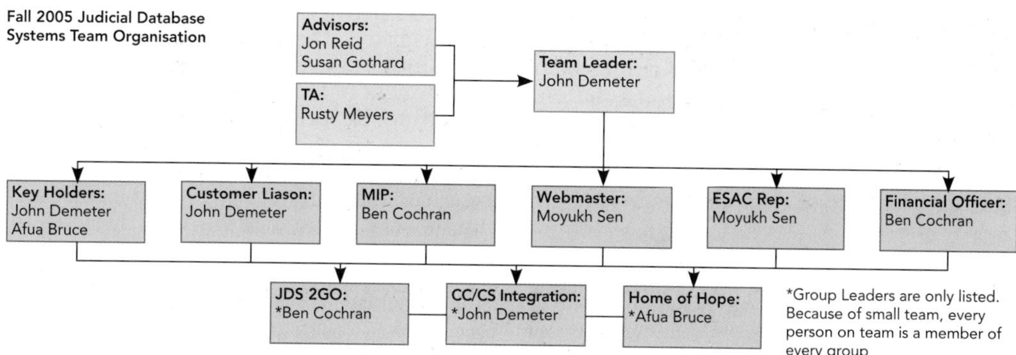


Figure 4.3 Roles and responsibilities

## Evidence activity 

### 2.2 Where to get additional support and advice

This activity helps demonstrate that you know where to get additional support and advice about how to resolve dilemmas.

In your workplace ask about the hierarchy of roles. Who is responsible for what? Draw a diagram or map illustrating key roles and functions. Do you think the individuals you provide care for know all of this?

# LO3 Know how to respond to complaints

## 3.1 Know why it is important that individuals know how to make a complaint

### What is a complaint?

A complaint is an expression of dissatisfaction about employees' actions, lack of actions or the standard of service provided. A complaint could be one of the following:

- An expression of unhappiness about the service provided.
- Action or lack of action by the organisation affecting an individual or group.
- An allegation that the organisation has failed to observe proper procedures.
- An allegation that there has been an unacceptable delay in dealing with a matter or about how an individual has been treated by a member of staff.

Within the health and social care sector a complaint is an expression of dissatisfaction that requires an investigation and a response. Complaints that are to be dealt with under the NHS and Social Care Complaints Procedure need to be made by complainants. Where there is doubt as to whether a complaint is a 'formal' complaint or a concern, the 'complainant' should be asked whether they wish the matter to be dealt with through the Primary Care Trust (PCT) NHS complaints process leading to a formal response from the Chief Executive.

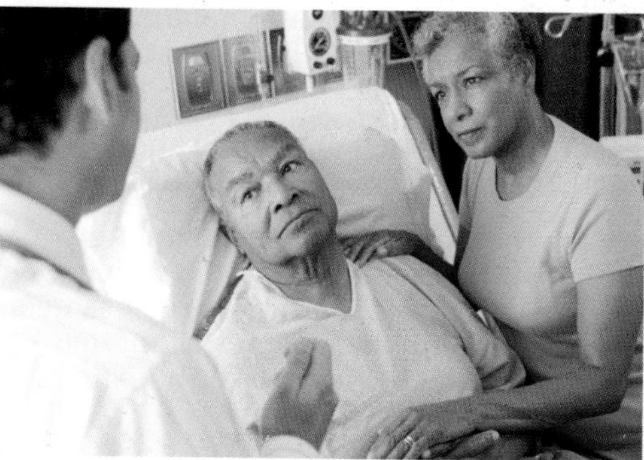

Figure 4.4 A complaint to make?

### The importance of complaints

From 1 April 2009, there is a single approach to dealing with NHS complaints. It gives organisations the flexibility they need to deal with complaints effectively. It also encourages a culture that seeks and then uses people's experiences to make services more effective, personal and safe.

Prevention is most definitely better than cure in relation to complaints. A well-organised setting with sound and effective procedures in place covering a wide range of service delivery and safety expectations will receive fewer complaints. Good communication with people ensures they have the information they need as they enter the setting and during their time with you. Policies regarding health and safety, patient care and so on will all help the smooth running of your setting. They will also reduce the likelihood of misunderstandings or dissatisfaction leading to complaints.

### Time to reflect

**Complaints**

Reflect upon a time when you complained about a service or product you received. How did you go about this? What was the outcome? Were you happy with the outcome?

## The legal framework

The legislation applies to NHS bodies, statutory or independent providers of NHS care (primary, secondary and tertiary care) and local authorities that provide adult social services. The new regulations came into force on 1 April 2009 and the law requires organisations to:

- Publicise their complaints procedure.
- Acknowledge receipt of a complaint and offer to discuss the matter within three working days.
- Deal efficiently with complaints and investigate them properly and appropriately.
- Write to the complainant on completion of a complaint investigation explaining how it has been resolved, what appropriate action has been taken, and reminding them of their right to take the matter to the Health Service Ombudsman if they are still unhappy.
- Assist the complainant in following the complaints procedure, or provide advice on where they may obtain such assistance.
- Ensure that there is a designated manager for complaints.
- Have someone senior who is responsible for both the complaints policy and learning from complaints.
- Produce an annual report about complaints that have been received, the issues they raise, and any matters where action has been taken or is to be taken to improve services as a result of those complaints.

If the complaint involves two or more organisations, the person complaining should get a single, coordinated response. The Department of Health has produced a guide 'Listening, Responding, Improving' which provides a practical resource that complaints managers and their teams can use to help design excellent customer care systems locally and to support clinical and administrative staff in implementing change.

http://www.opsi.gov.uk/stat.htm

People wishing to make complaints:

- must do so within 12 months of an incident happening or of becoming aware of the matter complained about
- can choose to complain to a commissioner instead of the service provider.

### Research & investigate

**Dealing with complaints**

Have any complaints been dealt with at your work setting? What process was used?

## The Health Service Ombudsman – 'Principles of Good Complaints Handling'

From 1 April 2009 the Health Service Ombudsman takes over responsibility for investigating NHS complaints that can't be resolved locally, and the new approach to complaints is based on the Health Service Ombudsman's Six Principles of Good Complaints Handling. In summary, good complaint handling means:

1. getting it right
2. being customer focused
3. being open and accountable
4. acting fairly and proportionately
5. putting things right
6. seeking continuous improvement.

## 3.2 The main points of agreed procedures for handling complaints

The complaints arrangements for health and social care have been reformed. Reports frequently identified that some complaints took too long to resolve and services did not systematically try to learn from the important feedback that complaints offer. In addition, there is strong evidence that some people do not complain because they either do not know how to or believe doing so will not result in any action.

Since 1 April 2009, a single complaints system covers all health and adult social care services in England. These revised arrangements will encourage an approach that aims to resolve complaints more effectively and ensure that opportunities for services to learn and improve are not lost. The Department of Health's new system for handling complaints about adult social care services aims to secure a first on two fronts.

Not only does it mean there will be a single process to deal with both health and social care-related complaints but the new legislation promises to deliver a more customer-focused approach. In addition the introduction of a single complaint route removes the difficulties many people claim they encounter navigating separate complaint systems for health and social services.

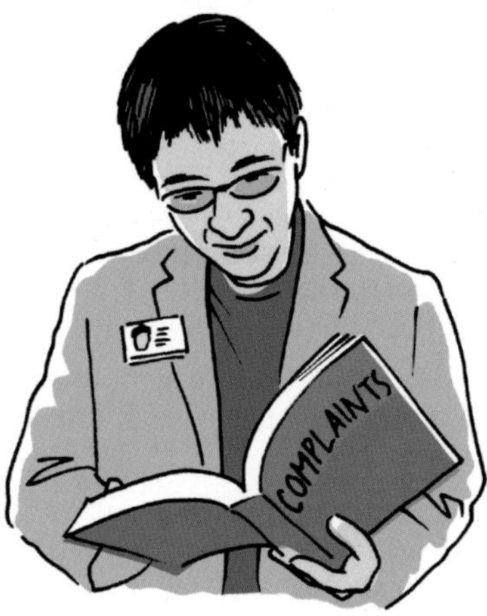


Figure 4.5 Monitoring complaints

The new arrangements have three main components:

1. First, new regulations that enable local organisations to develop more flexible and responsive complaints handling systems that focus on the specific needs of the complainant, seek to reach speedy local resolution, facilitate coordinated handling of across-boundary complaints, and learn from people's experiences to help improve services.
2. Second, the introduction of a single local resolution stage, replacing the tiered stages prescribed by the old local authority social care regulations.
3. Third, a new single system for independent review by the Parliamentary and Health Service Ombudsman for healthcare.

**Practice activity** 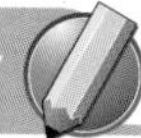

**3.2 The main points of agreed procedures for handling complaints**

This activity will demonstrate your knowledge of agreed procedures for handling complaints. Ask where and how complaints are recorded in your workplace. Make notes about the level of detail and how it is written.

## 3.3 Own role in responding to complaints as part of own duty of care

If a person wishes to make a complaint it is part of a health and social care worker's role to support them to do this and to ensure the complaint is directed to the right person. At all times agreed policies and procedures must be followed.

### Who is a complaint made to?

It is important that workers have a thorough understanding of their organisation's complaints procedure and their role in this. On occasions, it might be appropriate for the worker to assist the service user to initiate a complaint, particularly if the service user has no knowledge of the complaints procedure or if the service user is disadvantaged by language or disability. In this situation the worker may be acting as an 'advocate'. The GSCC Code of Practice refers to this activity as:

'3.1. Helping service users and carers to make complaints, taking complaints seriously and responding to them or passing them on to the appropriate person.'

Complaints about rights may also be made by workers. This is known as 'whistleblowing'. For example, the GSCC Code of Practice encourages social care workers to:

'3.2 Use established processes and procedures to challenge and report dangerous, abusive, discriminatory or exploitative behaviour and practice.'

The GSCC Code of Practice also encourages social care workers to:

'3.4. Bring to the attention of your employer or appropriate authority operational difficulties that might get in the way of the delivery of safe care.'

'3.5. Inform your employer or appropriate authority where the practice of colleagues may be unsafe or adversely affect standards of care.'

**Practice activity** 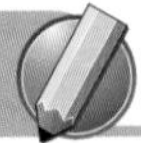

 **Your own role in responding to complaints**

This activity helps demonstrate your knowledge of your own role in responding to complaints.

Look for the GSCC Code of Practice. How does it impact on your role? Write down what you think you need to do to follow the Code.

## Dealing with conflict and disputes

Any situation that involves close and prolonged contact with others has the potential to create conflict and disputes. It is important that health and social care workers remain non-judgemental in their attempts to resolve disputes between individuals. If you encounter this situation, as a worker you should:

- Remain calm and speak in a firm, quiet and controlled voice.
- Be quite clear that neither verbal nor physical abuse will be tolerated.
- Listen attentively to both sides of the argument, without any interruption.
- Identify ways in which a compromise might be achieved without either party losing face.
- Be clear that compromise is the only means to achieving a resolution.

Complaints can be made to the organisation providing care, for example to a hospital or GP surgery, or direct to the commissioning body, usually the PCT or social services. If the PCT or social services receives a complaint about a provider, and they consider that they can deal with the complaint, they must seek consent from the complainant so that they can send details of the complaint to the provider. On receiving consent, the details must be sent as soon as possible. If, however, the PCT or social services consider it more appropriate for the provider to answer the complaint, and the complainant consents, the complaint can be passed to the provider for a response.

Complainants must choose at the outset whether to make a complaint to a primary care provider or the PCT. A complainant who makes an initial complaint to a provider and who does not agree with the provider's response cannot then seek a review from the PCT. Complainants who are dissatisfied with the response they receive from a primary care provider can refer the complaint to the Ombudsman.

If a complaint is made to any responsible body (the first body) which considers that the complaint should have been made to another responsible body (the second body), and the first body sends the complaint to the second body, the second body can respond to the complaint as if it had received it first. The second body must acknowledge the complaint within three working days.

The complaints procedure excludes:

- complaints made by one NHS body against another
- complaints made by employees in relation to their work for an NHS body
- complaints that were first made orally and which were resolved to the complainant's satisfaction within one working day
- complaints about the same subject matter as a complaint that has previously been made and resolved
- complaints alleging failure by a public body to comply with a request for information under the Freedom of Information Act 2000
- complaints about care solely provided by the independent healthcare sector, which has its own procedures.

If a responsible body considers that it is not required to consider a complaint, it must inform the complainant in writing of the decision and the reasons for it.

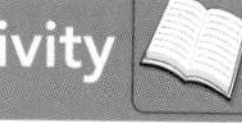

## Evidence activity

### 3.3 Responding to complaints

This activity demonstrates your knowledge of your own role in responding to complaints.

Locate a flow chart of how complaints are dealt with in your work setting. Make a copy of this for your own evidence.

## The complainant

Complainants should normally be current or former patients or nominated representatives, which can include a solicitor or a patient's elected representative, for example an MP. Never assume that someone complaining on behalf of a patient has authority to do so. The investigation of a complaint does not remove the need to respect a patient's right to confidentiality. Patients over the age of 16 whose mental capacity is unimpaired should normally complain themselves. Children under the age of 16 who are able to do so may also make their own complaint.

If someone other than the patient makes a complaint, you will need to make sure they have authority to do so. If patients lack capacity to make decisions for themselves, the representative must be able to demonstrate sufficient interest in their welfare and be an appropriate person to act on their behalf. This could include a partner or relative or someone appointed under the Mental Capacity Act 2005 with lasting power of attorney. If the power of attorney covers the person's welfare, this could include making complaints at a time when that person lacks capacity. In certain circumstances, the regulations impose a duty upon the responsible body to satisfy itself that a representative is an appropriate person to make a complaint. For example, if the complaint is about a child, the responsible body must satisfy itself that there are reasonable grounds for the representative to make the complaint, and not the child concerned. If the patient is a child or a patient who lacks capacity, the responsible body must also be satisfied that the representative is acting in the best interests of the person on whose behalf the complaint is made. If the responsible body is not satisfied that the representative is appropriate, it must not consider the complaint and must give the representative reasons for the decision in writing.

## Time limits

The regulations require a complaint to be made within 12 months from the date on which the matter occurred, or from when the matter came to the attention of the complainant. The regulations state that a responsible body should consider a complaint outside that time limit if the complainant has good reason for not making the complaint within that limit and, despite the delay, it is still possible to investigate the complaint fairly and effectively. It is often the practice to consider complaints made outside the time limit if it is possible to investigate them. If there are any difficulties, for example if the relevant information is no longer available, it would be advisable to discuss this with complainants as soon as possible so they know what steps, if any, can reasonably be taken to

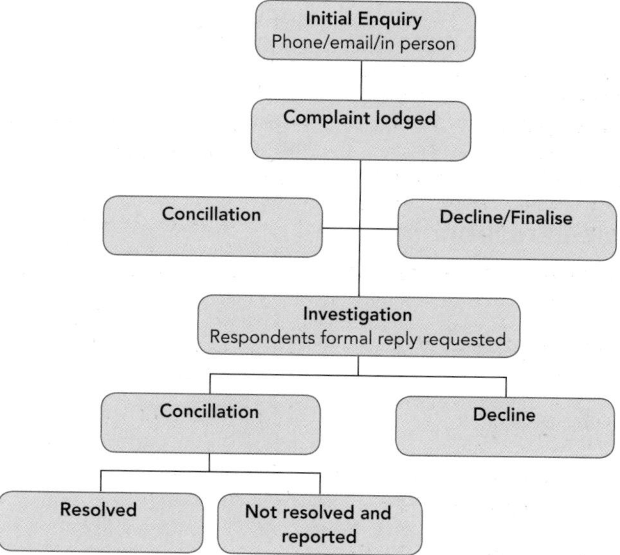


Figure 4.6 The complaints process

investigate a complaint outside the time limit. While the regulations do not set timescales for the procedure itself, they do require a timely, appropriate response. If a response is not provided within six months from the date the complaint was made, or a later date if one was agreed with the complainant, the complaints manager has to write to the complainant and explain why it is delayed. The complaints manager must ensure the complainant receives a response as soon as possible.

## Disciplinary and criminal procedures

The complaint's procedure is a means for addressing patient complaints and does not have a disciplinary function. Inevitably some complaints will identify matters that suggest a need for disciplinary investigation. This might result in action via local procedures or referral to the practitioner's regulatory body. Complainants have no role in decisions to initiate disciplinary investigations (though they can refer serious concerns directly to the GMC, NMC or other regulatory body). Disciplinary procedures are confidential between an employer and employee, or a contracting body and a contractor, and complainants have no right to know the details or the outcome of such procedures.

In very rare cases a complaint might relate to a matter under police investigation.

## Negligence claims

The regulations do not require a complaint to be stopped if there is a claim for negligence. If complainants are provided with a response setting out full details of the investigation and conclusions reached, this may help them and their legal adviser to decide whether there has been negligence.

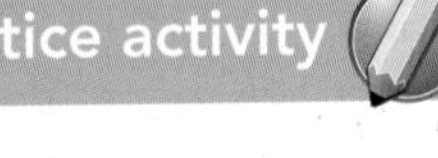

### Your own role in responding to complaints as part of your own duty of care

This activity will allow you to practise what you would do when responding to a complaint made at your setting.

If a complaint is made at your work setting what action would you take? When you have decided this, look at the complaints procedure to check you were correct.

## Relevant legislation and guidance

**The Local Authority Social Services & NHS Complaints (England) Regulations 2009** – came into force on 1 April 2009 and introduced a revised procedure for the handling of complaints by local authorities, in respect of complaints about adult social care, and by NHS bodies, primary care providers and independent providers in respect of provision of NHS care. The regulations align adult social care and health complaints processes into a single set of arrangements. These Regulations revoke the National Health Service (Complaints) Regulations 2004 and the National Health Service (Complaints) Amendment Regulations 2006.

**The Children Act 1989/2004** – provides a statutory basis for social care complaints.

**The Data Protection Act 1998** – governs the protection and use of person identifiable information (personal data). The Act does not apply to personal information relating to the deceased.

**The Human Rights Act 1988** – Article 8.1 provides that 'everyone has the right to respect for his private and family life, his home and his correspondence.' Article 8.2 provides that 'there shall be no interference by a public authority with the exercise of this right except as in accordance with the law and if necessary in a democratic society in the interest of national security, public safety or the economic well-being of the country for the prevention of crime and disorder, for the protection of health or morals, or for the protection of the rights and freedoms of others.'

**The Freedom of Information Act 2000** – the Act creates rights of access to information (rights of access to personal information remain under the Data Protection Act 1998) and revises and strengthens the Public Records Act 1958 and 1967 by reinforcing records management standards of practice.

## Assessment summary

Your reading of this chapter and completion of the activities will have prepared you to demonstrate your learning and understanding of the principles of duty of care in health, social care or children's and young people's settings. To achieve the unit, your assessor will require you to:

| Learning Outcomes | Assessment Criteria |
|---|---|
| Learning outcome 1: Understand the meaning of duty of care by: | 1.1 defining the term 'duty of care'<br><br>See Research and investigate activity 1.1 p. 52. |
| | 1.2 describing how the duty of care affects own work role<br><br>See Research and investigate activity 1.2 p. 54 and Evidence activity 1.2 p. 55. |
| Learning outcome 2: Be aware of dilemmas that may arise about duty of care and the support available for addressing them by: | 2.1 describing dilemmas that may arise between the duty of care and an individual's rights<br><br>See Research and investigate activity 2.1 p. 56. |
| | 2.2 explaining where to get additional support and advice about how to resolve such dilemmas<br><br>See Evidence activity 2.2 p. 57. |
| Learning outcome 3: Know how to respond to complaints by: | 3.1 explaining why it is important that individuals know how to make a complaint<br><br>See Research and Investigate activity 3.1 p. 58. |
| | 3.2 explaining the main points of agreed procedures for handling complaints<br><br>See Practice activity 3.2 p. 59. |
| | 3.3 describing own role in responding to complaints as part of own duty of care<br><br>See Practice activity 3.3 p. 60. |

Good luck!

## Weblinks

| | |
|---|---|
| Skills for Health | www.skillsforhealth.org.uk |
| Skills for Care and Development | www.skillsforcareanddevelopment.org.uk |
| Care Quality Commission | www.cqc.org.uk |
| General Social Care Council | www.gscc.org.uk |
| Nursing and Midwifery Council | www.nmc-uk.org |

# 5 Principles of safeguarding and protection in health and social care

## For Unit HSC024

### What are you finding out?

We all have a responsibility to help keep people safe and free from abuse. People who use health and social care services are vulnerable, because of their age, health, mental, physical or intellectual ability, and so are particularly at risk of neglect, harm or exploitation. Health and social care service providers have a duty to comply with legislation set up to safeguard vulnerable people, and health and social care workers have a responsibility to recognise and respond promptly and appropriately to suspicions or allegations of abuse.

The reading and activities in this chapter will help you to:

- Know how to recognise signs of abuse
- Know how to respond to suspected or alleged abuse
- Understand the national and local context of safeguarding and protection from abuse
- Understand ways to reduce the likelihood of abuse
- Know how to recognise and report unsafe practices

## LO1 Know how to recognise signs of abuse

Abuse is defined as a violation of someone's human rights by another person. Abusers include friends and relatives, health and social care workers and professionals, personal assistants, volunteers, other service users, people who deliberately exploit vulnerable people, and strangers. It can be physical, sexual, emotional or psychological, financial, or institutional neglect. Whatever the abuse, it causes significant harm to the person involved and must never be **condoned.**

No secrets: Guidance on developing and implementing multi-agency policies and procedures to protect vulnerable adults from abuse

www.dh.gov.uk

**Key term**

To condone means to ignore, excuse, forgive, make allowances for.

### 1.1 Different types of abuse

Physical abuse is pain, suffering or injury that is **wilfully** inflicted , including:

- Slapping, pushing and rough handling, for example during a moving and handling procedure.
- Forcing someone to do things that are inappropriate or against their wishes, such as being sent to their room as punishment.
- Hiding medication in food or giving it inappropriately, for example to control or calm someone down.
- Restraint, such as tying someone to a chair or toilet.
- Keeping the environment too hot or too cold.
- Denying food and drink.
- Failing to follow health and safety procedures.

**Key term**

Wilful means deliberate, intentional.

Sexual abuse is sexual assault, sexual harassment and making someone take part in sexual activity to which they haven't agreed or don't fully understand. It includes:

- Inappropriate kissing or touching, for example of the breasts and genitals.
- Vaginal, anal or oral rape, including penetration with objects.
- Using sexually-explicit language.
- Exposing someone to pornography.

Emotional/psychological abuse is mental suffering caused by someone in a position of trust, for example:

- Humiliation and intimidation, through blaming, harassment, verbal abuse, isolation.
- Bullying, such as taking control and pressurising someone to do something they don't want.
- Threatening harm, abandonment and withdrawal of services.
- Failing to prevent mental suffering caused by somebody else.

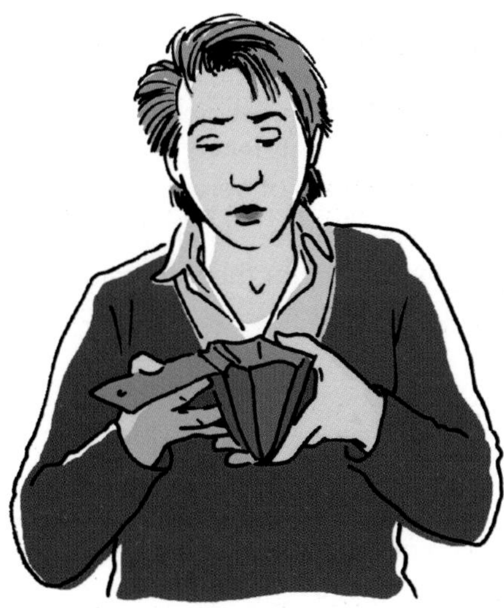

Figure 5.1 Financial abuse

Financial abuse is theft or the misuse of someone's money, property or belongings by someone in a position of trust, for example through:

- Threats and pressure, in connection with wills, inheritance and financial matters.
- Deceiving or swindling someone out of their savings and benefits.

Institutional abuse is the crushing of people's needs and choices because of poor professional practice and priority being given to rigid organisational procedures. It takes place, for example, when:

- There is no choice about what to eat and drink and when to get up, go to bed, or go to the toilet.
- Clothing and toiletries are shared.
- People are not allowed to make their own decisions.
- Medication isn't given at the right time.
- When someone's personal information is shared without their permission.

Neglect is the failure to give the necessary care to a vulnerable person. It includes:

- Ignoring their physical care needs, such as help with personal hygiene and toileting, prevention of pressure sores and protection from health and safety hazards.
- Failure to provide access to health and social care services.
- Depriving them of life's necessities, such as adequate nutrition, warmth, shelter and social contact.

Self-neglect is defined as the failure, usually of an adult, to care for themselves properly. It includes:

- Living in unsanitary, hazardous conditions.
- Not eating properly and not maintaining their personal hygiene.
- Not seeking help when ill and not taking prescribed medication.

## Time to reflect

### 1.1 Self-neglect

Health and social care workers have a hard job. They need to be fit, eat a nutritious diet and have enough rest and relaxation. If they neglect their health in any way, they can't do their job properly, which puts their and other people's safety at risk. Do you look after yourself properly?

## 1.2 The signs and symptoms associated with different types of abuse

A sign is an indication of health that can be:

- seen, for example **skin pallor**
- heard, for example when blood pressure is measured using a sphygmomanometer
- touched, for example feeling for a pulse.

Symptoms are the way someone feels when they are ill, such as in pain, confused, depressed.

**Key Term**

Skin pallor means paleness or rosiness of the skin.

Table 5.1 Signs and symptoms of abuse

| Type of abuse | Signs include | Symptoms include |
|---|---|---|
| Physical | Cuts, scratches, bite-marks; bruises; burns from cigarettes, rough handling, use of restraint; pressure ulcers; scalds and blisters; fractures; withdrawal. | Fear, belittled, anger; loss of self-confidence and self-esteem; pain due to injuries. |
| Sexual | Love bites; injuries to the mouth, genitals or anus; blood stained underwear; urinary tract and sexually transmitted infections; pregnancy; withdrawal; inability to develop normal sexual relationships; overtly sexual behaviour. | Fear, shame, guilt; loss of dignity and self-respect; pain due to injuries and infection. |
| Emotional/ psychological | Rocking, flinching; self-harm; comfort eating; tearfulness; withdrawal; aggression. | Embarrassment, fear, humiliation, resignation; loss of self-confidence, self-esteem and sense of belonging. |
| Financial | Unexplained loss of money and personal possessions; missing receipts; insufficient money for bills; being bought products that don't match ability to pay; care workers and carers benefiting from 'buy one get one free' offers when doing the shopping; dependency on others; diminishing health status due to reduced quality of life. | Anxiety about financial affairs and fears for the future; loss of independence and control. |
| Institutional | Loss of interest in the environment and loss of ability to make choices, act independently, communicate; loss of clothing and personal possessions; withdrawal; aggression. | Loss of independence and control over own life; anger; frustration; depression; despair; hopelessness. |
| Neglect and self-neglect | Dirty, smelly; under/overweight; poor health; poor living conditions; inadequate clothing; loss of interest; withdrawal. | Symptoms associated with poor health status, such as pain due to pressure ulcers, hunger, cold; loneliness. |

## Evidence activity

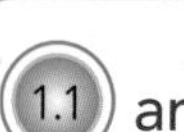

### 1.1 and 1.2 Define the different types of abuse and associated signs and symptoms

This activity enables you to demonstrate your knowledge of the different types of abuse and associated signs and symptoms.

Produce a set of cards to which everyone at your workplace can refer in order to help them recognise abuse. Your cards should:

- say what is meant by physical, sexual, emotional/psychological, financial and institutional abuse, and neglect and self-neglect
- describe the signs associated with each type of abuse and neglect
- describe the symptoms associated with each type of abuse and neglect.

## 1.3 Factors that may contribute to an individual being more vulnerable to abuse

Social isolation increases vulnerabity to abuse. For example living alone, isolated from family and friends can make people welcoming of company or help but unable to weigh up whether it is trustworthy. Tales of elderly people being exploited for this reason abound in the media. Social isolation also means restricted access to services such as health and social care, transport and the police. As a result, signs of abuse are less likely to be detected, giving free rein to **perpetrators**.

### Key term

A perpetrator is someone who carries out an act of abuse.

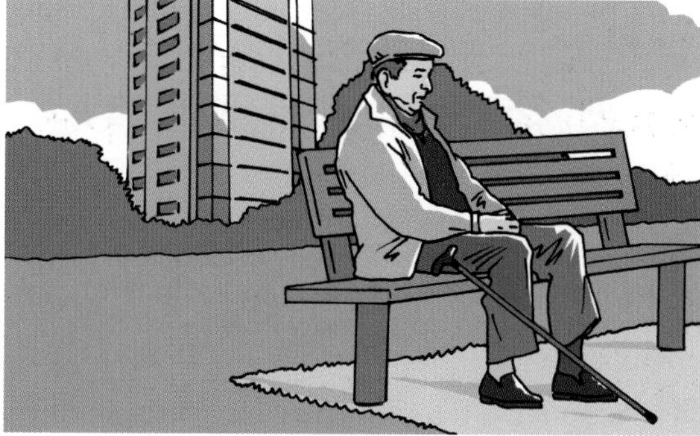

Figure 5.2 Social isolation and vulnerability

Poor housing and overcrowding can trigger aggression. Aggressive neighbours can be abusive, and there may be no escape. In addition, shared accommodation increases the risk of having to live with people you wouldn't choose to live with because of their potential to be abusive.

Using health and social care services is not without risk of abuse. People who have been abused themselves, which includes workers and people using the services, are at risk of becoming abusers. Care work gives people power and authority, which an abuser can use to their own advantage. In addition, work practice that fails to give the necessary care to a vulnerable person amounts to neglect. For these reasons, safeguarding legislation is in place which health and social care workers have a duty to obey.

Shocking as it may seem, depending on family or friends for care is not without risk. The needs of vulnerable people often exceed the ability and **empathy** of their **carers**, who usually have to change their lifestyle to carry out their caring role and, in doing so, can become socially isolated and develop their own personal difficulties. The consequence is often a soured relationship, which unfortunately can lead to abuse.

www.carers.org

### Key terms

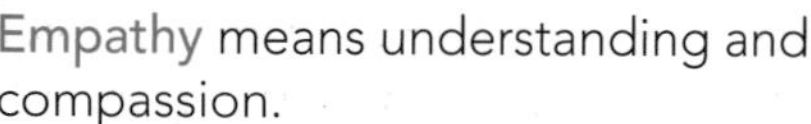

Empathy means understanding and compassion.
A carer is someone, who, without payment, provides help and support to a partner, child, relative, friend or neighbour, who could not manage without their help.

Some people are more vulnerable to abuse than others, for example, because they have:

- Limited life experience and sex education, so find it difficult to predict abusive situations.
- Learning, understanding and communication difficulties so are unaware of their rights, don't know how to deal with perpetrators and don't know how to complain.
- Personal, often intimate care needs, giving perpetrators an opportunity to commit sexual abuse.
- Low self-esteem, so lack power in relationships, enabling perpetrators to dominate and control them.
- A history of violent behaviour, alcoholism, substance misuse or mental illness, which a perpetrator can exploit with threats and use to their advantage.
- Money problems, such as debt and low income and are therefore vulnerable to self-neglect as well as perpetrators who would exploit them financially.

In addition, people's age, physical ability, for example their frailty, and strength of character, for example low levels of self-confidence and assertiveness, can **predispose** them to abuse.

**Key term**

To be predisposed to a situation means to be inclined to it.

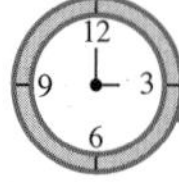

**Time to reflect**

**1.3 Vulnerability to abuse**

Think about the people at school who were bullied. Why do you think they were emotionally abused in this way? Was it, for example, because they had learning or physical difficulties, low self-esteem or were poor? How do you think they felt? How would you feel if you were a victim? How do you feel now if you were a perpetrator?

**Evidence activity**

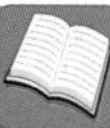

**1.2 Describe factors that may contribute to an individual being more vulnerable to abuse**

This activity enables you to demonstrate your knowledge of the factors that can make an individual more vulnerable to abuse.

Think about three individuals where you work who you think are especially vulnerable to abuse. What is it about these individuals that makes them more vulnerable? Is it, for example, where they live, the setting in which they are supported, their particular needs? It is important that you are able to identify individuals who are especially vulnerable, and why, in order to safeguard them effectively.

## LO2 Know how to respond to suspected or alleged abuse

### 2.1 Actions to take if there are suspicions that an individual is being abused

If you suspect that someone you support is being abused, discuss your concerns politely with the person you suspect. Never ignore your suspicions but never accuse anyone of abuse until you understand the reason for their behaviour. For example, asking someone to walk to the toilet when they've requested a wheelchair may not seem quite right to you but they may simply be encouraging independence and the ability to walk. On the other hand, they may not be aware that their behaviour is causing suffering.

If you remain concerned, you have a duty to speak out. Your workplace will have a procedure telling you how to deal with suspicions of abuse but, in general:

- Discuss your concerns in private, without delay, with your supervisor or line manager or, in the case of suspected child abuse, with the Child Protection Officer. They will decide an appropriate course of action, for example whether to contact the police, health or social services and family. Never overstep your responsibilities – dealing with suspected abuse will be someone else's responsibility.
- Record your concerns on the appropriate report form. Records should be clear, easy to understand, concise, relevant and factual. Only state things as they appeared to you – don't make anything up for the sake of 'a good story'.
- Make every effort to preserve any evidence of abuse. You will read about this later.
- Ask to be kept informed about what is decided and why.

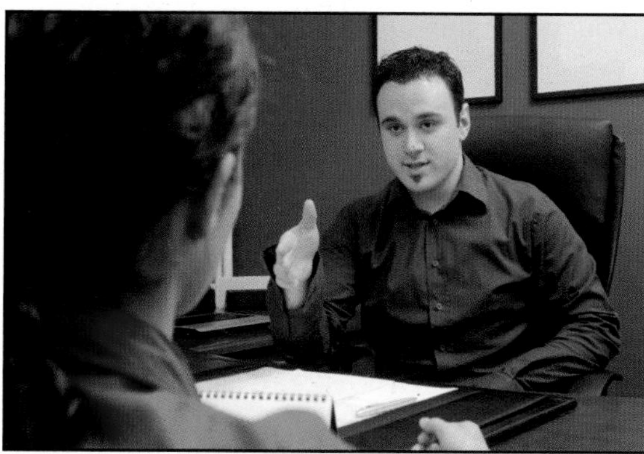

Figure 5.3 Responding to suspected or alleged abuse

If you suspect your supervisor or line manager of abuse, check with them so that you can understand the reason for their behaviour. If you remain concerned, talk things over with someone in a more senior position straightaway. If the person you suspect has seniority at your workplace, talk to the manager of your organisation or the body that regulates the quality of care in your part of the UK. Expect to make a record of your suspicions and ask to be kept informed about proceedings.

If you suspect that you have a tendency to be abusive, perhaps verbally because swearing is part of your everyday language or physically because you tend to handle people roughly in order to finish a task quickly, share your concerns with a trusted colleague or your line manager. If talking things through confirms your suspicions, request extra training and supervision. Ask to be relieved of working with people with whom you don't get on or of tasks that you know you don't perform well. At the end of the day, you are responsible for your behaviour, so it's up to you to make the necessary changes. As you read earlier, abuse must never be condoned, particularly when you are the perpetrator.

**Evidence activity** 

**2.1 Explain actions to take if there are suspicions that an individual is being abused**

This activity enables you to demonstrate your understanding of what to do in the event of suspicions of abuse.

- Check out your workplace's procedure about how to deal with suspicions of abuse. What are the reasons for following the various actions it describes?
- What should you do if you suspect that your own behaviour isn't all it should be?

## 2.2 Actions to take if an individual alleges that they are being abused

There are a number of ways in which abuse can be alleged. It could be that a victim tells you – discloses – that something has happened to them or an observer makes an accusation. It takes a great deal of courage for someone to allege abuse because, by doing so, they may worry that things will get worse or that they'll get blamed. They might also think that no one will believe them.

**Time to reflect** 

**2.2 Alleging abuse**

What might stop you making an allegation of an abuse, either of yourself or of someone else? Can you understand why people hesitate to do so?

Your workplace should have a procedure that describes how you must deal with a disclosure or allegation of abuse. However, when someone makes a disclosure to you, as a general rule:

- Accept what they say and reassure them that you believe them and take them seriously. Different people have different ideas about what makes for abuse. You might take no notice of sexually explicit language whereas others might be offended or deeply distressed. Don't let your views and emotions prevent you treating the victim with dignity and taking what they say seriously.
- Don't 'interview' them and don't interrupt. Listen calmly to what they say, avoid asking lots of questions and be comfortable with silences. Silences provide thinking time. Try to remember what they say so that you can record it afterwards, before you forget.
- Don't promise to keep things confidential. Explain that you will have to tell your line manager because they need to know so that they can help.
- Take steps to make them safe.
- Make every effort to preserve any evidence of abuse.

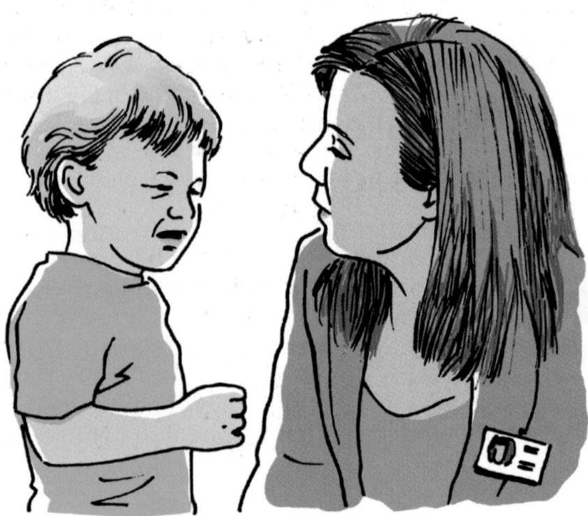

Figure 5.4 Listening to a disclosure

Records of disclosure should include:

- When the disclosure was made.
- Who was involved and the names of any witnesses.
- What happened – what you were told, facts only, no interpretations.
- Any other relevant information, for example details of previous incidents that have caused concern.

Use the relevant report form and keep it safe and confidential until you can give it to the appropriate person. Avoid the alleged perpetrator and don't discuss the incident with anyone as this could breach the victim's confidentiality and alert the perpetrator that suspicions have been aroused. It could also complicate any internal or police investigations. Ask to be kept informed about what is decided and why.

**Evidence activity** 

### 2.2 Explain actions to take if an individual alleges that they are being abused

This activity enables you to demonstrate your understanding of what to do in the event of an individual alleging that they are being abused.

Check out your workplace's procedure about what to do if an individual tells you they are being abused. What are the reasons for following the various actions it describes?

## 2.3 Ways to ensure that evidence of abuse is preserved

Because the police could be involved in a suspected or alleged case of abuse, it's important to preserve any evidence that relates to the incident. Failure to preserve evidence is often described as 'contamination'. If you're in any doubt about how to preserve evidence, such as footprints, fingerprints, blood, semen and anything else that the suspect may have left, check with the police on the telephone before they arrive.

10 Top Tips to ensure that evidence of abuse is preserved.

1. Don't remove or alter documentation relating to the incident and preserve security camera videotape. You will be held accountable if you destroy evidence.
2. Don't allow anyone except medical staff to enter the scene of the incident until the police arrive. A medical examination should only take place to assess injury, provide first aid or arrange for transfer to hospital.
3. Make a note, before you forget, of the state of the victim and alleged perpetrator's

clothing, their physical and emotional condition and of any obvious injuries.

4 Don't let the victim and alleged perpetrator come into contact with each other once the allegation has been made.

5 In the event of alleged sexual abuse, don't allow anyone to have physical contact with either the victim or the alleged perpetrator.

6 Don't move anything.

7 Don't touch anything unless you have to. If anything is handed to you, take care not to destroy fingerprints.

8 Don't clean up and don't wash anything, for example to remove blood or semen.

9 Don't throw anything away. If sexual abuse has been alleged, keep hold of any items that might provide evidence, for example used condoms.

10 Don't assume that it's too late if an allegation is made days after the alleged offence. It may still be possible to collect forensic evidence. Let the police decide.

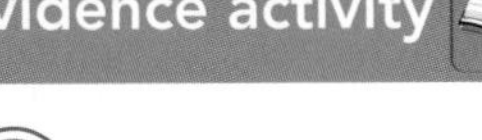

**Identify ways to ensure that evidence of abuse is preserved**

This activity enables you to demonstrate your knowledge of how to preserve evidence in the event of abuse.

Use a search engine such as Google or research local and national newspapers for reports of abuse. If you, as a worker, had been associated with these incidents, how would you have preserved evidence in order not to impair any police investigations?

## LO3 Understand the national and local context of safeguarding and protection from abuse

### 3.1 National policies and local systems that relate to safeguarding and protection from abuse

Following the murders of Jessica Chapman and Holly Wells by Ian Huntley, a school caretaker, the government commissioned the Bichard Inquiry (2002). One of the issues this Inquiry looked at was the way employers recruit people to work with children and vulnerable adults.

**Research & investigate**

**Recruitment where you work**

Find out how your organisation goes about recruiting staff to work with vulnerable people.

The Inquiry's recommendations led to the Safeguarding Vulnerable Groups Act 2006 and the Vetting and Barring Scheme, which is run by the Independent Safeguarding Authority (ISA). The ISA works closely with the **Criminal Records Bureau (CRB)** and uses information in the **PoVA** (Protection of Vulnerable Adults) and **PoCA** (Protection of Children Act) lists and in **List 99** to assess or vet anyone who wants to work or volunteer with children or vulnerable adults. As a result of vetting, the ISA either:

- gives them ISA registration, which demonstrates that they're able to work with children or vulnerable adults or
- puts them on one of the ISA Barred Lists. One list records people prevented from working with children and the other records people prevented from working with vulnerable adults.

www.isa-gov.org.uk; www.crb.homeoffice.gov.uk

**Key terms**

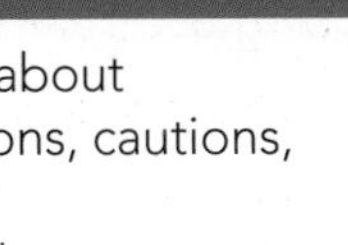

The CRB holds information about individuals, such as convictions, cautions, reprimands and warnings.

List 99 is a list of teachers who are considered unsuitable or banned from working with children in school.

The PoVA and PoCA schemes were replaced by the Vetting and Barring Scheme in October 2009.

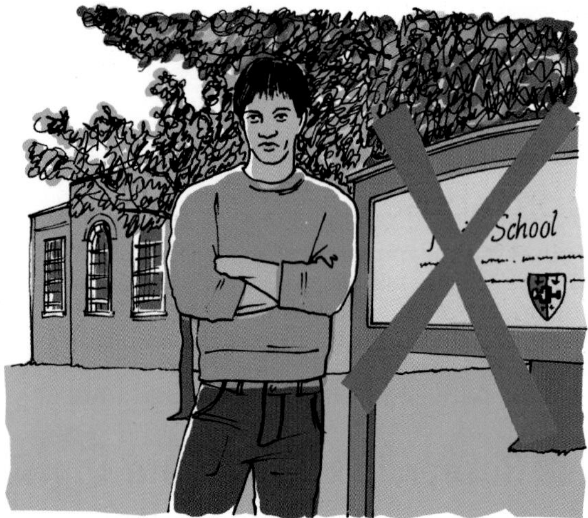


Figure 5.5 You can't work here!

At the time of writing (October 2010), the new coalition government has halted the Vetting and Barring Scheme for review. However, the following safeguarding regulations continue to apply:

- A person who is barred from working with children or vulnerable adults is breaking the law if they work or volunteer, or try to work or volunteer, with these groups.
- An organisation that knowingly employs someone who is barred from working with these groups is breaking the law.
- Organisations that work with vulnerable groups have a legal duty to give ISA information about people who they believe have harmed or may pose a risk of harm to children or vulnerable adults.

Following the report into the death of Victoria Climbié, who was horrifically tortured and eventually killed by her great aunt and her partner, the government published the **Green Paper** 'Every Child Matters' (2003). This Paper prompted wide consultation about services for children, young people and families. As a result, the government passed the Children Act in 2004, which ensures the safety and protection of children, young people and families.

## Key term

A Green Paper is a consultation document issued by the government that contains policy proposals for debate and discussion before a final decision is taken on the best policy option.

'Every Child Matters' spells out how professionals must work together to provide children's care. It is based on five outcomes, which Local Authorities use to write their 'Children and Young People's Plans'. These plans describe how services are to be developed and delivered and are used to measure their success. One of the outcomes is that children 'Stay Safe', in other words that they have security, stability, are cared for and that they are safe from:

- maltreatment, neglect, violence and sexual exploitation
- accidental injury and death
- bullying and discrimination
- crime and anti-social behaviour in and out of school.

In March 2010, the government published the guidance document 'Working Together to Safeguard Children'. This document describes the roles of the different organisations or agencies that are involved in safeguarding and protecting children and young people. They include:

- **public sector** organisations such as healthcare providers, police, probation services, Youth Offending Teams, schools, Connexions, early years services, Children and Family Court Advisory and Support Service (Cafcass) and the UK Border Agency (UKBA)
- **voluntary sector** organisations, such as the NSPCC and Barnardo's
- parents, carers and faith communities.

## Key terms

The public sector consists of organisations that are controlled by national and local government.

The voluntary sector, also known as the third sector, consists of charitable, non-profit-making organisations.

Children's Trusts consist of all the agencies working to safeguard and protect children within a locality. Children's Trust Boards oversee the **inter-agency working** agreements made between the different agencies. Local Safeguarding Children Boards (LSCBs) have a legal responsibility to agree how agencies will work together to put local 'Children and Young People's Plans' into practice.

## Key terms

**Inter-agency working**, also known as multi-agency working, means involving two or more agencies.

The media continues to report tragedies caused by a lack of protection for vulnerable adults. The Human Rights Act 1998 promotes everyone's right to freedom from abuse, and public sector health and social care providers have a responsibility to comply with the Act in their work with vulnerable adults. However, unless providing services on behalf of the public sector, private providers don't have any such responsibility. In addition, people who provide services to **direct payment** users don't have any responsibility to comply with the Act although the government is considering a review of this situation.

## Key term

**Direct payments** are local council payments to people who have been assessed as needing help from social services, and who would like to arrange and pay for their own care and support services instead of receiving them directly from the local council.

www.equalityhumanrights.com; communitycare.co.uk

## Research & investigate

### 3.1 Legislation relating to abuse

The Human Rights Act is one of a number of pieces of legislation that aims to protect vulnerable people from abuse. Find out which ones shape your work.

In its publication 'No secrets', the government describes its requirement for multi-agency working to protect vulnerable adults against abuse. To comply with 'No secrets' and with National Minimum Care Standards and professional body standards, such as the General Social Care Council Codes of Practice, local agencies have developed Safeguarding Adults Boards and Vulnerable Adults Safeguarding Policies and Procedures.

No secrets: Guidance on developing and implementing multi-agency policies and procedures to protect vulnerable adults from abuse. Dept of Health.

www.dh.gov.uk; www.gscc.org.uk

Safeguarding Adults Boards bring together local agencies that work with vulnerable adults and monitor their work. Agencies include:

- public sector organisations such as healthcare providers; learning disability teams; residential, sheltered and supported housing; police and DSS Benefits Agency
- voluntary sector organisations such as MIND, Age UK, the Alzheimer's Society, mencap and the CAB
- carer support groups and user groups
- private organisations such as lawyers
- multi-agency groups such as Local Authority Safer Community Partnerships.

www.mind.org.uk; alzheimers.org.uk; www.ageuk.org.uk; www.citizensadvice.org.uk; www.mencap.org.uk; www.carersuk.org

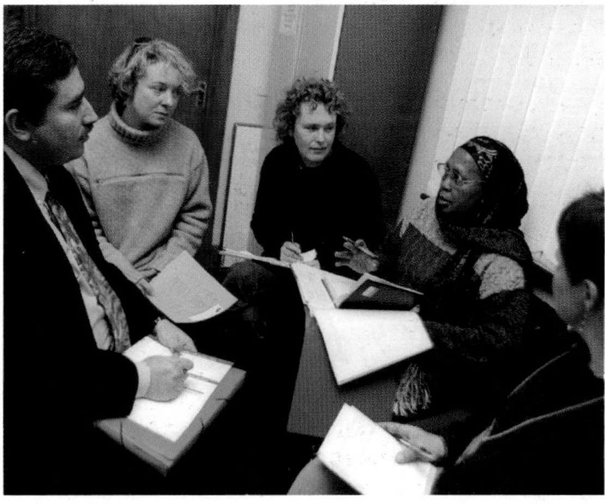

Figure 5.6 Multi-agency working

**Evidence activity** 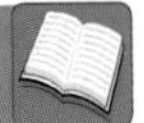

### 3.1 Identify national policies and local systems that relate to safeguarding and protection from abuse

This activity enables you to demonstrate your knowledge of national and local safeguarding and protection policies and systems.

Explore a variety of information sources, such as websites (try googling the title of this activity), your Local Authority, health service providers, the police and voluntary organisations that work with vulnerable people, to find out what safeguarding and protection policies and systems are at work in your area and what influence national government has had on shaping their existence.

## 3.2 The roles of different agencies in safeguarding and protecting individuals from abuse

As you read earlier, Safeguarding Children Boards have a responsibility to agree how agencies will work together to put 'Children and Young People's Plans' into action. In sum, it is the responsibility of everyone involved to:

- Be alert to potential abuse or neglect.
- Be alert to the signs and symptoms of abuse.
- Respect the children they work with, see situations from their perspective, and make sure the child's wishes and feelings underpin their work with them.
- Share information with other agencies so that an assessment can be made of whether a child is suffering, is likely to suffer, their needs and circumstances.
- Work cooperatively to safeguard and promote the child's welfare, including with parents as far as is appropriate.
- Take part in reviews that assess outcomes for the child against plans for their welfare.

Working Together to Safeguard Children – A guide to interagency working to safeguard and promote the welfare of children, Crown copyright 2010

Safeguarding Adults Boards bring together and monitor the work of local agencies that support vulnerable adults. In sum it is the responsibility of everyone involved to work cooperatively, share relevant information and to:

- Empower and promote the well-being of vulnerable adults.
- Support their rights to be independent and make choices but also to recognise when they are unable to make decisions and give appropriate advice, support and protection.
- Help them understand the hazards associated with any risks they want to take and minimise those risks as far as possible.
- Ensure their safety by following procedures.
- Ensure that they receive the protection of the law.

**Evidence activity** 

### 3.2 Explain the roles of different agencies in safeguarding and protecting individuals from abuse.

This activity enables you to demonstrate your understanding of the roles of different agencies in safeguarding and protecting individuals from abuse.

Think about the group of individuals with whom you work. It may be children, elderly people, people with mental health problems or people with learning difficulties. What agencies, apart from the one you work for, are involved in supporting these people? What is their particular role in providing support and why do they have this role?

## 3.3 Reports into serious failures to protect individuals from abuse

Abuse may be perpetrated by carers; care workers, including professional staff and personal assistants; people who deliberately exploit vulnerable people; friends, neighbours and strangers. And it can take place in any context, for example in someone's own home, in nursing, residential or day care settings, in schools and hospitals.

You read above about the shocking deaths of Jessica Chapman, Holly Wells and Victoria Climbié; and you have also heard about Baby Peter. Each died at the hands of either family or people they trusted and because the potential for abuse had not been identified and properly assessed. According to NSPCC research, during 2009:

- 15,800 children and young people were the victims of neglect.
- 4,400 children and young people were the victims of physical abuse.
- 2,000 children and young people were the victims of sexual abuse.
- 9,100 children and young people were the victims of emotional abuse.

In other words, in excess of 30,000 children and young people suffered some sort of abuse, not counting the cases that went unobserved or unreported.

www.nspcc.org.uk

Failure to protect vulnerable adults is reported on a regular basis in the media. You may have witnessed it yourself. Search engines such as Google list endless reports of neglect, self-neglect and financial abuse of elderly people; sexual and emotional abuse of people with learning difficulties; self-neglect and institutional abuse of people with mental health problems; and physical and emotional abuse of people with disabilities. But tragically many incidents of abuse go unobserved or unreported.

### Evidence activity 

#### 3.3 Identify reports into serious failures to protect individuals from abuse

This activity enables you to demonstrate your knowledge of reports into serious failures to protect individuals from abuse.

The reports of Lord Laming and Sir Michael Bichard have spearheaded the reform of safeguarding and protection. Check out their reports (try googling the title of this activity) as well as those published by the CQC (Care Quality Commission); private, charitable and voluntary organisations; specialist health and social care journals; and health and social care providers in your locality/region.

What do you think? How much progress have we made when it comes to protecting individuals from abuse? Why does it still happen?

## 3.4 Sources of information and advice about your role in safeguarding and protecting individuals from abuse

Sources of information and advice about safeguarding and protecting individuals from abuse.
Training courses.
Users of health and social care services.
Organisational policies, practice guidance, protocols and procedures.
Specialist books and journals.
Role descriptions/ person specifications.
National telephone help-lines and websites.
Work colleagues, including Designated Safeguarding Officers, management and Human Resources staff.
Legislation/advice leaflets/guidance documents.
Professional body Codes of Practice.
The Care Quality Commission (CQC).
Colleagues working in partner agencies.

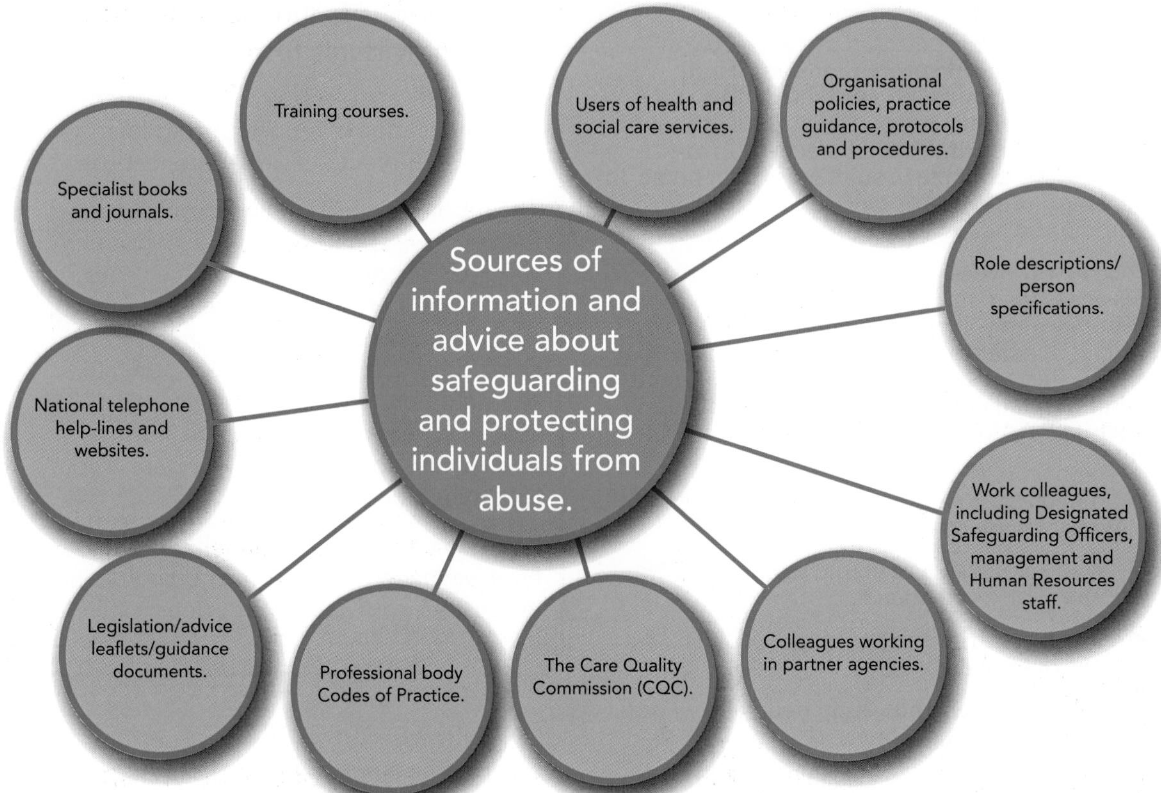

Figure 5.7 Where can you find information and advice about safeguarding and protecting individuals from abuse?

**Evidence activity** 

 **3.4 Identify sources of information and advice about own role in safeguarding and protecting individuals from abuse**

This activity enables you to demonstrate your knowledge of where you can find information and advice about your role in safeguarding and protecting individuals from abuse.

Make a list of five people and five places that you can use to find out what you should be doing to help protect people from abuse.

## LO4 Understand ways to reduce the likelihood of abuse

### 4.1 How the likelihood of abuse may be reduced

Abuse is either negligence or the result of deliberate intent to harm. It usually stems from the fact that perpetrators have little or no regard for their victims. They don't value them as people. Best practice in health and social care settings requires workers to use person-centred values in their work. By doing so, they demonstrate respect for:

- Personal values, beliefs, preferences and life experiences. A lack of respect for the value someone puts on family and treasured possessions, for their religious and political beliefs, for their likes and dislikes and their life history can be emotionally abusive.

- Choices. Denying a choice of food can be physical abuse and preventing someone from getting up and going to bed when they decide can be a form of institutional abuse.
- Rights. Failing to protect someone from danger and denying them medication can be physical abuse; unfair treatment and discrimination is emotional abuse; denying someone their pocket money or benefit payments is financial abuse; denying personal privacy could amount to sexual abuse; and not promoting dignity could be seen as neglect.
- Active participation and independence. We all have a need to be involved in everyday life and to maintain our independence. Failure to encourage people to participate in everyday activities and relationships and to live their lives as independently as possible may be both emotionally and institutionally abusive. In addition, preventing someone being an active partner in their care can be emotional abuse.

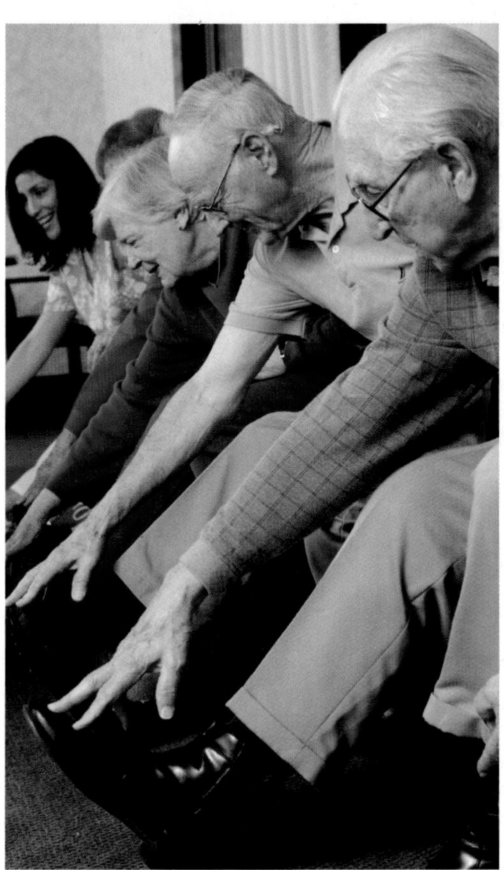

Figure 5.8 Active participation and independence

The likelihood of abuse is reduced by working with person-centred values, promoting choice and rights and encouraging active participation. Anything else is bad practice and the equivalent of abuse.

**Evidence activity** 

**4.1 Explain how the likelihood of abuse may be reduced by working with person-centred values, encouraging active participation and promoting choice and rights**

This activity enables you to demonstrate your understanding of how to reduce the likelihood of abuse.

Why do the following reduce the likelihood of an individual being abused?

- Demonstrating respect for their personal values, beliefs, preferences and life experiences.
- Promoting their rights to choice, safety, medical care, fair treatment, financial support, privacy and dignity.
- Actively involving them in their own care and day-to-day life.

## 4.2 The importance of an accessible complaints procedure for reducing the likelihood of abuse

Because abuse is a violation of an individual's human rights and illegal, it cannot be condoned. A complaint must be made and all health and social care providers are legally required to have a complaints procedure.

How does an effective complaints procedure benefit health
It helps them develop or preserve their good reputation as a service provider.
It shows that they are committed to providing a high quality service.
It shows that they are serious about listening to the people who use it.
It gives them an opportunity to identify poor working practices.
It helps them shape improvements to the way they work.
It helps them plan how to deliver services in the future.
It helps them identify where they need guidance from other agencies.
It provides them with an opportunity to deal with problems as they arise and tackle them before they become serious, avoiding staff discipline and criminal proceedings.
It can shed light on more serious issues.

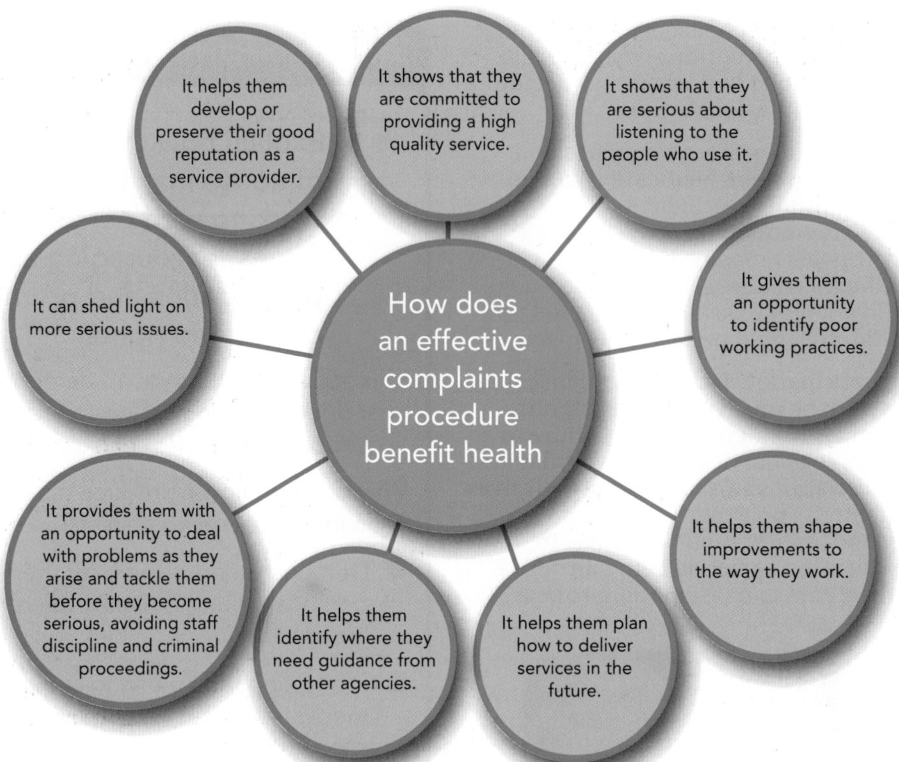

Figure 5.9 The benefits of complaints procedures

Complaints procedures need to be accessible. This is particularly important given the vulnerability of people using health and social care services. Accessibility means that they must:

- Be publicised and easy to get hold of, to advertise that people have a right to complain and to encourage them to do so. This includes everyone who suspects, has witnessed or is a victim of abuse.
- Be clear and understandable. Style and language are very important. For example, children, people with learning difficulties and speakers of foreign languages would have difficulty understanding a complaints procedure written for English adults, as would someone who uses Braille or who has a sight impairment. Complaints procedures must therefore be published in a variety of formats to reflect the age, understanding, ability and communication needs of the different people involved.
- Ensure confidentiality. Information leaks can have a serious impact on both the **complainant** and the alleged perpetrator. Unless confidentiality is ensured, people are anxious about making complaints.
- Ensure that complainants will be listened to, taken seriously and treated fairly, honestly and with respect.
- Reassure complainants that they will receive support while their complaint is being investigated and a response when the investigation is complete.

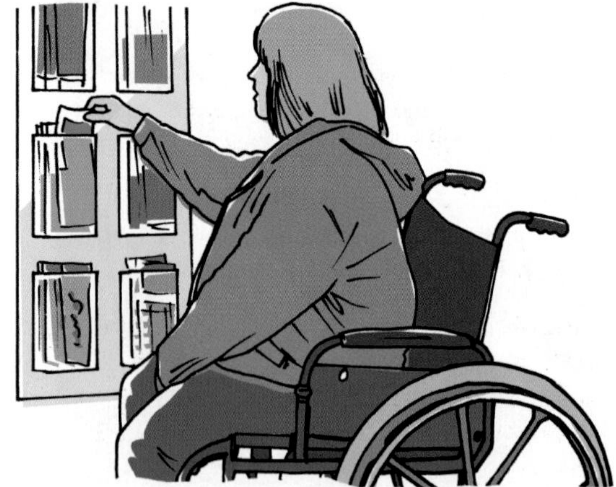

Figure 5.10 Accessible complaints procedures

## Key term

The complainant is the person making a complaint.

## Evidence activity

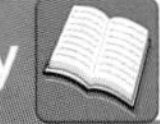

### 4.2 Explain the importance of an accessible complaints procedure for reducing the likelihood of abuse

This activity enables you to demonstrate your understanding of the need for an accessible complaints procedure.

Check out your organisation's complaints procedure.

- Does everyone who might want to use it know it exists?
- Is it easy to get hold of? Think in terms of its location – is it accessible by a wheelchair user? And is anxiety when asking for the procedure anticipated and dealt with?
- Is it clear and understandable – does it meet the communication needs of everyone?
- Does it reassure people that their complaint will be taken seriously and that confidentiality will be maintained?
- Does it describe what will happen once the complaint has been made and promise a response within a given time?

Hopefully your answers will all be positive. If not, talk the procedure over with your manager. It might not have occurred to them that the procedure is not fit for purpose.

# LO5 Know how to recognise and report unsafe practices

## 5.1 Unsafe practices that may affect the well-being of individuals

Unsafe, abusive work practices that can affect an individual's well-being include:

- Rough handling, for example pushing, pulling and dragging.
- Misuse of medication, for example hiding medication in their food or giving medication to control their behaviour.
- Ignoring their health needs, such as not attending to pressure ulcers; and not bothering to meet their **socio-emotional needs** such as helping them to maintain their appearance and personal hygiene.
- An environment that is too hot, too cold, drafty, stuffy.
- Not providing food and drink when requested and not taking them to the toilet when they need to go, leaving them in soiled, wet clothing or bedding.
- Inappropriate restraint, such as tying them down to a bed, chair or toilet.
- Dismissing their need for privacy and dignity, such as entering their room unannounced and helping them to wash or use the toilet in a less than private situation.
- Making people do things they don't want to do, for example eat or go to bed when they're not ready.
- Controlling them, making decisions for them, not allowing them to do as they wish.
- Abandoning and isolating them, for example to punish.
- Belittling people and using vulgar, sexually explicit language.
- Shopping for them and taking advantage of buy-one-get-one-free offers; collecting points for their purchases onto your club card; not giving them their receipts.
- Coercing them to buy from your personal shopping catalogue.

## Key term

Socio-emotional needs refers to someone's social and emotional needs.

## Time to reflect

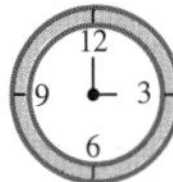

### Time to own up ...

Are you guilty of any of these abusive work practices? It could be that you have been unaware of your behaviour, that no one pointed it out to you, that nothing more was expected of you. Now you know what constitutes abuse, there is no going back. How can you ensure that you will work more safely in the future?

Resource and operational difficulties can also impact on well-being. Resources are the things you need in order to do your job safely and avoid abuse. They include:

- Health and safety training and supervision to ensure you work safely.
- Access to procedures and guidance documents, in particular safeguarding procedures that guide you in safe practice and enable you to report concerns.
- Safe, well-maintained equipment.
- Personal protective equipment and hand washing facilities.
- Safe disposal facilities.
- Time.

A lack of resources leads to unsafe practice and a threat to well-being.

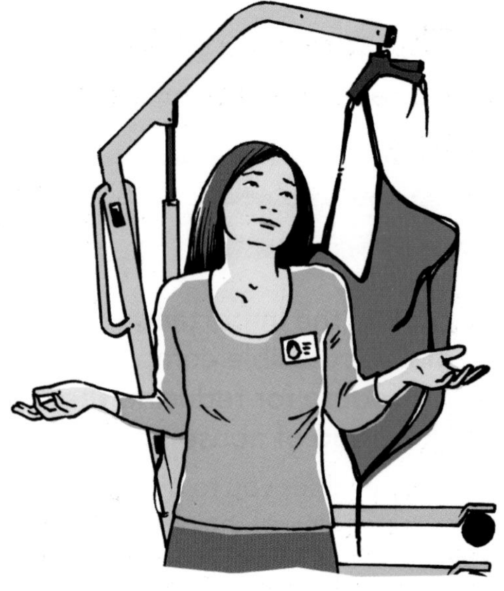

Figure 5.11 Resource and operational difficulties

Operational difficulties result from the way an organisation is managed. They too nurture unsafe practice and are a threat to well-being, for example:

- Understaffing, which means a stressed, time-poor workforce with a low morale, leading to neglect and accidents.
- A poorly trained and uncommitted workforce results in high staff turn-over, poor continuity of care and the possibility of abuse and neglect due to inexperience.
- Security issues, such as intruders and missing people, which create untold worry and concern.

## Evidence activity

### Describe unsafe practices that may affect the well-being of individuals

This activity enables you to demonstrate your knowledge of unsafe practices that can affect people's well-being.

Think about the way you and your colleagues carry out your work activities. Describe any unsafe practices that you feel could impact on safety and well-being.

## 5.2 The actions to take if unsafe practices have been identified

Health and social care providers are obliged to make sure their staff use safe practices and help them improve their performance. They must also have systems in place to enable staff to report inadequate resources or operational difficulties that could affect the delivery of safe care.

What should you do if you identify unsafe work practice? Initially, discuss your concerns with the person concerned.

Be discrete and sensitive – they may be unaware that their work is unsafe and pointing this out in public could be embarrassing and humiliating. If you feel that your discussion has been in vain, follow your workplace's procedure for reporting unsafe practice. Usually this involves discussing concerns with your manager and recording them on a specific report form.

What should you do if you experience resource or operational difficulties? Follow your workplace's procedure for reporting and recording your concerns. If, for example, an activity requires you to:

- use unsafe, ill-maintained equipment
- cut corners, because of time
- handle body fluids and contaminated waste without wearing protective clothing
- carry out an activity alone when the procedure says that a team is needed
- carry out an activity in which you haven't been trained, or work with a colleague who also lacks training

report and record your concerns as required and don't carry on with the activity until your concerns have been resolved. Not only would you be putting your safety at risk, you would also be compromising that of the people you work with.

**Evidence activity** 

**5.2 Explain the actions to take if unsafe practices have been identified**

This activity enables you to demonstrate your understanding of what to do when you identify unsafe practices.

Look back at your response to Evidence activity 5.1 where you identified work practice that could impact on safety and well-being. What actions should you take?

## 5.3 The action to take if suspected abuse or unsafe practices have been reported but nothing has been done in response

If you're concerned that a report you make of suspected abuse or unsafe practice is not acted upon, tell your manager. They must act on what you say and report back to you within an agreed timescale.

If you're concerned that management is involved in abuse or unsafe practice, speak to someone in authority on who you can rely to deal with the situation, for example your Trade Union Representative, someone in a more senior position than the manager concerned, or the organisation that regulates health and social care services where you work.

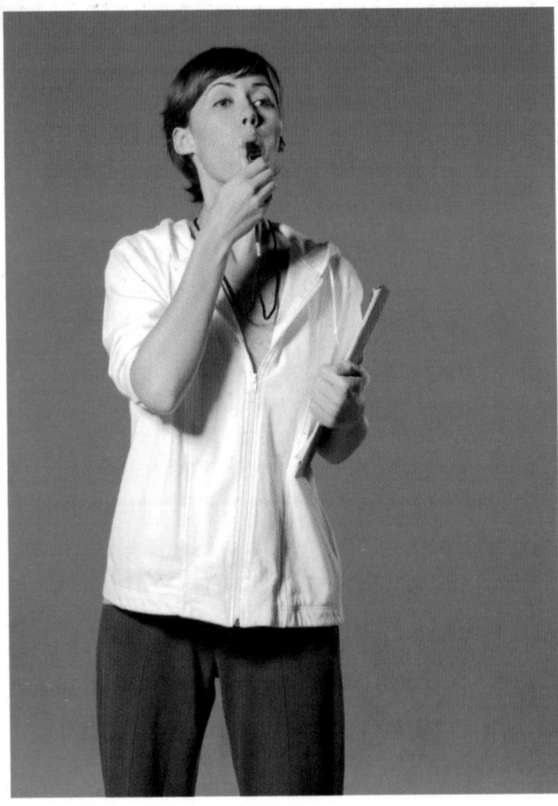

Figure 5.12 Whistle blowing!

Reporting or disclosing abusive or negligent behaviour in the interest of the people you work with is described as 'whistle blowing'. Many people are concerned that blowing the whistle on bad practice will affect their career. The Public Interest Disclosure Act 1998 protects workers who 'blow the whistle' from victimisation by their manager or employer, providing they follow the correct procedure.

You are protected as a whistleblower if you:

- are a 'worker'
- believe that bad practice is happening at work, has happened in the past or will happen in the future
- disclose information of the right type (a 'qualifying disclosure')
- disclose to the right person, and in the right way (making it a 'protected disclosure').

www.direct.gov.uk; www.hse.gov.uk

## Evidence activity 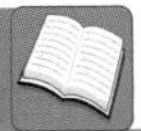

### 5.3 Describe the action to take if suspected abuse or unsafe practices have been reported but nothing has been done in response

This activity enables you to demonstrate your knowledge of what to do should a report of suspected abuse or unsafe practice not be acted on.

Check out what to do in the event that your employer fails to deal with a report of suspected abuse or unsafe practice. If there is no such procedure, check online for a whistleblowing procedure and produce a poster or information leaflet for everyone at work that describes what to do in the event that suspected abuse or malpractice is swept under the carpet.

## Assessment summary

Your reading of this chapter and completion of the activities will have prepared you to demonstrate your learning and understanding of the principles of safeguarding and protection in health and social care. To achieve the unit, your assessor will require you to:

| Learning Outcomes | Assessment Criteria |
|---|---|
| Learning outcome **1**: Show you know how to recognise signs of abuse by: | **1.1** defining the following types of abuse:<br>• physical abuse<br>• sexual abuse<br>• emotional/psychological abuse<br>• financial abuse<br>• institutional abuse<br>• self-neglect<br>• neglect by others<br>See Evidence activity 1.1 p. 67. |
| | **1.2** identifying the signs and/or symptoms associated with each type of abuse<br>See Evidence activity 1.2 p. 67. |
| | **1.3** describing the factors that may contribute to an individual being more vulnerable to abuse<br>See Evidence activity 1.3 p. 68. |
| Learning outcome **2**: Know how to respond to suspected or alleged abuse by: | **2.1** explaining the actions to take if there are suspicions that an individual is being abused<br>See Evidence activity 2.1 p. 69 |
| | **2.2** explaining the actions to take if an individual alleges that they are being abused<br>See Evidence activity 2.2 p. 70 |
| | **2.3** Identifying ways to ensure that evidence of abuse is preserved<br>See Evidence activity 2.3 p. 71 |
| Learning outcome **3**: Understand the national and local context of safeguarding and protection from abuse by: | **3.1** identifying national policies and local systems that relate to safeguarding and protection from abuse<br>See Evidence activity 3.1 p. 74 |

| Learning Outcomes | Assessment Criteria |
|---|---|
| Learning outcome **3**: Understand the national and local context of safeguarding and protection from abuse by: | (3.2) explaining the roles of different agencies in safeguarding and protecting individuals from abuse<br>See Evidence activity 3.2 p. 74 |
| | (3.3) identifying reports into serious failures to protect individuals from abuse<br>See Evidence activity 3.3 p. 75 |
| | (3.4) identifying sources of information and advice about own role in safeguarding and protecting individuals from abuse<br>See Evidence activity 3.4 p. 76 |
| Learning outcome **4**: Understand ways to reduce the likelihood of abuse by: | (4.1) explaining how the likelihood of abuse may be reduced by:<br>• working with person-centred values<br>• encouraging active participation<br>• promoting choice and rights<br>See Evidence activity 4.1 p. 77 |
| | (4.2) explaining the importance of an accessible complaints procedure for reducing the likelihood of abuse<br>See Evidence activity 4.2 p. 79 |
| Learning outcome **5**: Know how to recognise and report unsafe practices by: | (5.1) describing unsafe practices that may affect the well-being of individuals<br>See Evidence activity 5.1 p. 80 |
| | (5.2) explaining the actions to take if unsafe practices have been identified<br>See Evidence activity 5.2 p. 81 |
| | (5.3) describing the action to take if suspected abuse or unsafe practices have been reported but nothing has been done in response.<br>See Evidence activity 5.3 p. 82 |

Good luck!

## Weblinks

| | |
|---|---|
| Department of Health | www.dh.gov.uk |
| Princess Royal Trust for Carers | www.carers.org |
| Care Quality Commission (CQC) | www.cqc.org.uk |
| Scottish Commission for the Regulation of Care (SCRC) | www.carecommission.com |
| Independent Safeguarding Authority (ISA) | www.isa-gov.org.uk |
| Criminal Records Bureau | www.crb.homeoffice.gov.uk |
| Equality & Human Rights Commission | www.equalityhumanrights.com |
| Community Care website | Communitycare.co.uk |
| General Social Care Council | www.gscc.org.uk |
| Mind (mental health) | www.mind.org.uk |
| Alzheimer's Society | alzheimers.org.uk |
| AGE UK (Age Concern/Help the Aged) | www.ageuk.org.uk |
| Citizen's Advice Bureau | www.citizensadvice.org.uk |
| Mencap (learning disability) | www.mencap.org.uk |
| Carers UK | www.carersuk.org |
| National Society for the Prevention of Cruelty to Children | www.nspcc.org.uk |
| Office for Standards in Education, Children's Services and Skills | www.ofsted.gov.uk |
| Government website for public services | www.direct.gov.uk |
| Health & Safety Executive | www.hse.gov.uk |

# 6 The role of the health and social care worker

## For Unit HSC025

### What are you finding out?

Best practice in any work setting is underpinned by effective working relationships, an ability to follow agreed ways of working and an ability to work in partnership with others.

In health and social care settings, effective work relationships are based on professionalism and principles of care, which require workers to respect and promote the rights of everyone with whom they work. This includes team members, colleagues, other professionals, the individuals who need care and support and everyone who is important to them, for example their families, friends and advocates.

Ways of working in health and social care settings are described in an organisation's formal written policies and procedures, and more informally in records that have been agreed by all concerned and that allow needs to be met more flexibly. They are based on legislation, government reports and guidance documents, and professional body Codes of Practice. Workers are required to follow these ways of working to promote and maintain the health, safety and well-being of everyone in the workplace.

Collaborative or partnership working in health and social care settings requires input from all the relevant '**stakeholders**'. Team members, colleagues, other professionals and people working in voluntary agencies are all stakeholders in meeting the care and support needs of individuals, but equally important is the input of the individuals themselves, their families, friends and advocates. Partnership working through 'joined up' care ensures a best practice **holistic approach** to care needs.

The reading and activities in this chapter will help you to:

- Understand working relationships in health and social care
- Be able to work in ways that are agreed with the employer
- Be able to work in partnership with others.

**Key terms**

A stakeholder is a person or group having an interest in the success of an activity, enterprise etc.

A holistic approach is one that meets all aspects of an individual's care needs, including physical, intellectual, emotional, social and spiritual.

## LO1 Understand working relationships in health and social care

### 1.1 The difference between working and personal relationships

Relationships are probably the most involved and emotionally charged area of our lives. From the moment we're born we form relationships, each one requiring something different from us and giving us something different in return. We learn to identify people we like and don't like; we learn that we need to relate differently to different people; and we learn that some relationships are satisfying and rewarding whilst others are almost impossible to navigate! However, relationships are a basic human need and something which the majority of us strive to develop and maintain throughout our lives.

All relationships involve some level of **interdependence**. People in personal relationships, for example family members, friends, sexual and business partners, tend to influence each other, share personal and sometimes intimate thoughts and feelings, do things together and give and take emotional, physical and financial support. Because of this interdependence, things that impact on one member of the relationship will also impact on the other.

### Key term

Interdependence means dependence between two or more people.

According to the psychologist George Levinger, the natural development of a personal relationship follows four or five stages:

1. Acquaintance. This begins a relationship and can continue indefinitely, without any build-up.
2. Build-up. This is when people begin to trust and care about each other.
3. Continuation. This is when people commit to a long-term friendship or romantic relationship, perhaps marriage. Mutual trust is important for keeping a relationship going.
4. Deterioration. Not all relationships deteriorate, but in those that do, people become bored, resentful, dissatisfied and incommunicative. There is betrayal and a loss of trust.
5. Termination. This marks the end of the relationship, either by death in the case of a healthy relationship, or by separation.

When a personal relationship terminates because one or other of the people in it have become bored, resentful, dissatisfied or uncommunicative, we say it has lost its **integrity**. Because it's absolutely inconceivable that users of health and social care services should lose their trust in and feel betrayed by workers on whom they depend, best practice in a health and social care setting is built on the integrity of work relationships.

### Key term

Integrity means morally-upright, credible, trusting.

## Time to reflect

### 1.1 Personal relationships

Think about the personal relationships you have experienced during your life.

- Why did the person become more than an acquaintance?
- What sort of personal relationship did they become? Friendship? Romantic? Marriage?
- Which of them have survived?
- Of those that haven't survived, what was the reason for the termination?

## Case Study

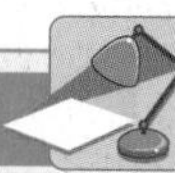

### 1.1 Betrayal of trust

The following is a synopsis of a report published in the *Telegraph* in 2007.

A teacher who had sex with one of his female pupils has been jailed for five years.

Mr X, a teacher for 21 years at the time of the offences – when the girl was 14 – was involved in after-school sports clubs at the school. The girl was a member of an after-school running club, and Mr X would go into the changing room to talk to her. The girl, who had never had sexual intercourse before but had been emotionally involved and not resisted, said they had sex four times in the store room and at his home, when contraception was not used.

Mr X told the court that he bitterly regretted his actions and had betrayed his professional principles, his position of responsibility and for that there was no excuse. He said he was unable to comprehend his actions, had lost his self-respect and dignity, and had shattered the lives of all the people he loved. *Contd.*

## Case Study *Continued*

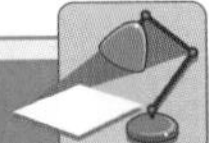

1. According to the paper, the girl was willing. Does this excuse Mr X's behaviour? If not, why not?
2. Mr X told the court that he had betrayed his professional principles. What do you think he meant by this?
3. What impact do you think this event will have on both people's lives?

**www.telegraph.co.uk**

A morally-upright work relationship in a health and social care setting is built on professionalism. Professionalism is a set of values, attitudes and behaviours that underpin best practice and help shape positive outcomes for the individuals you work with.

Whilst it's not appropriate to make personal disclosures in a professional working relationship, some individuals you support may need to relax in your company, especially if you help them with personal care needs. Letting work relationships become more personal doesn't mean you need to disclose personal things about yourself or ask personal questions. But, for example, mentioning holiday plans, remembering birthdays and asking after grandchildren can create a deeper relationship which helps you get to know each other better, making working together easier and more efficient. It also shows that you are approachable and that you're human!

Finally, and as you read earlier, effective work relationships are based on principles of care. This means that, whatever your job role, when you support individuals with health and care needs, you must:

- Show respect for their beliefs, opinions, life experiences and social, cultural and ethnic backgrounds.
- Shape the way you work around their wishes, expectations and preferences.
- Support their rights to dignity, choice, privacy, independence, confidentiality, equality and fair treatment.
- Protect them from harm whilst supporting their right to take risks.
- Communicate using a method of their choice.
- Care for them in such a way that meets their specific needs.

## Evidence activity

### 1.1 How working relationships differ from personal relationships

This activity enables you to demonstrate your understanding of the differences between a working relationship and a personal relationship.

Use the following table to compare aspects of the relationships you have with a friend and someone you support and care for at work.

| Behaviours | My friend | The person I support at work | Reasons for the differences in my behaviour |
|---|---|---|---|
| How I communicate | | | |
| How I show respect | | | |
| What I tell them about me | | | |
| What I ask them about | | | |
| What we do together | | | |

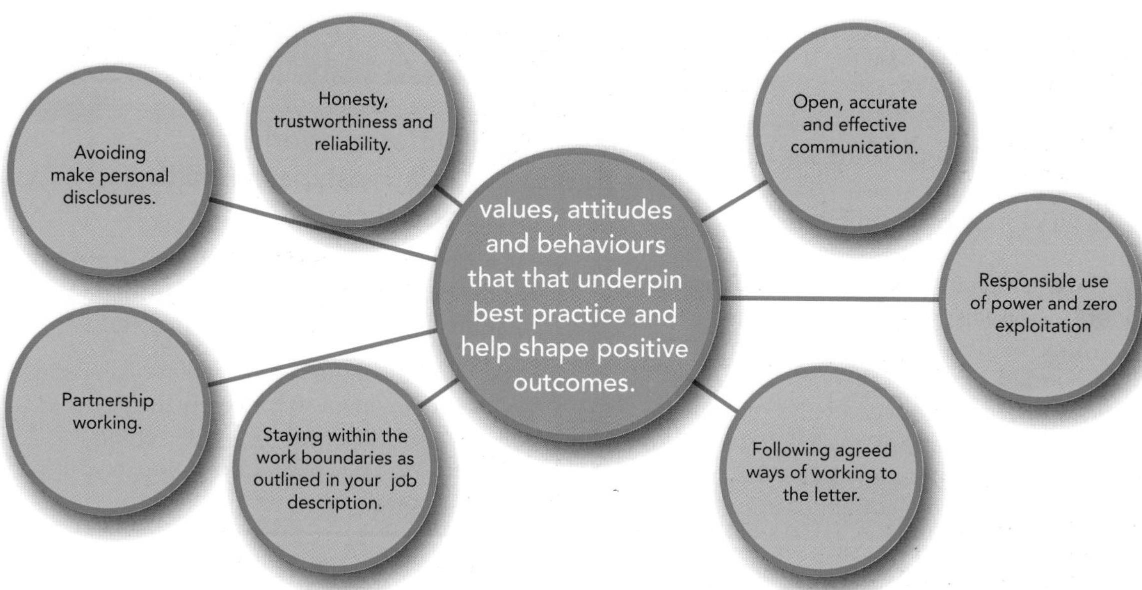


Figure 6.1 Professional practice

## 1.2 Different working relationships in health and social care settings

Everything you do as a health and social care worker involves joint working, with individuals at your workplace and with people from other agencies (inter-agency working). As a result you're required to develop working relationships with:

- the individuals you support
- their carers, family, friends and advocates
- everyone at your workplace, including colleagues, members of work teams, your manager
- professionals from other agencies
- voluntary organisations including faith groups, and voluntary workers, including members of support groups
- people with whom you liaise about your work, for example inspection agencies, manufacturers and suppliers of equipment, and maintenance and repair staff.

See Working Together to Safeguard Children: A guide to inter-agency working to safeguard and promote the welfare of children (www.dcsf.gov.uk) and your Local Authority's Inter-Agency Policies and Procedures for working with vulnerable adults, for example.

Each working relationship will have different requirements of you but in general you need to be:

- a clear communicator, both verbally and in writing
- courteous, reliable, trustworthy, responsible, well organised and a good time-keeper
- able to get on with and cooperate with others,
- able to use your initiative and work under pressure
- able to take, follow and give instructions
- willing to learn new skills and develop your understanding.

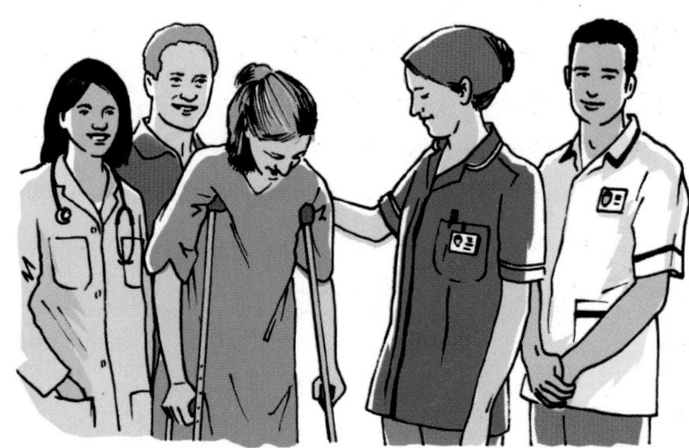

Figure 6.2 Working relationships

It's worth mentioning here that the general public depends on professional working relationships for support and care both for themselves and their loved ones. Health and social care workers are therefore perceived to be in a working relationship with the public. Unfortunately, events continue to undermine public trust in health and social care services. You therefore have a responsibility to behave, both at work and outside, in such a way as to develop and maintain public trust and confidence in the profession.

## Research & investigate

### 1.2 A loss of public trust

You will be familiar with the video footage of Ian Tomlinson, showing him being struck on the leg and pushed to the ground by a police officer. Prosecutors were unable to prove beyond reasonable doubt that there was any link between his death and the alleged abuse. As a result, an intense debate continues about the deteriorating trust and confidence that the public have in the police force.

Check the internet, local and national **media** and family, friends and colleagues for information about other events that have rocked public trust and confidence in different sectors and professions. What impact do you think a decline in trust and confidence in the health and social care sector has in the short and long term on everyone concerned?

## Key term

**Media** is the means of communication, such as radio, television, newspapers and magazines that reach or influence people widely.

## Time to reflect

### 1.2 What about you?

Is your behaviour likely to influence how people think about:

- you as a professional?
- the organisation you work for?

Do you think it matters that people have respect for you in your work role? What could be the outcome if people didn't have respect for you in your work role?

## Evidence activity

### 1.2 Different working relationships in health and social care settings

This activity enables you to demonstrate your knowledge of the range of working relationships in which you are involved.

Make a list of all the working relationships in which you are involved, identify the people you work with and describe the personal qualities and skills expected of you in your role as a working partner.

# LO2 Be able to work in ways that are agreed with the employer

## 2.1 The importance of adhering to the agreed scope of your job role

The scope of your job role consists of the different tasks or activities that you need to carry out to get your job done. It describes:

- what activities you have to do
- when you need to do them
- how you must do them
- who you must work with
- where you must work.

Because it also includes details about what you're aiming to achieve, your job scope is also used to judge your performance. So the more detail it contains, the better chance you have of success!

The scope of your job role should also describe what you must not do! This could include activities that:

- you haven't yet been trained to do
- you're not capable of doing, because of your health status, lack in seniority, lack of experience and so on

- your age, sex and understanding prevents you from carrying out, such as helping someone of the opposite sex with intimate care needs
- you're not allowed to carry out because of a criminal record.

Working in ways that are clearly defined as 'no go' puts the health, safety and emotional well-being of all concerned at risk.

Given that the scope of your job role is used to measure your performance, it's important that you're consulted about what's expected of you. Informal supervision, for example, observation, enables your supervisor to identify your strengths and limitations and chat with you about how you could improve. Formal supervision, such as appraisal, gives you an opportunity to discuss your work with your manager and how you could:

- improve your learning, understanding and performance
- adapt activities, to make them more successful.

It's also an opportunity for you to discuss situations you find difficult to handle and personal, resource and operational difficulties that impact on your performance.

The aim of supervision is to reach a mutual agreement about the scope of your job role. It should ensure you have a clear remit of what you can and can't do, an improved understanding of your work activities and how you can improve your performance, and an up-dated Continuous Personal Development (CPD) plan that describes your learning and performance needs and how and when they will be met.

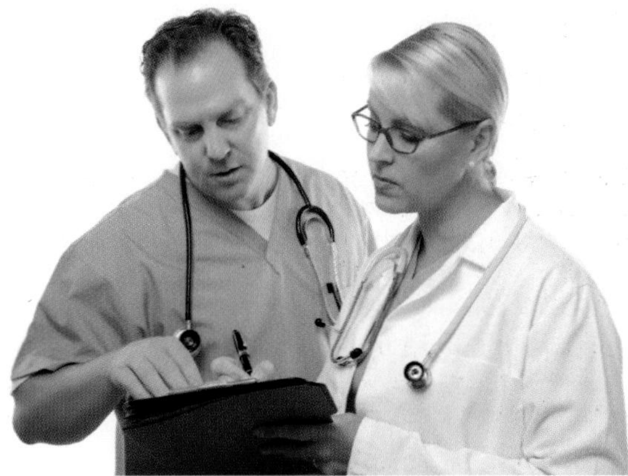

Figure 6.3 Agreeing your job scope

**Evidence activity** 

### 2.1 The importance of adhering to the agreed scope of your job role

This activity enables you to demonstrate your knowledge of the importance of adhering to the agreed scope of your job role.

- Make a list of all the activities for which you have a responsibility. What is the purpose of each? What could happen if you failed to carry them out as required?
- What activities aren't you allowed to undertake? Why not? What could happen if you carried them out?

## 2.2 Access full and up-to-date details of agreed ways of working

Workplace policies set out the arrangements that a workplace has for complying with legislation. For example, in order to comply with the Health and Safety (First Aid) Regulations, every workplace should have a policy that describes how it manages first aid.

Procedures describe the ways of working that need to be followed for policies to be implemented. They record who does what, when and how in order to maintain health, safety and well-being at all times. For example, first aid procedures describe the roles of first aiders, the people responsible for maintaining first-aid equipment and facilities, when and how to call the emergency services and when and how to complete an accident report form.

Most workplace procedures are extremely rigid and prescriptive. However, because the people you work with have their own individual needs and capabilities, and because the environments in which you work are so diverse, some procedures have to be more flexible. For example, fire evacuation procedures will differ according to where people live – a purpose-built residential care home will be equipped with fire doors and fire-fighting equipment, but not so the family home in which your grandmother wants to live out her remaining days. Similarly, a purpose-built residential care home will be equipped with hoists and stair lifts whereas your grandmother's house may not have room for moving and handling equipment. In such situations, ways of working have to be devised and agreed by all concerned.

## Case Study

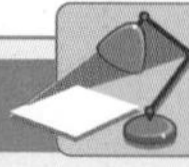

### 2.2 Meeting needs flexibly

Dorrie, aged 9, has spastic cerebral palsy, which means she has stiffness, problems with mobility and impaired sight and hearing. She lives in a residential care home during the week, where she has therapy to help with movement, balance and coordination, eating, drinking and swallowing, and lives at home with her mother, father and baby sister at weekends. Dorrie has a care plan that describes her needs but obviously the care home is equipped to meet them in a different way from her family, at home.

Identify four of Dorrie's needs, including a physical, an intellectual, an emotional and a social need, and compare how they might be met differently in the care home than at home with her family.

All workplaces have procedures and agreed ways of working in place to ensure that work practice conforms to a vast array of legislation. Because health and social care settings vary in the type of work they do, their procedures and agreed ways of working will also vary. However, in general, health and social care settings have procedures and agreed ways of working that address:

- safeguarding and protection
- equal opportunities
- confidentiality
- record keeping
- medicines administration
- first aid
- concerns and complaints
- missing persons
- emergency evacuation.

It is a legal requirement that you follow procedures and agreed ways of working to the letter. They promote and maintain safe work practice and failure to follow them jeopardises the health, safety and well-being of everyone concerned. It could also mean the loss of your employer's reputation as a well-regarded service provider and the end of your career in health and social care.

Workplace procedures and agreed ways of working are usually stored centrally, where they are accessible to everyone who needs to know their content and a responsibility to keep them updated. Updates are made in response to, for example:

- Changes in legislation. Failing to amend a procedure or agreed way of working to allow for a change in legislation results in illegal practice.
- Government and **Sector Skills Council (SSC)** initiatives, such as the changes in work practice recommended in the government guidance document 'Working Together to Safeguard Children'. Failure to work according to such initiatives means failure to use best practice.
- Technological advances that result in more effective and efficient ways of working, for example day surgery.

## Key Term

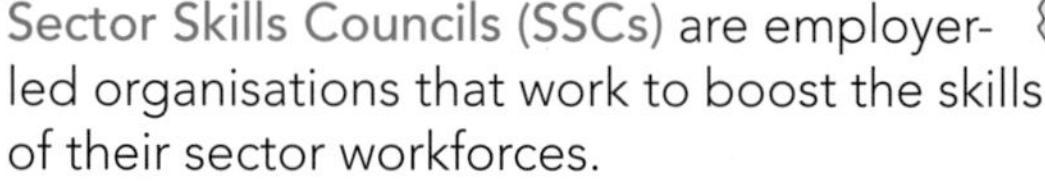

Sector Skills Councils (SSCs) are employer-led organisations that work to boost the skills of their sector workforces.

Updates to agreed ways of working are also made in response to changes in the condition and needs of the individuals you support. This ensures that care needs continue to be met appropriately.

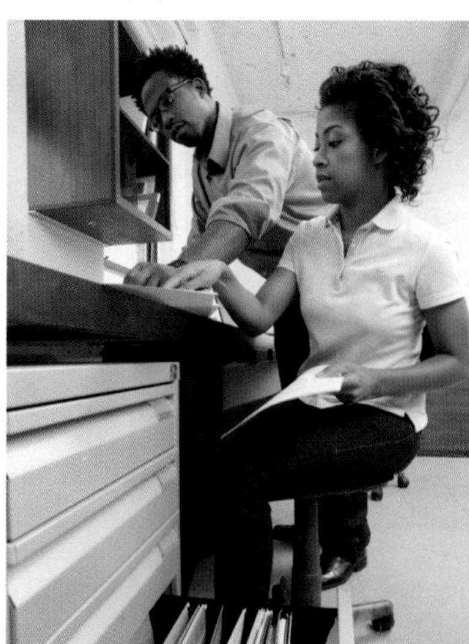

Figure 6.4 Accessing agreed and up-to-date ways of working

Practice activity 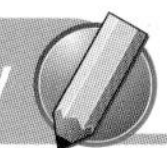

### 2.2 Accessing full and up-to-date details of agreed ways of working

This activity gives you an opportunity to practise accessing full and up-to-date details of agreed ways of working.

- Where does your organisation store procedures and agreed ways of working? Why is it important that you know this?
- Identify three activities that you carry out on a regular basis and, for each, check the procedure or agreed way of working to make sure you work as required. What is likely to happen if you don't fulfil your duties?
- How do you know that the procedure or agreed way of working is up to date? What can you do to check that it is up to date? Why is it important to ensure that agreed ways of working are up to date?

## 2.3 Implement agreed ways of working

Ten Top Tips for implementing procedures and agreed ways of working.

1. Only carry out a procedure or agreed way of working if it is included in the scope of your job role and you have had the relevant training.
2. Make sure you know and understand what you have to do before you start working. If there is anything you don't understand, ask for help.
3. If you identify operational problems, such as short-staffing, or problems with resources, such as faulty equipment, tell the appropriate person and don't proceed until you are confident that the problem has been solved.
4. Constantly monitor the activity for hazards. If anything happens that could put health, safety and well-being at risk, stop working and get help.
5. If the activity provides care and support to an individual, give them clear and accurate information about what you have to do and encourage them to work with you.
6. If the activity involves team work, accept and follow the team leader's instructions. If you are the team leader, give clear, authoritative instructions.
7. Take responsibility for your own actions and those of the people to whom you give directions.
8. Accept responsibility for and learn from your mistakes so that you don't repeat them.
9. Accept and use feedback from others to help you improve your understanding and performance.
10. Report and record any problems with the activity and be prepared to suggest how the activity could be improved.

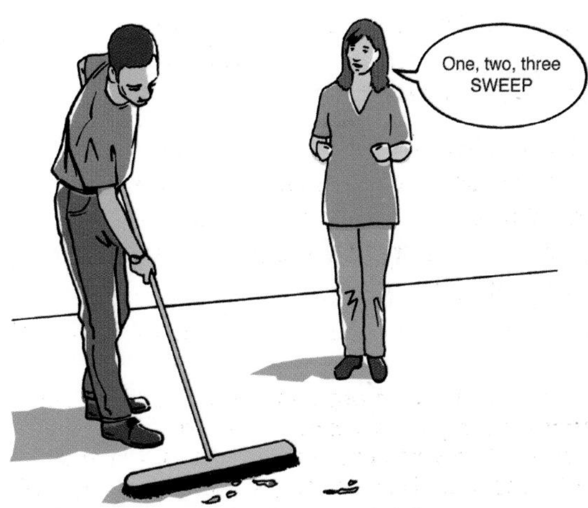


Figure 6.5 Give clear, authoritative instructions

Time to reflect 

###  2.3 Working as required?

Look at the 'Ten Top Tips for implementing procedures and agreed ways of working'. Can you honestly say you bear each of them in mind when carrying out your activities? Are there any Top Tips you would add to the list?

## Practice activity 

### 2.3 Implement agreed ways of working

This activity gives you an opportunity to practise putting agreed ways of working into action.

Ask for supervision as you carry out your activities and for feedback regarding how well you perform. Keep a diary to show how you are developing professionally. The entries you make will be useful for appraisals and for completing your CPD plan, the document in which you record your learning and performance needs and how and when they will be met.

# LO3 Be able to work in partnership with others

## 3.1 The importance of working in partnership with others

Partnership working in health and social care is the coming together of agencies that have a share in the support of people who have care needs. The key principles of partnership working are shared values, agreed goals or outcomes for the individuals they support, and regular communication.

## Evidence activity 

### 3.1 Why it is important to work in partnership with others

This activity gives you an opportunity to demonstrate your understanding of the importance of working in partnership with others.

Make a list of all the people you work with, both individually and in a team. Why is it important to work with each of these people? What are the benefits to all concerned? What might be the outcome if you failed to work with them?

## 3.2 Ways of working that can help improve partnership working

Partnership working is spread right across the public, private and voluntary sectors. The partners or 'stakeholders' that you work with will include the individuals you support, their carers, family and friends; your colleagues and team members; other professionals; and people who are important to the individuals you support, such as advocates and members of faith and support groups.

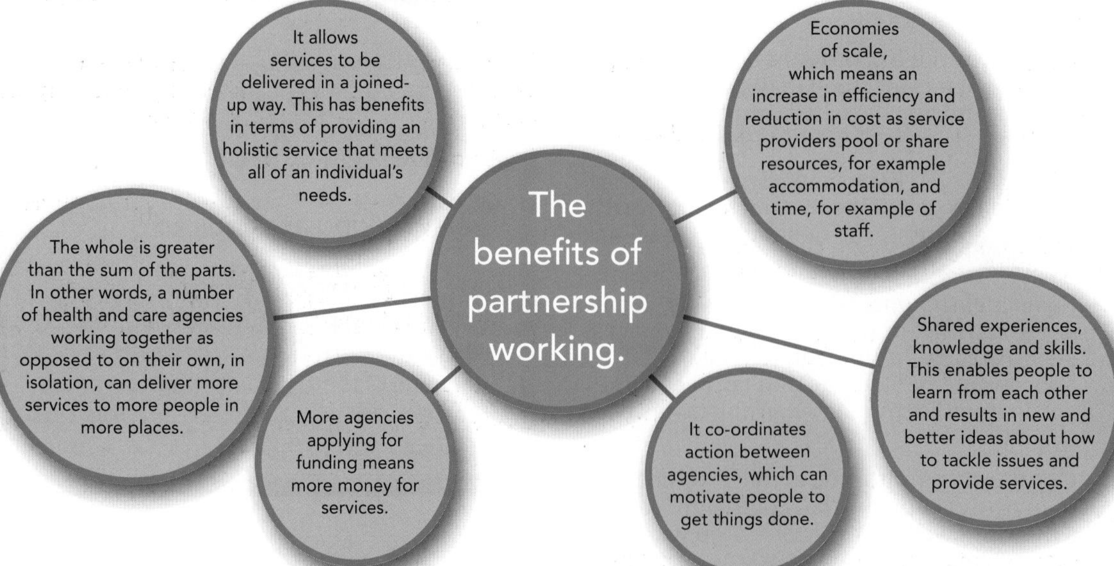


Figure 6.6 The benefits of partnership working

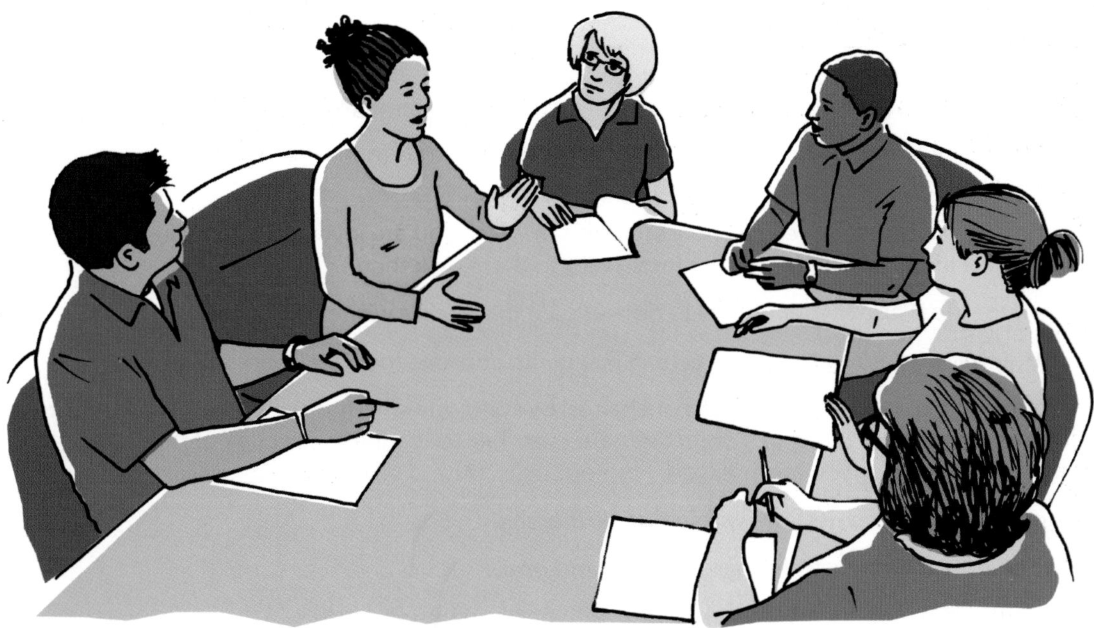

Figure 6.7 Partnership working

You can help encourage and improve partnership working by promoting the three key principles: shared values, agreed goals or outcomes for the individuals you support, and regular communication.

Shared values:

- Have a genuine desire, commitment and enthusiasm for working with other people.
- Be open, trustworthy, honest and professional in order to gain the confidence of everyone concerned.
- Always have the interests of the individuals you support at the heart of your work.
- Be prepared to learn new things and adapt the way you work.

Agreed goals or outcomes:

- Understand what goals or outcomes the partnership is trying to achieve, and by when. If you don't understand, ask.
- Understand exactly what is expected of you in achieving goals or outcomes but remember not to act beyond your job scope. If you have any concerns about what is expected of you, talk to your manager.
- Understand exactly what is expected of everyone else. If you're not sure, ask.
- Keep people informed about what you have been doing. The more you inform, the more satisfied people will be.

Regular communication:

- Make sure you attend all meetings and appointments; be punctual and well-presented.
- Use **jargon**-free communication. The individuals you support, their carers, family and friends, volunteers and people working in other agencies may not understand the language of your workplace, so using it would put them at a disadvantage.
- Listen actively to others and show that you value their contribution.
- Be sensitive to and supportive of each other's well-being, and acknowledge and respect their perceptions and points of view.
- Ensure confidentiality.
- Remain positive if communication becomes tense and conflicts develop.

## Key term

Jargon is the specialist or technical language of a trade or profession.

Practice activity 

## 3.2 Ways of working that can help improve partnership working

This activity gives you an opportunity to practise demonstrating that you can help improve partnership working.

The most important people in any partnerships in which you are involved are the individuals you support and the people that are important to them. Ask them:

- how they feel about your efforts to deliver care that meets wishes and needs
- if they have any suggestions as to how you could improve their situation.

Working partnerships are usually led or chaired by someone who has the ability and authority to ensure that the partnership's objectives are met. Talk to the leader or chair of the partnerships in which you are involved. Find out:

- how they think you perform within the partnership
- whether you demonstrate shared values and goals
- whether your communication skills promote partnership working
- if they have any suggestions as to how you could improve your ways of working.

## 3.3 Skills and approaches needed for resolving conflicts

### Time to reflect

#### 3.3 Rocky relationships ...

Think about a meeting you recently attended. How did it go? Was it obvious that everyone had shared goals and values? Was communication positive? Was there agreement about the way forward? Or was there disagreement? Did people go away from the meeting unconvinced and irritated? If so, why?

Because partnership working requires individual people and agencies to set aside their own agendas and work towards a common goal, there can be a risk of conflict. Conflict is not necessarily a bad thing. If it is dealt with effectively, we can learn from it and develop personally and professionally. However, if it is not resolved effectively, the results can be damaging. Conflicts can cause personal dislike; teamwork breaks down; talent is wasted as people remove themselves from the partnership; and in a health and social care scenario, individuals fail to receive appropriate care and support.

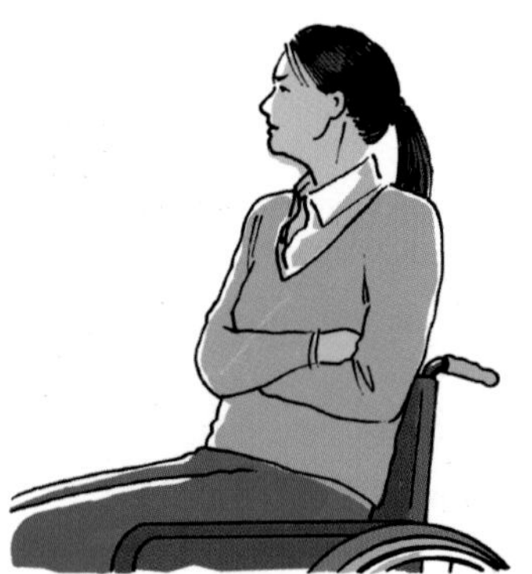

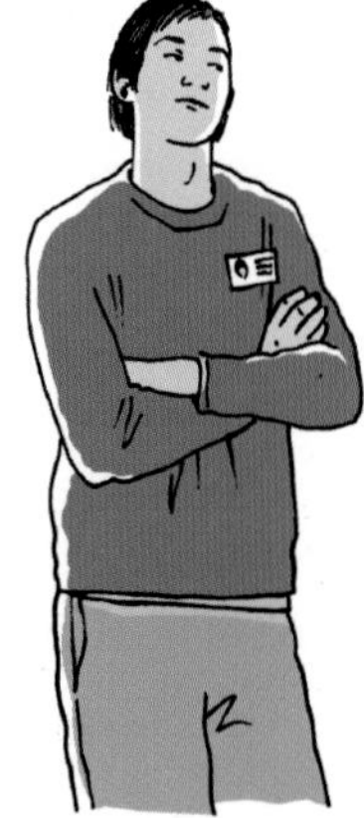

Figure 6.8 Conflict!

The guiding principles behind successful conflict resolution are mutual respect, effective communication, an open mind and a desire to understand different points of view, an enthusiasm to work cooperatively with others, and a willingness to consult, negotiate and compromise.

## Five steps to conflict resolution

### Step One: Effective communication

Effective communication is far more successful at resolving conflict than aggression. People who are involved in a conflict must be given an opportunity to express their view of the problem, and active listening ensures they are heard and understood.

- Show that you are interested in what the other person is saying, for example by maintaining eye contact.
- Show that you are trying to understand their point of view, for example by mirroring their facial expressions and tone of voice; by using appropriate body movements, such as head nods; and by making affirmative noises such as 'mmm' and 'yes'.
- Check your understanding by asking questions, **paraphrasing** what they tell you and summarising what you understand them to have said.

And make sure that when you talk, you are calm, courteous and assertive rather than confrontational and aggressive.

**Key term**

Paraphrasing is rephrasing what you have been told in your own words.

### Step Two: Research

Everyone has their own interests, needs and concerns. Conflict arises when someone feels that theirs are being ignored or not taken into account. Try to understand how the partnership's way of doing things is affecting them, for example is it affecting their work performance, or is it affecting the way an individual feels cared for or supported? Be objective – focus on work issues and leave personalities out of the discussion.

### Step Three: Identify the problem

Everyone needs to have a clear understanding of the problem. As you read above, different people have different needs, interests and concerns, and as a result they see problems differently. You need to reach an agreement about what the problem is before you can find a mutually acceptable solution.

### Step Four: Negotiate a win-win solution

If everyone is to feel comfortable with the way a problem is solved, they need to be involved in identifying possible solutions. Involvement means being open to all ideas, including the ones they hadn't thought of. If agreement can't be reached, consider making a compromise.

### Step Five: Problem solving

Action the agreed or compromise solution, and monitor the situation to make sure that it does resolve the problem. And be prepared to try out any of the other proposed solutions, to see whether they are more effective.

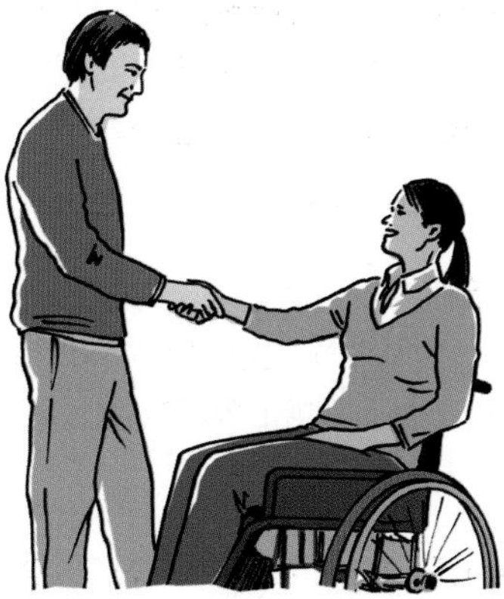

Figure 6.9 Problem solved!

**Evidence activity**

**3.3 Skills and approaches needed for resolving conflicts**

This activity gives you an opportunity to demonstrate your knowledge of how to behave in order to resolve a conflict.

Produce a poster for display in the staff room entitled 'Conflict Resolution' that describes the skills and approaches needed to get to the bottom of and settle a conflict.

## 3.4 Accessing support and advice about partnership working and resolving conflicts

Working with other people can present hazards. For example, there may be a personality clash or you may be asked to carry out an activity that:

- is outside the scope of your job role
- is within the scope of your job role but for which you have yet to be trained, or, because of inexperience, you are not confident you could do well
- is not written into an individual's care plan
- would compromise your integrity, for example if you are asked to disclose confidential information
- would compromise the professional boundaries between you and an individual you support, for example if you were asked to use your position to exploit them in some way.

Where can you go for advice and support if you have concerns about partnership working or conflict is rearing its ugly head? First of all, talk to the person concerned as soon as possible and before things get any worse. Be assertive but not confrontational. Tell them how you feel and why and don't make accusations!

If talking doesn't resolve the problem, or if the person you find it difficult to work with or with whom you have a dispute is your manager, get advice or support from a higher level. Most organisations have procedures in place to deal with disputes and conflicts. They may require you to speak with someone in Human Resources, a union representative or an outside agency, such as a mediator or the Advisory, Conciliation and Arbitration Service (Acas) www.acas.org.uk

## Key terms

A **mediator** is an intermediary third party, which is neutral and helps negotiate agreed outcomes.

**Acas** provides confidential and impartial advice to assist workers in resolving issues in the workplace.

If you want to complain about being a victim of a dispute or conflict, keep a record of what happened, when and where it happened, as well as anything else you think might be relevant, for example emails, texts, notes and letters. If it gets as far as a hearing, you'll need these as evidence.

Disputes and unresolved conflicts affect people professionally and personally, so should never be ignored.

Dealing with conflict can be difficult if you have a problem:
Seeing things from another point of view.
Understanding someone else's problem.
Communicating calmly in tense situations.
Defending your position when you are being criticised.
Co-operating with people for whom you have little or no respect.
Negotiating, perhaps because you are stubborn.
Compromising, because you think you are always right.
Saying no.

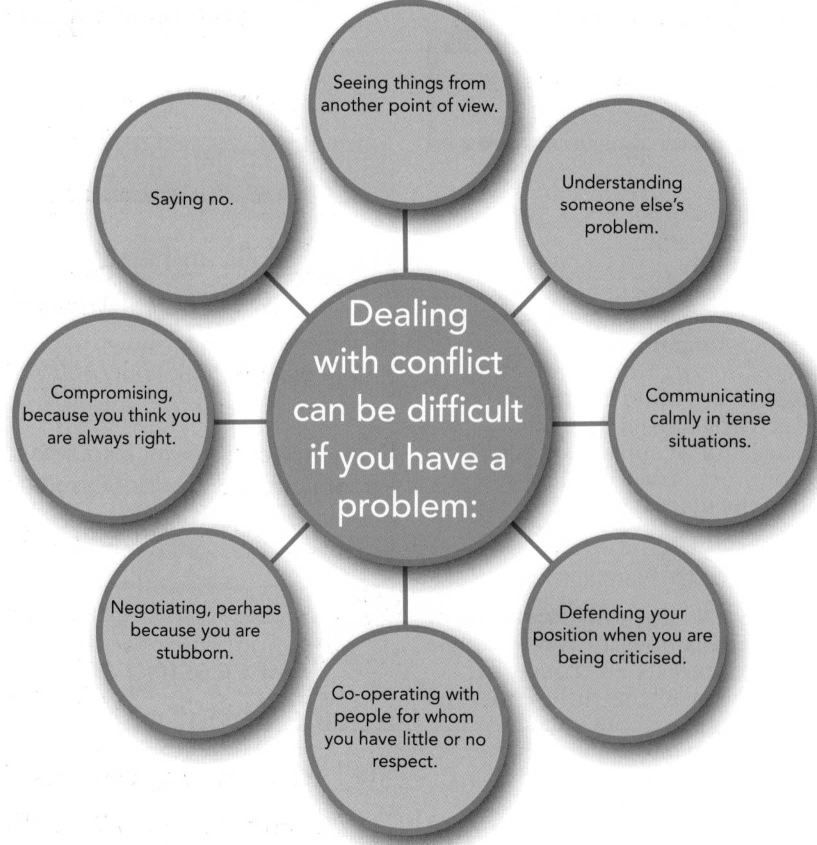

Figure 6.10 Difficulties in dealing with conflicts

Practice activity 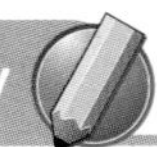

### 3.4 How and when to access support and advice about partnership working and resolving conflicts

This activity gives you an opportunity to practise demonstrating how and when to access support and advice about partnership working and resolving conflicts.

- Talk to your manager about what you should do and when if there is a conflict or you experience difficulties in working within a partnership.
- Check out your workplace procedures and agreed ways of working in the event that talking doesn't resolve a problem.
- Research Acas and mediators in your locality. Find out how they can help in the event of a dispute.
- Produce an information sheet for circulation within your workplace that details your findings.

## Assessment summary

Your reading of this chapter and completion of the activities will have prepared you to demonstrate your learning and understanding of the role of the health and social care worker. To achieve the unit, your assessor will require you to:

| Learning Outcomes | Assessment Criteria |
|---|---|
| Learning outcome 1: Understand working relationships in health and social care by: | 1.1 explaining how a working relationship is different from a personal relationship<br><br>See Evidence activity 1.1 p. 88. |
| | 1.2 describing different working relationships in health and social care settings.<br><br>See Evidence activity 1.2 p. 90. |
| Learning outcome 2: Be able to work in ways that are agreed with the employer by: | 2.1 describing why it is important to adhere to the agreed scope of the job role<br><br>See Evidence activity 2.1 p. 91. |
| | 2.2 accessing full and up-to-date details of agreed ways of working<br><br>See Practice activity 2.2 p. 93. |
| | 2.3 implementing agreed ways of working<br><br>See Practice activity 2.3 p. 94. |

| Learning Outcomes | Assessment Criteria |
|---|---|
| Learning outcome 3: Be able to work in partnership with others by: | 3.1 explaining why it is important to work in partnership with others<br>See Evidence activity 3.1 p. 94. |
| | 3.2 demonstrating ways of working that can help improve partnership working<br>See Practice activity 3.2 p. 96. |
| | 3.3 identifying skills and approaches needed for resolving conflicts<br>See Evidence activity 3.3 p. 97. |
| | 3.4 demonstrating how and when to access support and advice about:<br>• partnership working<br>• resolving conflicts.<br>See Practice activity 3.4 p. 99. |

Good luck!

## Weblinks

| | |
|---|---|
| The Department for Education, previously the Department for Children, Schools and Families and Schools | www.dcsf.gov.uk |
| Care Quality Commission (CQC) | www.cqc.org.uk |
| Scottish Commission for the Regulation of Care (SCRC) | www.carecommission.com |
| Advisory, Conciliation and Arbitration Service | www.acas.org.uk |

# 7 Implement person-centred approaches in health and social care

## For Unit HSC026

### What are you finding out?

In care, it is vital that people have the right care to meet their needs. It is therefore important that procedures are followed to ensure needs are met. It is equally vital that individuals are at the centre of this process so that they feel like they are actively involved in their own care. Good, effective care planning can ensure all these needs are met. Care packages should never be made for the ease or convenience of care workers. The reading and activities in this chapter will help you to:

- Understand person-centred approaches for care and support
- Be able to work in a person-centred way
- Be able to establish consent when providing care or support
- Be able to encourage active participation
- Be able to support the individual's right to make choices
- Be able to promote the individuals' well-being.

## LO1 Understand person-centred approaches for care and support

### 1.1 Define person-centred values

Person-centred care is best practice in health and social care. It is vital that the individual is at the centre of all health and social care matters. Whether it is the planning of services, the delivery, treatment or communications, all these activities need to ensure the individual is at the hub. To do this, it is crucial that care workers have certain values.

#### Individuality

Individuals are unique, and should never be treated as a 'number', a 'patient', a 'pupil', a 'resident', or a 'service user'. Everyone is different and this should be recognised in health and social care.

#### Rights

Individuals have rights, which are what we are entitled to. The rights range from legal rights to 'everyday' rights. Care workers need to ensure that all their practice ensures these rights are met.

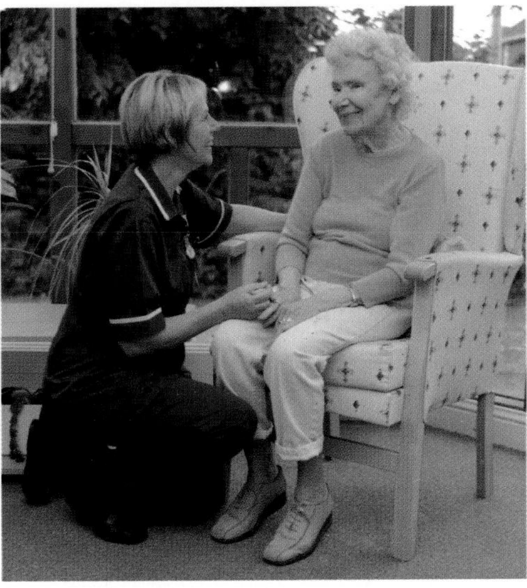

Figure 7.1 See the person inside

#### Choice

Care workers need to make certain that individuals have choice in all care provision. This is **empowering** for individuals as it allows them to feel in control over their own life and care.

> **Key term**
>
> Empowering means allowing individuals to have control over their own lives.

## Privacy

Treating individuals in a way that guarantees their privacy is essential. Privacy can fall into three categories. First, individuals must be protected from any private information being overheard. Second, individuals must be protected from being seen by anyone when not needed, for example when dressing. Third, information about individuals must be kept private.

## Independence

Everyone has the right to do for themselves what they are able to do. Encouragement, provision of equipment, patience and so on will all allow an individual to remain as independent as possible. Being dependent on others can be frustrating if an individual wants to and is able to carry out tasks for themselves.

## Dignity

All individuals have rights to be treated in a way which is not humiliating, degrading or embarrassing. Care workers need to ensure that all their care is provided in a dignified way, for example in how they treat, speak to and care for individuals.

## Respect

Every individual should be treated with respect and valued. An individual's age, sex, religion, abilities or disabilities, appearance and so on should have no bearing on an individual being treated respectfully. Being disrespectful is discourteous and impolite.

## Partnership

Partnership involves working with and valuing the contribution of all agencies who can work to provide services. This could be health services, social services, education services, early years services, informal carers, family and friends, as well as obviously the individual themselves.

### Research & investigate

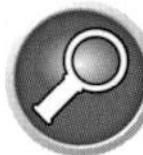

**Our rights**

Find out about some of the legal rights we have. You may examine the Human Rights Act, discrimination laws, confidentiality laws and so on.

### Case Study

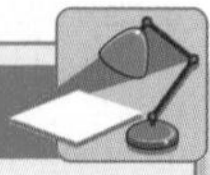

**Steven**

Steven is 38 and has severe learning difficulties and requires care. At his residential home, the care workers don't bother to brush his hair as 'he doesn't know how he looks'. He wears 'hand-me-down' clothes from other residents which don't fit him properly. When helping him to eat, they put a baby style bib on him, and do 'train noises' to encourage him. When he spills food on his face and clothes, they rarely clean him and leave him with food on himself. He has to go to bed at 9pm along with all the other residents and his bedding has cartoon characters on although he has no idea who they are.

1. What person-centred values are the care workers not providing here?
2. What suggestions would you make to Steven's care?

### Time to reflect

**The right to privacy**

How would you feel if, when you were being cared for in hospital, the doctor didn't pull the curtain fully around so others could see when any examinations were taking place, and spoke in loud tones so other patients could hear what they were saying?

**Evidence activity** 

### 1.1 Person-centred values

This activity enables you to demonstrate you can define person-centred values.

Produce a poster, defining all the person-centred values.

## 1.2 Explain why it is important to work in a way that embeds person-centred values

Embedding person-centred values has many benefits. Being person-centred is about listening to and learning about what individuals want from their lives and helping people to think about what they want now and in the future.

The benefits of this are significant.

- Empowering – individuals will feel they have power and control over their own lives, that they are the ones driving the care they receive.
- Promotes confidence and self-esteem – working in a way that is person-centred will lead to individuals having an increased belief that they are able to confidently contribute to discussions. This will help individuals to feel good about themselves and value the contribution they can make.
- Provides tailor-made care – individuals participating in their care will lead to care that is more suited to their needs, views and preferences. Care will be better matched and hence will be more effective.
- Encourages feelings of being valued and respected – if individuals feel they are encouraged to participate it will develop feelings of a sense of worth and make them feel that their contributions and ideas are important.

The consequences of not embedding person-centred values are significant and could be felt in both the short term and the long term:

**Withdrawn:**
if individuals feel they don't have a voice they may withdraw from communication and interaction altogether

**Disempowered:**
if individuals feel unimportant, like a burden, then they may feel they have no control over their lives

**Anger:**
Feelings of frustration may result in challenging behaviour and resentment

**Apathy:**
If individuals feel let down or disapointed with their care they may give up trying to participate

Figure 7.2 Consequences of ignoring person-centred values

## Key term

**Apathy** means lack of interest, indifference.

## Evidence activity

### 1.2 The importance of working in a way that embeds person-centred values

This activity enables you to demonstrate you understand why it is important to work in a way which embeds person-centred values.

Write a short report explaining how you would feel if you were cared for in a way which ignored person-centred values.

## 1.3 Explain why risk taking can be part of a person-centred approach

We all take risks in life; everyday risks, such as not wearing a coat when it's cold outside, to larger risks such as bungee jumping. It's part of what makes us human; it helps us to feel 'alive'. Often these challenges provide **adrenaline** rushes and provide us with a 'buzz'. Individuals requiring health and social care also have the right to take risks.

Some individuals take part in risky behaviour such as smoking, alcohol, sunbathing, eating unhealthy food and so on. As free-willed individuals, everyone has a right to make these choices and hence so do individuals requiring health and social care.

Not allowing an individual the right to take risks is denying them the right to choose how to live their life.

Parents increasingly allow their children to take more risks as they get older. This can be a difficult time, but parents are aware that it is necessary as it is part of growing up, as we often learn from our mistakes, and it helps children be equipped for later life.

## Time to reflect

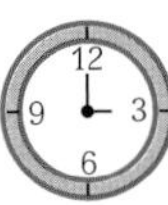

### 1.3 Risk-taking

How would you feel if you were told you couldn't ever go shopping without supervision, you were never allowed to eat anything unhealthy, never allowed to 'stay up late' as a treat?

## Key term

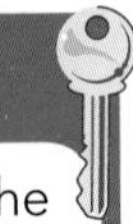

**Adrenaline** is a hormone that stimulates the nervous system, stimulating the heart and breathing, and causes a sense of alertness and excitement.

## Case Study

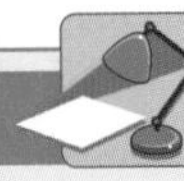

### 1.3 John

John has recently had a car accident and after suffering serious brain injuries is attending sessions for rehabilitation. John is baking; he will need to use knives, a hot oven and a food processor. Although, there is no evidence to show that John cannot cope, his care worker is hovering over him, doing everything for him, fussing. John is 'allowed' to mix the ingredients together with a spoon and then watch as the care worker does the rest.

1. How could the care worker's actions be disadvantageous to John?
2. What suggestions would you make to balance safety and independence?

Taking risks is part of life – hence person-centred care would allow this.

Their age – younger or older
Physically disabled
Learning difficulties
Memory problems
Lifestyle issues
Bereavement
Addiction issues
Mental health issues
Family issues or breakdowns
Reasons why individuals may need care

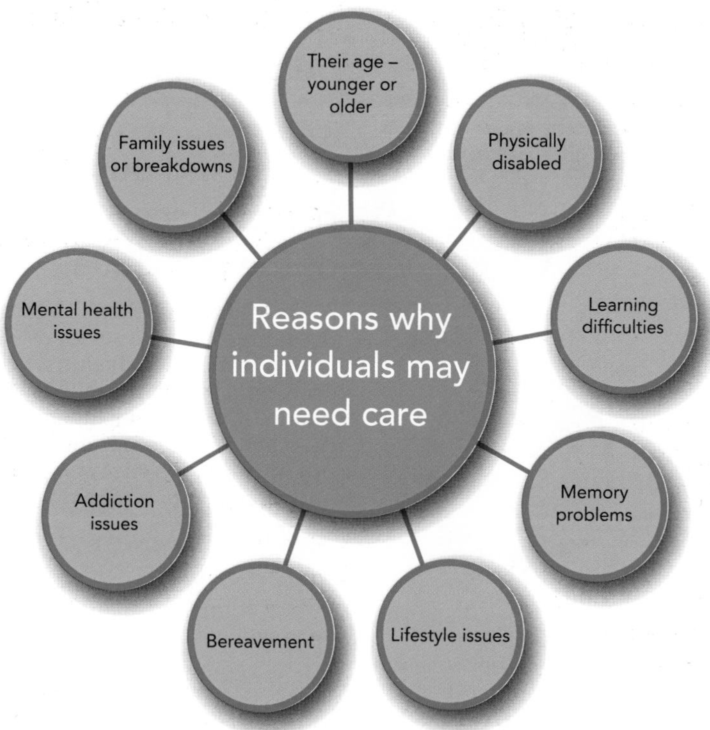

Figure 7.3 Reasons why individuals may need care

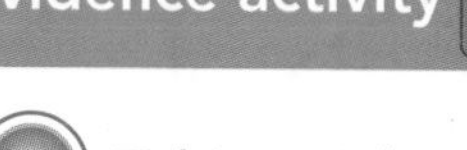

## Evidence activity

### 1.3 Taking risks as part of a person-centred approach

This activity enables you to demonstrate that you understand why risk taking is part of a person-centred approach.

Produce a report explaining why John in Case study 1.3 needs to partake in risk taking activities.

## 1.4 Explain how using an individual's care plan contributes to working in a person-centred way

Individuals may need care at times in their life; Figure 7.3 shows some of the reasons why this could be.

Because there is such a range of individuals, there is such a range of needs. To meet all these individually specific needs, person-centred care planning is vital.

The NHS & Community Care Act (1990) states that individuals are entitled to have their needs assessed and a care plan produced. A **care plan** may be known by other names, such as a support plan or individual plan. It is the document where day–to-day requirements and preferences for care and support are detailed.

To be person-centred, the individual concerned in the care should be involved in every stage of the planning process. Usually the planning process involves the following stages:

1. Assess – the individual and the care professionals will assess the needs that currently are and are not being met in the individual's life.
2. Plan – the individual and the care professionals will put together a plan of care to meet the needs identified.
3. Implement – the care 'package' is put into action.
4. Monitor – the individual and the care professionals will routinely check to consider if the care 'package' is actually meeting the needs identified.
5. Evaluate and adapt – the individual and the care professionals will decide what revisions need to be made based on any changing needs of the individual or failings in the current care 'package'.

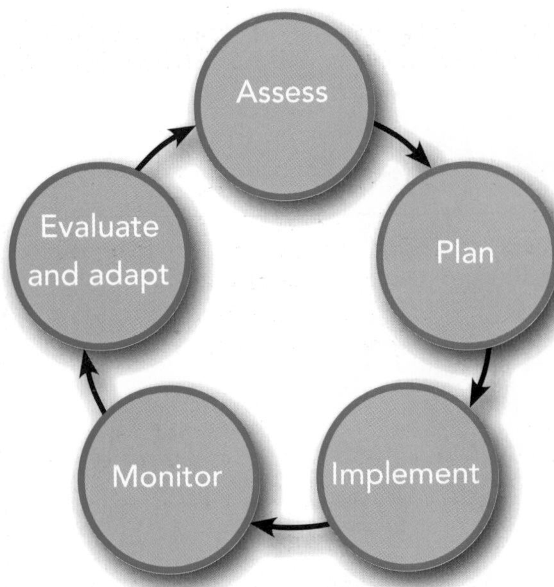


Figure 7.4 Stages of care planning

This cycle must have the potential to be continuous as needs change (maybe because the individual no longer has unmet needs or has increasing, or different, needs). A care plan which is meeting needs fully when first implemented may not still be doing so six months later.

At all stages of the planning process, it is vital that the individual leads the process. Although this sounds obvious, it is surprising how often this is overlooked and care professionals may think they 'know what is best' for the individual. Care workers have to remember that the individual is at the foundation of care planning; it is their body, their life, their discomfort, their pain. Care planning which is not person-centred is meaningless.

It is best practice to respect the individual's role in this process. It is a key way of empowering people in their own care.

# LO2 Be able to work in a person-centred way

## 2.1 Find out the history, preferences, wishes and needs of the individual

An individual is more than the needs presented to care services. They are a person, with a past, with dreams, with feelings and opinions. Ignoring these ignores the person inside. It will never matter how 'good' the care provided is if it does not take into account the individual's history, preferences, wishes and needs. It is vital that care workers find these out!

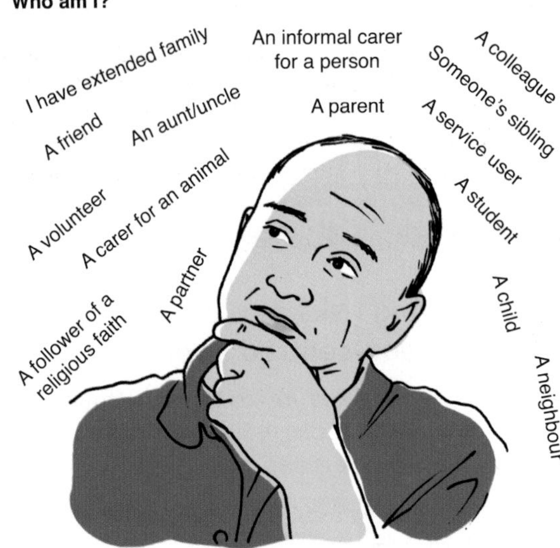


Figure 7.5 See the individual beneath

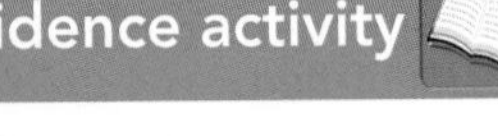

Evidence activity

### 1.4 Explain how using an individual's care plan contributes to working in a person-centred way

This activity enables you to demonstrate your knowledge of how using an individual's care plan contributes to working in a person-centred way.

Imagine that you required a care plan. How would using this provide you with person-centred care?

## Case Study

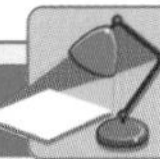

### 2.1 Becky

Becky is an able woman who uses a wheelchair. Her carer is assessing her; he asks Becky about all the things she cannot do. Becky explains these are certain personal hygiene matters, washing clothing, housework (e.g. hovering, sweeping), transport and so on that she struggles with. These are noted. Becky is never given the opportunity to say the things she can do, such as ironing, doing her own hair and makeup, dusting and polishing her house. Becky also loves dancing and watching dance programmes like 'Strictly Come Dancing'; she would love to be in a dance group or go to watch dance acts.

All the services that Becky's carer believes she requires to meet her unmet needs, such as personal hygiene matters, washing clothing, housework, transport and so on are put into place.

1. How might Becky feel when **domiciliary** carers iron her clothes for her, dust and polish her house or do her hair?
2. Becky never manages to go to any dance classes, or go to see any dance shows. How could this affect her health and well-being?

## Key term

Domiciliary means at home.

## Practice activity

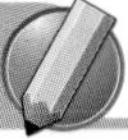

### 2.1 Find out the history, preferences, wishes and needs of the individual

This activity enables you to demonstrate you can find out the history, preferences, wishes and needs of an individual.

Consider Becky in Case study 2.1 and prepare a list of questions you would ask her to provide person-centred care and establish her history, preferences, wishes and needs.

## 2.2 Apply person-centred values in day-to-day work taking into account the history, preferences, wishes and needs of the individual

We know from section 1.1 that the following person-centred values are vital:

- individuality
- rights
- choice
- privacy
- independence
- dignity
- respect
- partnership.

Hence it is also important to apply these values when taking into account history, preferences, wishes and needs of the individual.

This could be for small things, as in the case of Margaret in Case study 2.2 below, or more significant issues such as accommodation issues, living arrangements, finances and so on.

Some examples of applying person-centred values to care issues are provided in Table 7.1.

Table 7.1 Examples of applying person-centred values to care issues

| Care need | How can provision promote person-centred values? |
|---|---|
| Living arrangements | • Ensure individuals have access to all the information regarding different options.<br>• Arrange visits to allow individuals to see for themselves.<br>• Work with all agencies involved to consider the **logistics** of various options.<br>• Provide living aids and promote independence whichever option is decided upon.<br>• Wherever the individual resides, they are allowed to have their own style, decor, ornaments etc. |
| Food | • Ensure individuals can express their dietary requirements and nutritional needs.<br>• Consider religious requirements for food.<br>• Allow individuals to express likes and dislikes about food.<br>• Allow individuals to eat for themselves if they can (and if they can't, ensure all support is not demeaning or belittling, e.g. the wearing of a bib, or 'feeding' someone).<br>• Allow individuals to eat where and how they prefer. |
| Clothing | • Consider religious requirements for clothing.<br>• Promote an individual's right to wear what they want.<br>• Encourage individuals to dress on their own, but if this is difficult aids and support should be provided.<br>• Provide options for clothing, which are clean, appropriate and of the individual's taste.<br>• Wash clothing with respect to the preferences of the individual.<br>• Ensure individuals are allowed privacy and dignity when they are dressing. |
| Personal hygiene arrangements | • Allow individuals to wash how they prefer, i.e. shower, bath or bed bath.<br>• Ensure choices are given, e.g. whether soap or shower gel, and which brand, fragrance etc.<br>• Provide choice as to when individuals prefer to wash, e.g. morning, evening.<br>• Even if individuals need support, do this with dignity and privacy in mind. |

## Key term

**Logistics** means the organisation of services, supplies, resources.

## Case Study

### 2.2 Margaret

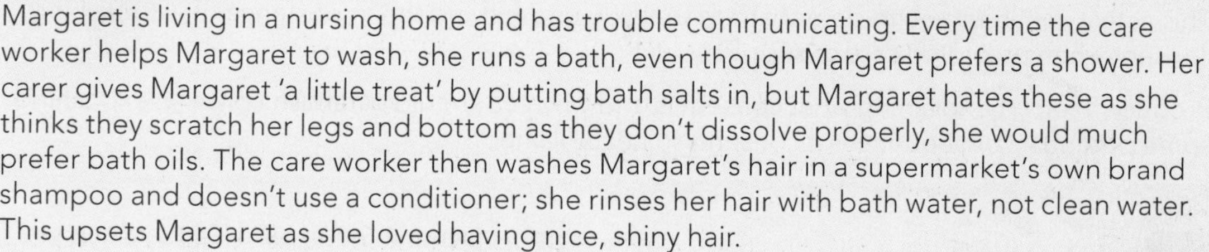

Margaret is living in a nursing home and has trouble communicating. Every time the care worker helps Margaret to wash, she runs a bath, even though Margaret prefers a shower. Her carer gives Margaret 'a little treat' by putting bath salts in, but Margaret hates these as she thinks they scratch her legs and bottom as they don't dissolve properly, she would much prefer bath oils. The care worker then washes Margaret's hair in a supermarket's own brand shampoo and doesn't use a conditioner; she rinses her hair with bath water, not clean water. This upsets Margaret as she loved having nice, shiny hair.

1. Consider how something as simple as this washing practice is not respecting Margaret's history, preferences, wishes and needs.

## Practice activity

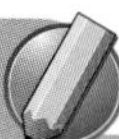

### 2.2 Apply person-centred values in day-to-day work

This activity enables you to demonstrate that you can apply person-centred values in day-to-day working.

Consider three of the day-to-day activities you carry out; using the values identified in 1.1, how would you want them to be provided?

# LO3 Be able to establish consent when providing care or support

## 3.1 Explain the importance of establishing consent when providing care or support

The majority of care requires consent. Consent means **informed** agreement to an action or decision. The process of establishing consent will vary according to an individual's assessed ability to consent. Only in exceptional circumstances is consent not required.

## Key term

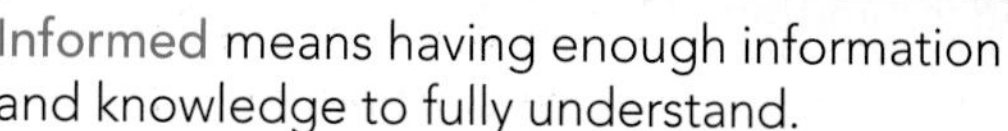

Informed means having enough information and knowledge to fully understand.

For care to be person-centred, the individual has to have given their consent. Whether this is for an examination, a treatment, an operation, or support from care workers, the individual needs to have 'allowed' for it to have happened. However, all information needs to be given for this to happen – including *all* possible outcomes. For example, in preoperative discussions, a surgeon must explain the risks of a procedure before the patient can give consent; therefore consent has to be informed.

For informed consent, the individual must be able to competently receive and understand all facts. There are circumstances when individuals may be deemed not able to give informed consent due to their health, intellectual or emotional abilities or age. In which cases, often another individual (such as parents, legal guardians) or the courts may decide. In cases of an emergency, decisions may need to be made in the individual's best interests as there may not be time to gain consent from them or others.

## Time to reflect

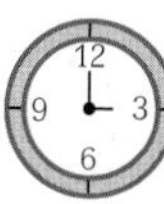

### 3.1 Informed consent

How would you feel if you had no say over care or treatment, if no one asked you to consent?

## Practice activity 

### 3.1 The importance of establishing consent when providing care or support

This activity enables you to demonstrate that you understand the importance of establishing consent when providing care or support.

Produce a report explaining what consent is and why you should establish consent, explaining some potential consequences if consent isn't established.

## 3.2 Establish consent for an activity or action

The General Medical Council provides guidance in their publication *Consent: Patients and Doctors Making Decisions Together* and this is certainly worth looking at for a full understanding of consent.

In particular though, it advises that:

Whatever the context in which medical decisions are made, you must work in partnership with your patients to ensure good care. In so doing, you must:

**(a)** listen to patients and respect their views about their health

**(b)** discuss with patients what their diagnosis, prognosis, treatment and care involve

**(c)** share with patients the information they want or need in order to make decisions

**(d)** maximise patients' opportunities, and their ability, to make decisions for themselves

**(e)** respect patients' decisions.

These are good general guidelines for establishing consent in any care service.

## Research & investigate 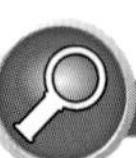

### 3.2 Getting consent right

Access the General Medical Council's website and read the report Consent: Patients and Doctors Making Decisions Together to fully understand consent in medical care.

Individuals may consent verbally, in writing or by compliance (as they fully cooperate). Non-written forms are usually acceptable in certain circumstances, for example when you go to the dentist you are implying by your actions that you are consenting to the dentist examining your mouth and teeth. However, if treatment is more risky, costly or lengthy, then written consent should be sought formally through a consent form. This is just as important if an individual refuses to consent. It is vital in both cases, should individuals or next of kin later question the care received.

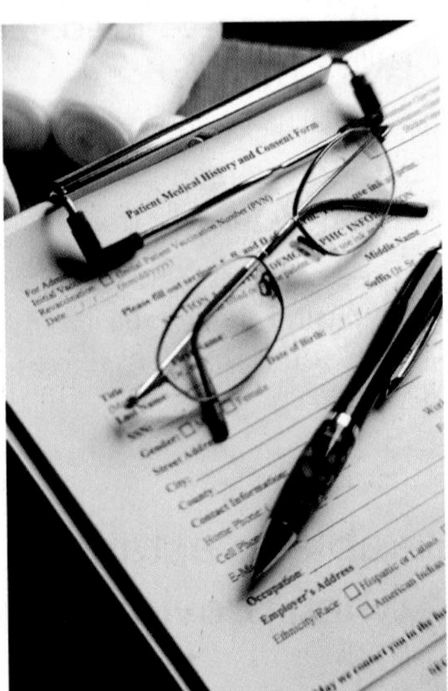


Figure 7.6 A consent form

## Practice activity 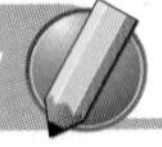

### 3.2 Establishing consent for an activity or action

This activity enables you to demonstrate knowledge of how consent is established

Produce a mock consent form for individuals to complete. The form should include all the key questions and areas to be covered for establishing consent.

## 3.3 Explain what steps to take if consent cannot be readily established

Sometimes, it may not be clear if consent is given, or if it is that it is informed. There may be some issues which care workers need to resolve.

- Competency. Care workers may question the ability of the individual to give informed consent, that is how competent they are. And whilst the need to respect the individual's wishes at all time is **paramount**, if care workers doubt competency in any way, they need to seek clarification. This assessment does not need to be the responsibility of the care worker, but care workers have a responsibility to request and discuss.
- Is it an emergency? If the condition is life-threatening, treatment may be given to preserve life (unless the individual has stated before that they refuse treatment). However, if a delay to care isn't life threatening, then consent should be sought from the individual or next of kin when that opportunity arises. However, sometimes individuals give an advanced directive detailing the care they should or shouldn't receive in the event that they cannot consent to treatment, this could mean that medical care is not given to preserve life.
- Next of kin. It may be that care workers need to seek guidance from next of kin or family. They may be aware of consent arrangements or may be legally responsible for consent.
- Courts. It may be that care workers need to seek guidance from the courts. If there are serious questions over consent to care or disagreement between care workers and individuals or next of kin and family, legal clarification may be sought.
- Professional Councils. It may be that care workers need to seek guidance from their respective Professional Councils. Each Professional Council which professionals are registered with will have guidance and support if there is uncertainty.
- Clarification. If care workers are still unsure, they could seek advice from their line manager or supervisor as they are responsible for care workers' decisions and have increased authority to make decisions.

### Key term

**Paramount** means of the utmost importance.

### Research & investigate

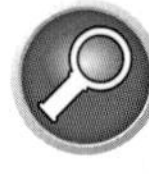

**3.3 Professional Councils**

Find out what you can about Professional Councils for the following professions:

- teachers
- doctors
- nurses and midwives
- health professionals
- social workers
- dentists.

### Practice activity

**3.3 Explain what steps to take if consent cannot be readily established**

This activity enables you to demonstrate that you understand the steps to take if consent cannot be readily established. Produce a PowerPoint slide show explaining all the steps a care worker could take to establish consent.

# LO4 Be able to encourage active participation

## 4.1 Describe how active participation benefits an individual

Active participation is a way of working that recognises an individual's right to participate in the activities and relationships of everyday life as independently as possible; the individual is regarded as an **active** partner in their own care or support, rather than a **passive** recipient. Active participation allows the individual more control over their support.

## Key terms

**Active** means involved, taking part.
**Passive** means uninvolved, having things 'done to'.

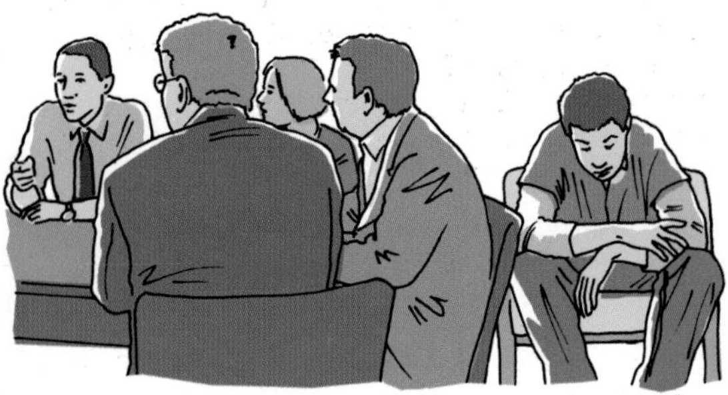

Figure 7.7 Actively participating?

The benefits of active participation are numerous:

- improved confidence and self-esteem
- improved ownership and a sense of control over one's own care
- provides more individualised, more tailored care
- improved independence.

Fundamentally, active participation is a key way of providing person-centred care.

## Time to reflect

### 4.1 Involved?

Anthony is a busy care worker; he has lots of individuals to see in his schedule. Often he has to help individuals apply for things; car tax rebate, housing benefit, applications for new equipment or adaptations. There are times when Anthony is so rushed, he just takes the forms and completes them himself. 'No problems', he says, 'at least they get done!'.

Why is Anthony's practice a problem?

## Practice activity

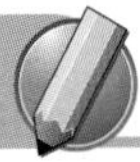

### 4.1 Describe how active participation benefits an individual

This activity enables you to demonstrate you understand how active participation benefits an individual.

Prepare a mock speech to deliver to a new care worker about why they should encourage active participation.

## 4.2 Identify possible barriers to active participation

Although active participation is vital, there are certain aspects which may at times make it more difficult.

- Shortage of time. Although staff may have best intentions to encourage active participation, if they are busy, short staffed, or with other individuals to see, it may be that active participation is not a priority.
- Poor knowledge and experience. If staff are not aware of the need for active participation, or do not know how to encourage it, then it will make it more difficult for it to happen.
- Ability. If individuals have learning difficulties, emotional or behavioural issues, or have poor health, then their ability to actively participate may be hindered, even if care workers have all the best intentions to do so.
- Confidence. If individuals are not confident to actually actively participate then they will not be able to do so, even if care workers do everything they can to encourage active participation.
- Communication issues. If individuals have issues communicating, then they will not be able to actively participate. Sensory impairments such as hearing or visual, or speech problems could all act as a barrier to active participation.

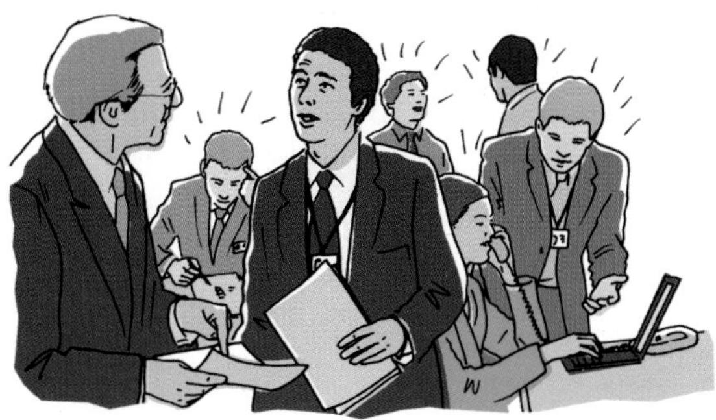

Figure 7.8 Able to actively participate?

Practice activity 

4.2 Identify barriers to active participation

This activity enables you to demonstrate you can identify possible barriers to active participation.

Consider a character from soap or someone you know who has care needs. Identify some of the barriers which may act as barriers for them to actively participate.

## 4.3 Demonstrate ways to reduce the barriers and encourage active participation

A good care worker will always be aware of, and aim to reduce barriers to active participation.

- Advocacy. **Advocates** will not make decisions on an individual's behalf, but will seek information, ask questions, present the information to the individual in an unbiased way, allowing the individual to be informed and hence make decisions. Advocates ensure that the individual's rights and interests are supported. Advocates can help individuals to actively participate in all their care issues.
- Time and patience. Care workers will help to promote active participation if they give enough time and have enough patience to allow active participation to occur. Individuals will not feel rushed and will feel respected enough to relax and get fully involved. Sometimes individuals need time to think and reflect before making comments on their care.
- Training. It is of great use to care workers to receive training on how to promote active participation properly. Regular **continuous professional development** is best practice to ensure staff are all best skilled to actively promote participation.
- Provide communication equipment. If individuals are provided with communication methods which meet their needs then active participation will be easier. Braille, sign language, audio formats, Makaton, photosymbols, signs, symbols, signers and interpreters can all help individuals be fully involved and actively participate.

**Key term**

An advocate is someone who represents another.

Continuous professional development is the process of lifelong training and development to ensure skills and knowledge are up to date.

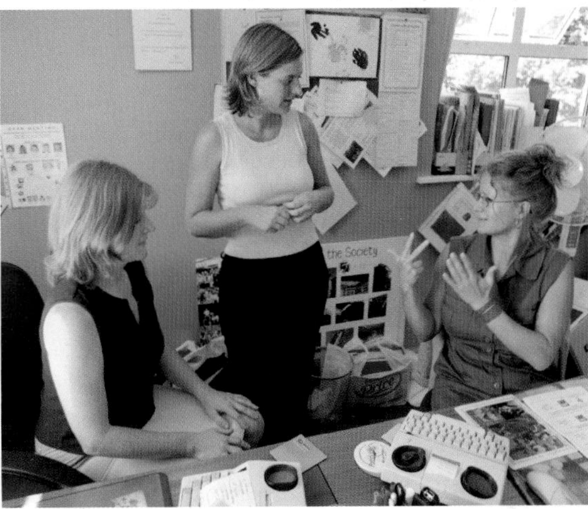

Figure 7.9 Using a signer

Research & investigate 

4.3 Advocacy

Find out about advocacy, what is it, what is its purpose?

**Practice activity** 

### 4.3 Demonstrate ways to reduce the barriers and encourage active participation

This activity enables you to show you can demonstrate ways to reduce the barriers and encourage active participation.

Consider the same individual you used for Practice activity 4.2, suggest ideas to reduce the barriers and encourage active participation.

# LO5 Be able to support the individual's right to make choices

## 5.1 Support an individual to make informed choices

Informed choices are made when:

1. All the options are made available to fully guarantee choice. There is little point only giving one or two options, all viable options need to be presented.
2. The advantages and disadvantages are explicitly discussed. All issues need to be discussed with their strengths and weaknesses. Issues could be around:
   - cost
   - staff
   - health risks
   - health benefits
   - health and safety
   - distance travelled
   - waiting involved.

   Care workers should never:
   - try to manipulate decisions
   - provide information in a biased way
   - judge any decisions which are made or be disrespectful about them
   - withhold information from individuals
   - pressure individuals into a quick or cheaper decision.

Care workers can support individuals by providing resources for research such as books, brochures, guides, prospectuses or computers and internet access. Care workers could also help to arrange visits to services and also arrange for the individuals to speak to experts to get other opinions and advice.

Okay, I think I prefer Copper Hill Residential home, can we arrange to visit?
No problems, I'll call them now to arrange.

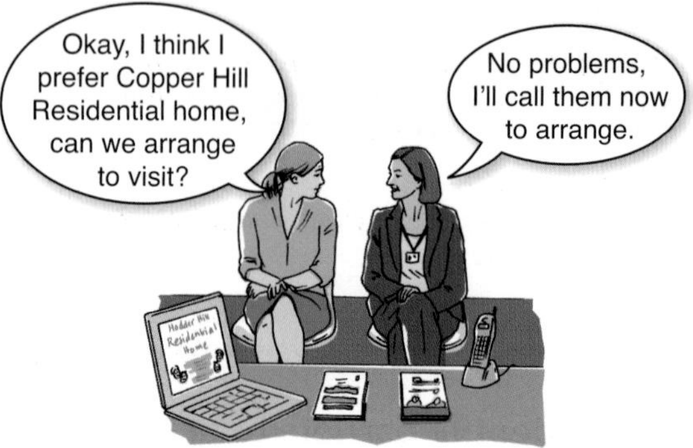

Figure 7.10 Informed choice

**Practice activity** 

### 5.1 Support an individual to make an informed choice

This activity enables you to demonstrate your understanding of how to support an individual to make informed choices.

Imagine you were at a time of your life when you needed residential care support, what information would you want, and how could you find this out?

## 5.2 Use agreed risk assessment processes to support the right to make choices

Risk assessment is the process of identifying risks and then implementing procedures to minimise or eliminate those risks. If an individual desires an outcome which is associated with risks, a good care worker would identify the risks and then take actions to minimise risks or make them safer.

Risks can be associated with everyday activities, not just 'high risk' ones, and they need to be dealt with consistently. For someone who is vulnerable, frail or confused, an everyday activity could be exceptionally risky. For example, a task of making a cup of tea could have many associated risks.

A variety of techniques could be put in place to reduce risks.

- Guides/Prompt sheets for individuals to follow.
- Adapted equipment to reduce risks.
- 'Trial periods' to gauge how significant the risk is.
- Pre-prepared resources to minimise the risks, such as precooked meals which just need heating up.
- Reducing supervision over a period of time to increasingly allow more independence.

## Case Study

### 5.2 Adele

Adele is 30 and has severe learning difficulties. She lives with her parents and her dog. When her parents go to work, a rota of her aunts, uncles, neighbours and care workers all help with her care. Adele is getting increasingly frustrated at being unable to complete tasks for herself. She has requested that she be allowed to cope on her own during the day; make her own lunch, go to the shops, wash her own clothes and so on.

1. Identify some of the risks which could be associated with Adele's request.
2. What strategies could you put in place to help Adele and meet her request to be more independent while maintaining safety?

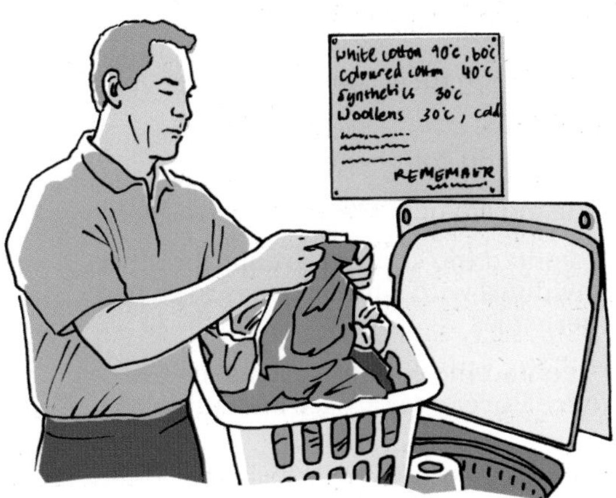


Figure 7.11 Using prompts to minimise risks

## Evidence activity

### 5.2 Using agreed risk assessment processes to support the right to make choices

This activity enables you to demonstrate you can use agreed risk assessment processes to support the right to make choices.

Consider your daily activities.

1. Identify what potential risks there could be.
2. Make suggestions for reducing those risks.

## 5.3 Explain why a worker's personal views should not influence an individual's choices

Just as individuals have their rights to their own opinions and views it is clear that care workers will also have their own opinions and views. However, it has to be remembered that care workers are at work and therefore need to behave professionally and objectively. At home, in their personal life and when not at work, care workers can express their own opinions more openly.

An individual making choices needs to make choices that are right for them. It is possible that, if care workers start to express their opinions openly, they may influence an individual's beliefs or, more worryingly, the individual may feel pressured to agree with what the care worker believes. Person-centred care will not work effectively if individuals are influenced by the personal view of care workers.

Furthermore some individuals, who may be more vulnerable or susceptible to persuasion by care workers, may see care workers as role models. Care workers need to be aware of the potential power they can have and act neutrally and **objectively** at all times.

## Key term

Acting objectively means not being influenced by personal feelings or opinions.

Care workers can have two types of influence:

1. Where they **consciously** try to influence an individual's decisions.
2. Where they **subconsciously** influence an individual's decisions.

## Key term

Conscious means aware, purposely.
Subconscious means not aware, oblivious.

## Time to reflect

### 5.3 Listened to?

How would you feel if you made a decision, had ideas about what you wanted, and a care worker tried to change your mind?

## Practice activity

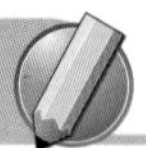

### 5.3 Explain why a worker's personal views should not influence an individual's choices

This activity enables you to demonstrate that you can explain why a worker's personal views should not influence an individual's choices.

Produce a report explaining the consequences if an individual were to be influenced by a worker's personal views.

## 5.4 Describe how to support an individual to question or challenge decisions concerning them that are made by others

Individuals need to be in a position to challenge and question decisions that are made for them. As mentioned earlier, individuals cannot just be passive in decisions about them. Individuals need to feel strong enough to say 'Why'? 'No' 'I disagree'. However there may be times when this may be difficult.

- Maybe the individual has low self-esteem, confidence issues or is naturally a shy, quiet passive person. If an individual feels devalued they may not be able to 'stand up for themselves'
- Maybe the care worker is intimidating. Even when care workers try not to be, their confidence, physical stature, verbal and non-verbal communication may develop a sense of intimidation in a relationship which they are neither aware of nor are encouraging.
- It may be that individuals view care workers as having all the power within the relationship which may translate into individuals assuming that 'the care worker knows best'. Care workers can hold a sense of 'professionalism' that many, (and, it could be argued, especially the older and the more vulnerable), hold in high esteem, as giving higher status and meaning they should not be questioned.

Clearly, this is not a situation that is person-centred. Hence care workers need to ensure they support any individuals to question or challenge decisions concerning them that are made by others and be aware of any influence they may have.

How can this be done? By:

- asking individuals
- allowing them time to consider, making notes
- building confidence
- using advocacy or self advocacy
- contacting support groups for other individuals with similar issues to share experiences
- contacting groups such as the Citizen Advice Bureau for advice and guidance.

Practice activity 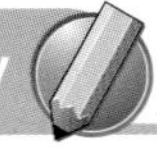

### 5.4 Describe how to support an individual to question or challenge decisions

This activity enables you to describe how to support an individual to question or challenge decisions concerning them that are made by others.

Imagine you are an advocate. Produce a booklet for individuals, entitled 'Finding your Voice' giving tips to an individual to question or challenge decisions concerning them made by others.

## LO6 Be able to promote individuals' well-being

### 6.1 Explain how individual identity and self-esteem are linked with well-being

**Well-being** is a **holistic** concept, meaning it is made up of many elements. These elements can affect how an individual feels; whether they feel in good health and prosperity or not.

Well-being may include aspects that are:

- spiritual
- emotional
- cultural
- religious
- social
- political.

**Key terms**

Well-being means in good health, happiness and prosperity.
Holistic means the 'whole'. In health this tends to mean the whole person and not just physical health.

An individual's identity is who they are. Self-esteem is how one values oneself. There are many factors which can affect an individual's identity and their self-esteem; one of these is well-being and vice versa. Figure 7.12 shows how identity and self-esteem are linked.

A sense of identity and good self-esteem can promote increased well-being as it can improve your physical, intellectual, emotional and social health.

Good well-being can promote a good sense of identity and improved self-esteem as it can make you feel better about who you are.

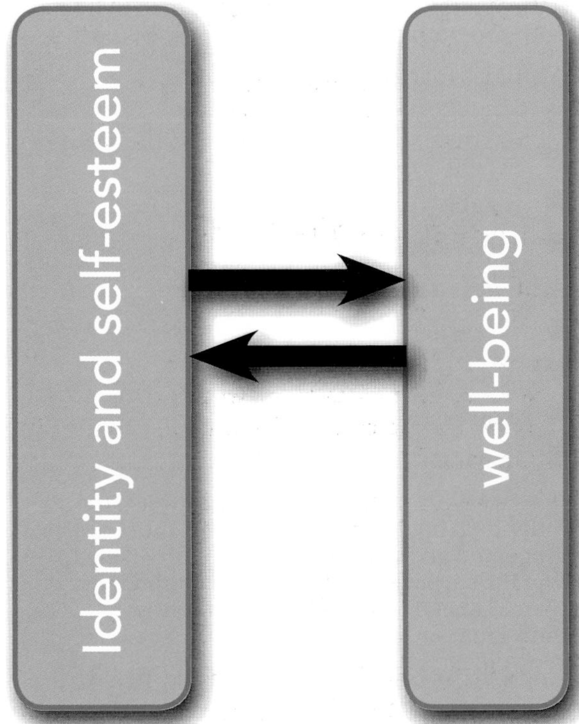


Figure 7.12 The link between identity and self-esteem and well-being

Practice activity 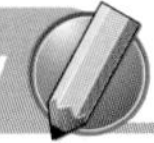

### 6.1 Demonstrate how individual identity and self-esteem are linked with well-being

This activity enables you to demonstrate you can explain how individual identity and self-esteem are linked with well-being.

Explain how an individual with a weak sense of identity and low self-esteem could therefore have poorer well-being.

## 6.2 Describe attitudes and approaches that are likely to promote an individual's well-being

Attitudes are a way of thinking or behaving.

Approaches are methods of dealing with something.

Care workers need to ensure that both their attitudes and approaches are not only consistent with person-centred care, but are also in line with promoting an individual's well-being.

Attitudes that would be positive are:

- friendly
- caring
- reliable
- professional.

Attitudes that would be negative are:

- sarcastic
- discriminatory
- aggressive
- impatient.

If a care worker displays good attitudes, the individual being cared for will feel more respected and valued. They are more likely to find the care worker approachable and trust them. This will assist in promoting the individual's well-being.

Approaches care workers could take to aid well-being are as follows:

- Encouraging approach – care workers could motivate and support individuals when they need it.
- Positive approach – care workers can show approval and give positive feedback and praise when appropriate.
- Disengagement approach – there may be times when care workers need to **disengage** temporarily, allowing an individual time to themselves to work through things, reflect, gather their thoughts or even regain composure.
- Challenging approach – care workers could set realistic targets for individuals to work towards, giving individuals a sense of purpose and incentive.
- Trustful approach – care workers need to develop trust with individuals. This works both ways; the care worker trusting the individual and the individual being able to trust the care worker.
- Distraction approach – there may be times when care workers need to offer a short-term diversion to deflect an individual from more negative concerns. In simple terms, 'taking their mind off it'.
- Observant approach – care workers need to be aware of the more subtle behaviours and actions of individuals to assess well-being and go beyond the face value of the picture. Observing may achieve a more realistic indication of an individual's feelings and needs.
- Partnership approach – care workers will have more success with individuals if care is less 'us and them' and more of a 'team effort'. Care workers modelling good behaviour, working alongside individuals, getting 'stuck' in and engaging in the same activity as the individual, will help individuals more.
- Safe approach – care workers need to manage an individual's safety and ensure that individuals are less at risk and all hazards reduced.

Care workers who display good attitudes and follow the above approaches are more likely to promote an individual's well-being.

### Key term

**Disengage** means to detach, withdraw from something.

### Time to reflect

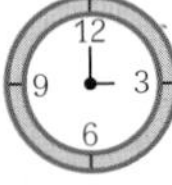

#### Approaches in action

Using the list above, consider how a good, effective care worker could use these approaches in a residential home to improve an individual's well-being.

### Practice activity

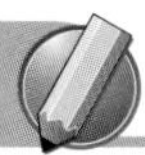

#### 6.2 Describe attitudes and approaches that are likely to promote an individual's well-being

This activity enables you to demonstrate your ability to describe attitudes and approaches that are likely to promote an individual's well-being.

Consider an effective teacher; describe the attitudes and the approaches they could use to improve an individual's well-being.

## 6.3 Support an individual in a way that promotes a sense of identity and self-esteem

A sense of identity (self-concept) and self-esteem develop from the communication we have had and the respect received. The saying, we are a 'product of our environment' simply means just that; we are who we partly are as a result of the interactions we have, therefore carers need to ensure that the actions they take, act as positives to both identity and self-esteem.

Care workers therefore need to consider:

- how they speak to individuals
- the language they use
- the choices they give
- the judgements they make
- the praise they give
- how they show disapproval
- that individuals need to make mistakes
- that individuals need to be allowed to experiment with their identity, for example with clothes and appearance.

All care workers should ensure that the care they provide promotes a sense of identity and self-esteem.

### Case Study

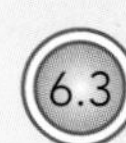

#### 6.3 Chris

Chris has learning difficulties as well as **dyspraxia**. He is sometimes clumsy and knocks things over. One day, he knocks a vase over and spills water and flowers on a carpet, the care worker shouts at him and says 'You stupid boy, will we ever be able to have nice things without you ruining them?!'.

1. How could what the care worker said damage Chris' sense of identity and self-esteem?

### Key term

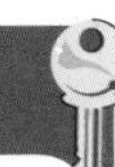

Dyspraxia is a condition which affects ability to perform coordinated movements.

### Practice activity

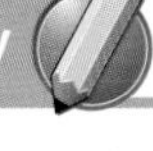

#### 6.3 How to support an individual in a way that promotes a sense of identity and self-esteem

This activity enables you to demonstrate your understanding of how to support an individual in a way that promotes a sense of identity and self-esteem.

Consider your work placement, describe how you would support an individual there to promote their sense of identity and self-esteem.

## 6.4 Demonstrate ways to contribute to an environment that promotes well-being

There is little point in care workers doing all they can to promote well-being if the environment around them is not considered too.

It is vital that any of the environments mentioned below promotes well-being:

- Education services – nurseries, primary schools, crèches.
- Health services – GP, hospitals, dentists, opticians, maternity, waiting areas for services.
- Social services – residential setting, **domiciliary care**, day care services, outreach, community.

## Key term

Domiciliary care is the provision of care in the individual's own home.

Carers need to consider:

### Physical comfort

Individuals need to have furniture and furnishings which are pleasant to use and pleasant to see. Items which are broken, uncomfortable, look unpleasant, are dirty or soiled will not contribute to good well-being. The temperature of the environment will also affect how comfortable an individual is; heating and cooling methods should be available.

### Anti-discriminatory resources

Resources in an environment need to be anti-discriminatory. Displays need to represent all of society; books, DVDs, toys, and so on all need to represent different ages, ethnic groups and abilities. Having an **inclusive** environment will promote well-being as individuals will have a greater sense of psychological security and feeling of belonging.

## Key term

Inclusive means not excluding any individual or section of society.

### Safety

Environments which are safe will promote feelings of well-being. Well-being will be promoted if individuals are in safe buildings, secure from intruders who may hurt them or take their property. Further, the environment needs to ensure it prevents abuse from staff. Feelings of being safe are just as important as being safe itself.

### Engaging atmosphere

Environments which are welcoming will be more beneficial to well-being. Living areas which are devoted to certain activities will help. Some areas devoted to being 'lively', with music, televisions, entertainment and so on will promote well-being. Also important are rooms which are quieter and more for reading, relaxing, arts and crafts and so on.

### 'Homely' atmosphere

Care environments which are too 'clinical' or institutional may disadvantage well-being. Soft furnishings, plants, animals, ornaments, pictures and so on may all help individuals feel welcomed into the care setting and make them feel that they are comfortable being there.

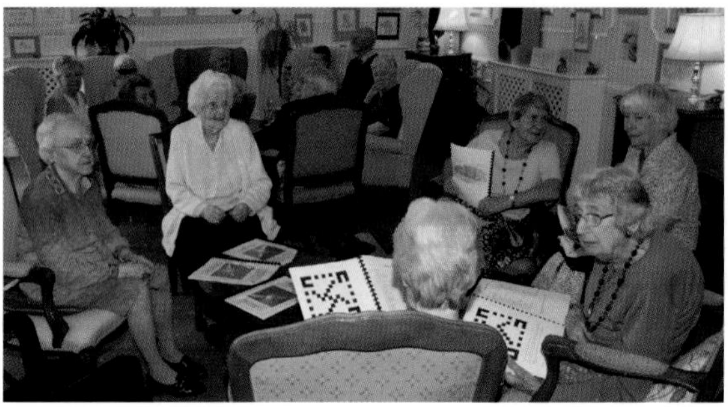

Figure 7.13 Promoting well-being

## Time to reflect

### 6.4 Promoting well-being?

Describe why the environment in Figure 7.13 is promoting well-being.

## Practice activity

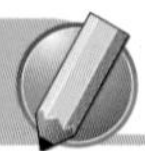

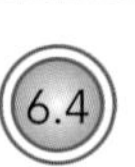

### 6.4 How to provide an environment that promotes well-being

This activity enables you to demonstrate your understanding of how to provide an environment that promotes well-being.

Produce a report on your work placement. What elements of the environment promote well-being, what elements may currently need to be developed?

From reading this chapter, you should understand that we are all individuals. No two people are the same; hence it is not appropriate to say that because two people have had a stroke they both have the same care needs. Person-centred care provides care that is centred around the person, and not just their care needs. It looks at understanding individual needs and the development of appropriate individual care plans, actively listening to individuals, helping individuals to make choices and aiming to promote their well-being and self-esteem.

## Assessment summary

Your reading of this chapter and completion of the activities will have prepared you to demonstrate your learning and understanding of the principles of implementing person-centred approaches in health and social care. Assessment of Learning Outcomes 2,3,4,5 and 6 must be assessed in a real work environment. To achieve the unit, your assessor will require you to:

| Learning Outcomes | Assessment Criteria |
|---|---|
| Learning outcome 1: Understand person-centred approaches for care and support by: | 1.1 defining person-centred values<br>See Evidence activity 1.1 on p. 103 |
| | 1.2 explaining why it is important to work in a way that embeds person-centred values<br>See Evidence activity 1.2 on p. 104 |
| | 1.3 explaining why risk-taking can be part of a person-centred approach<br>See Evidence activity 1.3 on p. 105 |
| | 1.4 explaining how using an individual's care plan contributes to working in a person-centred way.<br>See Evidence activity 1.4 on p. 106 |
| Learning outcome 2: Be able to work in a person-centred way by: | 2.1 finding out the history, preferences, wishes and needs of the individual<br>See Practice activity 2.1 on p. 107 |
| | 2.2 applying person-centred values in day-to-day work taking into account the history, preferences, wishes and needs of the individual.<br>See Practice activity 2.2 on p. 109 |

| Learning Outcomes | Assessment Criteria |
|---|---|
| Learning outcome **3**: Be able to establish consent when providing care or support by: | **3.1** explaining the importance of establishing consent when providing care or support<br>See Practice activity 3.1 on p. 110 |
| | **3.2** establishing consent for an activity or action<br>See Practice activity 3.2 on p. 110 |
| | **3.3** explaining what steps to take if consent cannot be readily established.<br>See Practice activity 3.2 on p. 111 |
| Learning outcome **4**: Be able to encourage active participation by: | **4.1** describing how active participation benefits an individual<br>See Practice activity 4.1 on p. 112 |
| | **4.2** identifying possible barriers to active participation<br>See Practice activity 4.2 on p. 113 |
| | **4.3** demonstrating ways to reduce the barriers and encourage active participation<br>See Practice activity 4.3 on p. 114 |
| Learning outcome **5**: Be able to support the individual's right to make choices by: | **5.1** supporting an individual to make informed choices<br>See Practice activity 5.1 on p. 114 |
| | **5.2** using agreed risk assessment processes to support the right to make choices<br>See Evidence activity 5.2 on p. 115 |
| | **5.3** explaining why a worker's personal views should not influence an individual's choices<br>See Practice activity 5.3 on p. 116 |
| | **5.4** describing how to support an individual to question or challenge decisions concerning them that are made.<br>See Practice activity 5.4 on p. 117 |

| Learning Outcomes | Assessment Criteria |
|---|---|
| Learning outcome **6**: Be able to promote individuals' well-being by: | 6.1 explaining how individual identity and self-esteem are linked with well-being<br>See Practice activity 6.1 on p. 117 |
| | 6.2 describing attitudes and approaches that are likely to promote an individual's well-being<br>See Practice activity 6.2 on p. 119 |
| | 6.3 supporting an individual in a way that promotes a sense of identity and self-esteem<br>See Practice activity 6.3 on p. 119 |
| | 6.4 demonstrating ways to contribute to an environment that promotes well-being<br>See Practice activity 6.4 on p. 120 |

Good luck!

## Weblinks

General Medical Council www.gmc-uk.org/index.asp

# 8 Contribute to health and safety in health and social care

## For Unit HSC 027

### What are you finding out?

For the years 2009/10, the **Health and Safety Executive (HSE)** reported that:

- 1.3 million people were suffering from an illness they believed was work-related.
- 152 workers were killed at work.
- 121,430 injuries to employees were reported under **RIDDOR.**
- 233,000 **reportable injuries** occurred.
- 28.5 million days were lost overall, 23.4 million due to work-related ill health and 5.1 million due to workplace injury.

Source: www.hse.gov.uk

Whatever your role within health and social care, you have a duty to contribute to health and safety within your workplace. On the surface, this sounds simple. However, when you start to think more deeply about health and safety, you begin to realise that this is quite a considerable and complex subject. Because of the nature of their job, health and social care workers are at an increased risk of accidents, illness and injury due to certain aspects of the role, for example: supporting service users with their moving and handling needs; coming into contact with bodily fluids; coming into close contact with people who sometimes may be ill and working in a **communal environment**. These tasks put health and social care workers at increased risk of stress, slips, trips, falls, **musculoskeletal disorders**, illness and infection, all of which can lead to accident, injury and ill health. If a health and social care worker sustains an accident or suffers an injury or ill health, this can seriously impact upon the delivery of health and social care services. Because health and safety is so important, there are laws in place which ensure that everyone within the workplace is protected from danger. For these reasons, we all have a duty to contribute to health and safety within the workplace.

The reading and activities in this chapter will help you to:

- Understand your own responsibilities, and the responsibilities of others, relating to health and safety
- Understand the use of risk assessments in relation to health and safety
- Understand procedures for responding to accidents and sudden illness
- Be able to reduce the spread of infection
- Be able to move and handle equipment and other objects safely
- Be able to handle hazardous substances and materials
- Be able to promote fire safety in the work setting
- Be able to implement security measures in the work setting
- Know how to manage stress.

### Key terms

A **communal** environment is an environment which is shared by a group of people.
The **HSE** is the national independent watchdog for work-related health, safety and illness, working to reduce workplace death and serious injury.
**Musculoskeletal disorders** happen when the musculoskeletal system is injured over time.
The **musculoskeletal system** is the system of muscles, tendons, ligaments, bones and joints and associated tissues that move the body and maintain its form.
**Reportable injuries** are those that need to be reported to the HSE through the RIDDOR reporting system.
**RIDDOR** stands for Reporting of Injuries, Diseases and Dangerous Occurrences Regulations.

## LO1 Understand own responsibilities, and the responsibilities of others, relating to health and safety

### 1.1 Legislation relating to general health and safety in a health or social care work setting

There are a number of important pieces of health and safety legislation that affect health and social care settings. The organisation in which you work is primarily governed by the Health and Safety at Work etc Act 1974. The Health and Safety at Work etc Act is an important piece of legislation, as it forms the basis of all current occupational health and safety within the United Kingdom. The Act is known as an 'enabling Act' which means that other legislation can be made under it.

Table 8.1 Summary of the key pieces of legislation relating to general health and safety in a health or social care work setting

| Legislation | Main purpose of the legislation |
|---|---|
| Health and Safety at Work etc Act (HASWA) 1974 | Provides a framework for ensuring the health and safety of everyone who may be affected by work activities |
| Management of Health and Safety at Work Regulations (MHSWR) 1999 | Requires employers and managers to assess and manage risks through the process of risk assessment within the workplace |
| Workplace, (Health, Safety and Welfare) Regulations 1992 | Concerned with minimising risks to health associated with the working environment |
| Manual Handling Operations Regulations (MHOR) 1992 (as amended 2002) | Concerned with minimising risks to health and safety associated with moving and handling activities |
| Provision and Use of Work Equipment Regulations (PUWER) 1998 | Concerned with minimising risks to health and safety associated with the use of work equipment |
| Lifting Operations and Lifting Equipment Regulations (LOLER) 1998 | Concerned with minimising risks to health and safety associated with the use of lifting equipment |
| Personal Protective Equipment at Work Regulations (PPE) 1992 | Concerned with minimising risks to health and safety whereever personal protective equipment may be required |
| Reporting of Injuries, Diseases and Dangerous Occurrences Regulations (RIDDOR) 1995 | Places a requirement on employers to report certain work-related injuries, diseases and dangerous occurrences to the HSE or local authority |
| Control of Substances Hazardous to Health Regulations (COSHH) 2002 | Provides a framework to minimise the risks to health and safety in association with hazardous substances |
| Electricity at Work Regulations 1989 | Places a duty on employers to assess risks associated with work activities involving electricity |

*Contd.*

| Legislation | Main purpose of the legislation |
|---|---|
| Regulatory Reform (Fire Safety) Order 2005 | Places a duty on employers to assess and manage risks associated with the risk of fire |
| Health and Safety (First Aid) Regulations 1981 | Places a responsibility on employers to ensure that everyone can receive immediate attention if they are injured or taken ill in the workplace |
| Disability Discrimination Act (DDA) 1995 | Places responsibility on employers to ensure people with a disability can safely access and exit the workplace in the event of needing to evacuate the premises |
| Food Safety Act 1990 and the Food Hygiene (England) Regulations 2006 | Place a duty on the organisation to minimise risks to health and safety associated with food handling |

**Evidence activity** 

### 1.1 Identify legislation relating to general health and safety in a health or social care work setting

This activity enables you to demonstrate your knowledge of the health and safety legislation that applies to your work setting.

Think about the needs of your service users and the type of service provided by your workplace. Make a list of the Acts and Regulations from Table 8.1 that you think apply to your work setting. Discuss your answer with your manager.

## 1.2 Health and safety policies and procedures

Health and safety policies set out the arrangements that your workplace has for complying with legislation. For example, in order to comply with the Health and Safety (First Aid) Regulations, every workplace should have a policy that describes how it manages first aid.

Health and safety procedures describe the activities that need to be carried out for the policies to be implemented. They explain who does what, when and how. For example, first aid procedures will describe the role of first aiders and the people responsible for maintaining first aid equipment and facilities. They will also explain when and how emergency services should be contacted, and when and how accident records should be completed.

**Time to reflect** 

### 1.2 Health and safety outside the work setting

The word 'procedure' is workplace terminology for a 'course of action'. We all follow courses of action in our everyday lives; if we didn't, our lives would be chaotic and we would lurch from one disaster to the next! Think about the course of action you would take if you were faced with an emergency situation outside the work setting. For example, a person falls and injures his head in the street. How would you deal with this health and safety emergency? What might happen if you didn't deal with it?

It is a legal requirement that you follow workplace health and safety procedures as dictated by your organisation's policies. Failure to do so could put others within your workplace at risk, which could lead to disciplinary procedures and ultimately dismissal from your job.

## Research & investigate

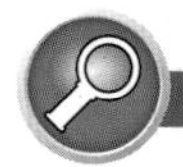

### 1.2 The consequences of failing to follow health and safety procedures

Check out the consequences of you failing to follow health and safety procedures within your organisation. Think about what could happen to:

- you
- service users
- your colleagues
- the organisation.

## Evidence activity

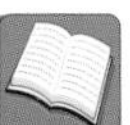

### 1.2 Describe the main points of health and safety policies and procedures agreed with the employer

This activity enables you to demonstrate your understanding of the reasons why policies and procedures shape the way you do your work.

- Make a note of two policies that govern practice within your workplace. Explain why it is necessary for these policies to be in place.
- Make a note of two procedures you must follow as you carry out your activities. Explain why it is necessary for you to follow these procedures.

## 1.3 Main health and safety responsibilities

Health and safety within the workplace is not the responsibility of just one person. It is a responsibility that is shared between yourself, your employer and your colleagues. The law places certain responsibilities on each of these people, and it is important that you know the boundaries of your responsibilities.

### The employer's responsibilities

Under the Health and Safety at Work etc Act 1974, your manager or employer has a responsibility to:

- ensure your workplace is safe and free from risks
- assess risks and take action to reduce them
- ensure health and safety policies are made available to employees
- provide information, training and supervision to support your health and safety
- provide adequate welfare and first aid facilities
- provide protective clothing and equipment free of charge
- set up emergency procedures
- take precautions against dangers and provide safety signs
- avoid the risk of injury from manual handling procedures
- report injuries, diseases and dangerous occurrences to the appropriate authorities
- make arrangements to ensure that substances hazardous to health are handled, stored and transported safely.

### The responsibilities of yourself and others in the work setting

Under the Health and Safety at Work etc Act 1974, whilst at work, you have a duty to:

- take reasonable care of yourself and anyone else who may be affected by your actions, including colleagues, the individuals you work with, their families, and any visitors or contractors who enter the premises
- cooperate with your employer or manager in relation to health and safety issues
- follow policies and practise safe procedures
- follow safe systems of work
- attend any training that has been provided
- use work items correctly and in accordance with instructions and training
- not interfere with or misuse anything provided in the interest of health and safety, for example first aid and firefighting equipment, health and safety notices
- report any changes or faults back to your employer or manager.

In addition, you have a responsibility to stay up to date with health and safety training, and not carry out any task in which you have not been trained.

Like you, your colleagues also have a duty to follow safe systems of work. Visiting families, carers and other people who enter the premises also have a part to play in maintaining health and safety, especially in relation to security issues, hand washing, adhering to 'no smoking' rules, and their general conduct.

**Evidence activity** 

### 1.3 Outline the main health and safety responsibilities of yourself, your employer or manager and others in the work setting.

This activity enables you to demonstrate your understanding of different people's responsibilities as you carry out your work.

Think of one work activity that you carry out on a regular basis, for example moving and handling. Outline the responsibilities of the following people in ensuring the task is carried out safely:

- yourself
- your colleagues
- your employer or manager
- any other people in the work setting.

## 1.4 Specific tasks in the work setting that should not be carried out without special training

Within health and social care settings it is essential that you only work within your sphere of competence. You should therefore never undertake any tasks for which you have not received training. Examples of these sorts of tasks include:

- moving and handling
- use of equipment
- administering first aid procedures
- administering medication
- food handling and preparation.

Training is essential in order that health and social care staff can deliver a safe level of care that is based on up-to-date information. You need to know why you are undertaking certain tasks, as well as the procedures for undertaking them. Some training is mandatory and should be refreshed on a regular basis, for example moving and handling training should be refreshed annually. This is because practices and legislation change from time to time.

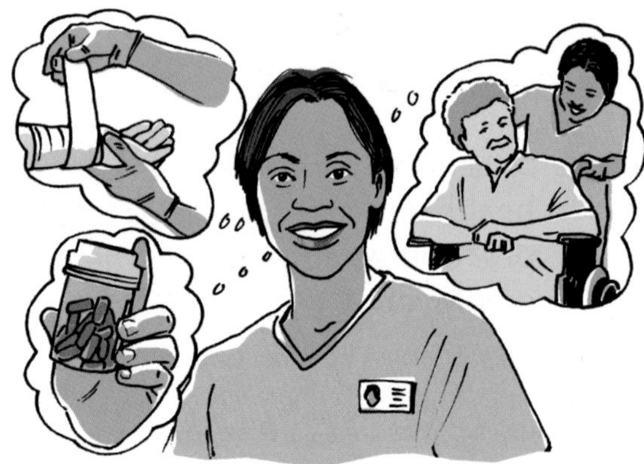

Figure 8.1 Mandatory training

If you have not received adequate training, you will not be equipped to undertake the task in a safe manner. This will increase risks associated with health and safety within the workplace. If you undertake a task without having received adequate training you are not only putting yourself at risk, but you are also putting service users and your colleagues at risk too.

Evidence activity 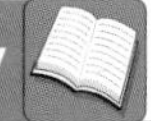

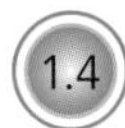

### 1.4 Identify specific tasks in the work setting that should not be carried out without special training

This activity enables you to demonstrate your knowledge of work activities that should not be undertaken prior to receiving training.

Make a note of any tasks you undertake within your work setting. Which of these activities required you to undertake special training?

## 1.5 Accessing additional support and information relating to health and safety

This chapter has pointed you in the direction of legislation, policies and procedures that identify your responsibilities for promoting health and safety. There are, however, other places where you can access further information. The internet is full of information. You only have to type 'health and safety' into your search engine and you will be presented with:

- official government websites, including HSE, which is an excellent source of information and has numerous free leaflets that you can download
- websites belonging to many different Sector Skills Councils and Trades Unions, which provide information about legislation relating to health and safety in their particular sector
- websites promoting training courses
- websites advertising books and journals
- organisations that provide support in resolving health and safety issues; and so on.

There may be a Trade Union Representative in your workplace or there may be a health and safety officer. Either will be able to provide you with health and safety information. They will also be able to support you with any concerns you may have, as will your manager or employer and the staff in your Human Resources department.

Libraries and community centres can provide information on a range of health and safety issues, as can fire stations, GP practices, hospitals, manufacturers of materials and equipment used in health and social care settings, and so on.

Practice activity 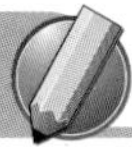

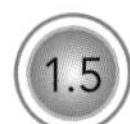

### 1.5 Access additional support or information relating to health and safety

This activity gives you an opportunity to practise showing that you can access additional support or information relating to health and safety.

Choose an aspect of health and safety that interests you and using as many sources of information as you can find, put together a portfolio of fliers, posters, computer print outs, course leaflets and so on to show your developing skills in accessing information and support.

Other places where additional support and information relating to health and safety can be accessed through:

- libraries and community centres
- fire stations
- GP practices
- hospitals
- manufacturers of materials and equipment

In addition, there may be a Trades Union Representative in your workplace or there may be a health and safety officer. Either will be able to provide you with health and safety information. They will also be able to support you with any concerns you may have, as will your manager or employer and where applicable, the staff in your Human Resources department.

# LO2 Understand the use of risk assessments in relation to health and safety

## 2.1 The importance of assessing health and safety hazards posed by the work setting or by particular activities

A health and safety hazard can be defined as any object or situation that has the potential to cause harm. Hazards can include chemicals and medication, faulty equipment, obstructions in passageways and on stairs, challenging behaviour, lack of security and unsafe food handling. The harm they cause ranges from burns, fractures, infection, illness, stress, asphyxiation (restriction of oxygen to the brain), through to death. Whilst it is not always possible to fully eliminate risks to health and safety, legislation requires employers to minimise them as far as possible. Your employer will fulfil this role through the process of risk assessment. Identification of the hazard is the first step in the risk assessment process. Risk assessments are vitally important in order to protect the safety of everyone within the workplace including the employer, staff and service users. If hazards are not identified, then the risk assessment process cannot take place. The risk assessment process contains five steps. The process of which should be seen as circular.

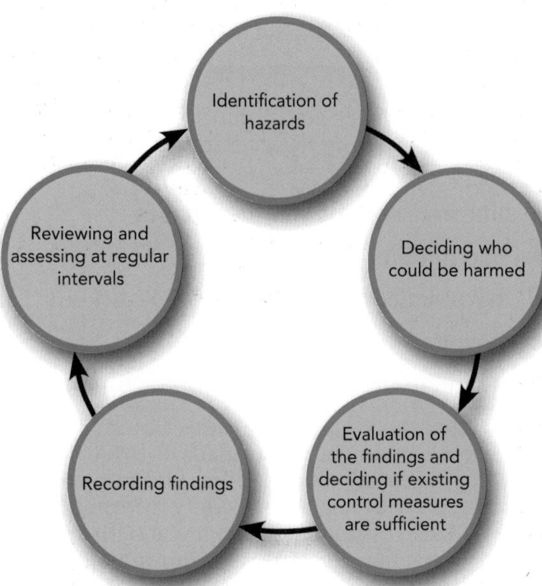


Figure 8.2 The risk assessment process

The following list is a guide to some of the hazards which should be considered when identifying hazards for the purpose of risk assessment.

- Slipping/tripping hazards.
- Fire hazards.
- Storage hazards.
- Manual handling hazards.
- Noise hazards.
- Chemical hazards.
- Electricity hazards.

## Evidence activity 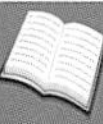

 2.1 **'Explain why it is important to assess health and safety hazards posed by the work setting for particular activities**

This activity will help you demonstrate that you can explain why it is important to assess health and safety hazards posed by the work setting for particular activities.

Identify activities that you undertake on a daily basis whilst at work. Make a note of any hazards which are known to accompany these activities. What control measures have been put in place to address the hazards? Finally, explain what could happen if these hazards are not identified.

## 2.2 How and when to report potential health and safety risks that have been identified

A health and safety risk can be defined as the likelihood that a **hazard** will cause harm. Health and social care workers are best placed to identify health and safety risks, because they are the ones who are undertaking the activities on a daily basis. The identification of hazards is not enough on its own. The risks associated with hazards need to be reported in order that the associated risk can be either eliminated, or minimised, and this should be done the moment the hazard is identified.

Practices for reporting risks vary between organisations but, initially, the risk should be reported verbally to your line manager, who will advise you of the appropriate records that need to be made. Finally, it is important to take steps to isolate the risk and warn others of the hazard, in order that no person is injured.

### Key term

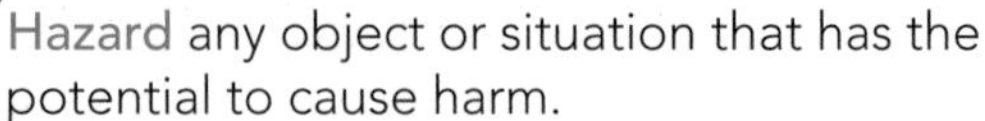

**Hazard** any object or situation that has the potential to cause harm.

## Evidence activity 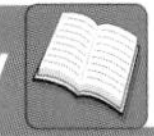

### 2.2 How and when to report potential health and safety risks that have been identified

This activity gives you an opportunity to explain how and when to report potential health and safety risks that have been identified within your workplace.

Explain the procedure for identifying and reporting potential health and safety risks within your workplace. Explain what might happen if you did not report these health and safety risks.

## 2.3 How risk assessments can help dilemmas between rights and health and safety concern

When you work in an environment where you provide care for people, there may be times when risks need to be managed and balanced against the rights of an individual. It's an all too familiar dilemma, as health and social care staff have a duty to protect the safety of service users, yet also have a duty to ensure service users are empowered to make decisions and take control of their lives; even if that means allowing them to take risks. Getting the balance right between safety and choice is never easy, and if not handled sensitively could lead to a situation of conflict. It is therefore essential that open channels of communication are maintained between care staff, service users and their relatives, in order that everyone is aware of the dilemmas that the organisation is faced with on a daily basis. Care organisations have a legal obligation to undertake risk assessments; however service users have a right to make decisions. Highlighting the hazards and risks within a risk assessment can assist individuals to balance risks against their wishes and preferences. Risk means different things to different people, and some people may not fully understand the extent of certain risks. We cannot stop service users from taking risks, but we can inform them of the dangers. Under no circumstances should you ever put yourself at risk to protect the rights of service users. It is also important to identify any decisions made through the care planning process. Every organisation will have its own policy surrounding the management of risks and care planning, and it is important that records concerning decisions are made as well as the outcomes.

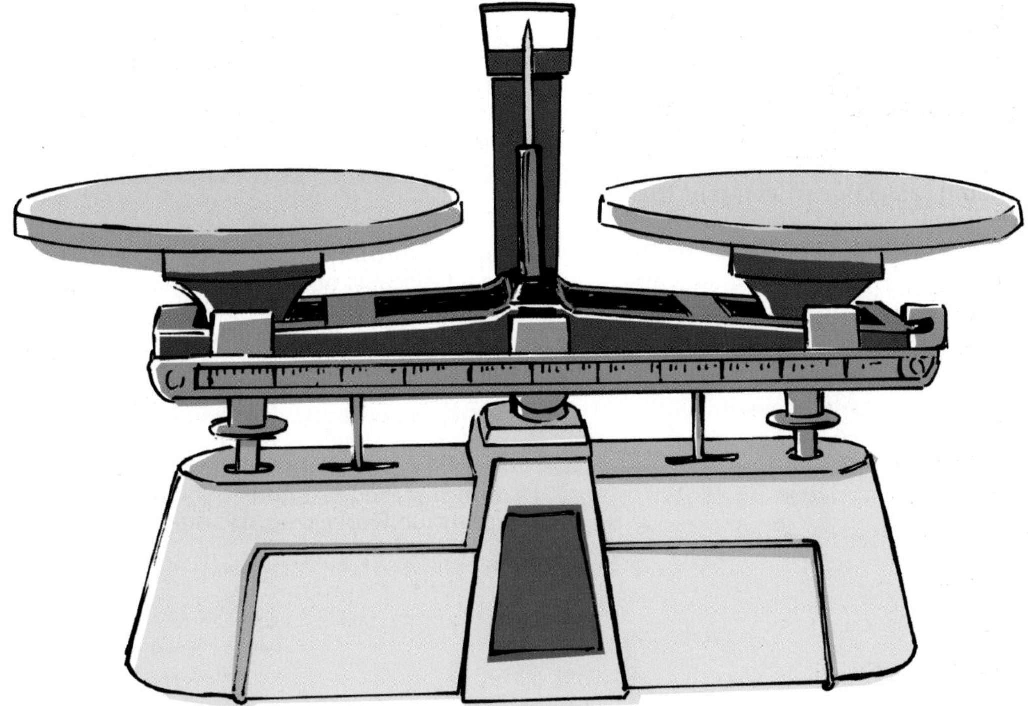

Figure 8.3 Balancing risks and rights

### Evidence activity 

#### 2.3 How risk assessments can help address dilemmas between rights and health and safety concerns

This activity gives you an opportunity to explain how risk assessments can help address dilemmas between rights and health and safety concerns.

Explain the procedure that should be followed within your organisation if decisions made by service users conflict with documented risk assessments. Why is it important to balance these decisions?

## LO3 Understand procedures for responding to accidents and sudden illness

### 3.1 Different types of accidents and sudden illness that may occur in your work setting

Workplace **accidents** can happen at any time to anybody and can range from minor to major. However, some types of accidents are more common than others, depending on the work setting.

#### Key term

An accident is an unforeseen incident that can result in a person being injured.

Musculoskeletal injuries – The Health and Safety Executive (HSE) report that musculoskeletal injuries are the most common cause of occupational sickness in Great Britain, affecting around one million people each year. Further to this, according to the most recent results of the Labour Force Survey (LFS), the frequency of musculoskeletal disorders in 2007/08 and 2008/09 was higher in the health and social care sector than in any other sector.

Violence and aggression – The HSE also report that health and social care workers can be as much as four times more likely to experience accidents caused by violence and aggression than any other workers. There are many reasons why violence may occur, for example, frustration, anxiety, resentment, feeling powerless, drugs, drink and medical conditions that can lead to unpredictability and lack of understanding.

Needle stick injuries – The main groups of workers at risk from a **needle stick injury** are those who work within healthcare. These injuries can occur at any time when people use, disassemble, or dispose of needles. When not disposed of properly, needles can become concealed in linen or household waste and injure other workers who encounter them unexpectedly. Needle stick injuries are hazardous because they can transmit infectious diseases, for example hepatitis B (HBV), hepatitis C (HCV) and Human Immunodeficiency virus (HIV).

#### Key term

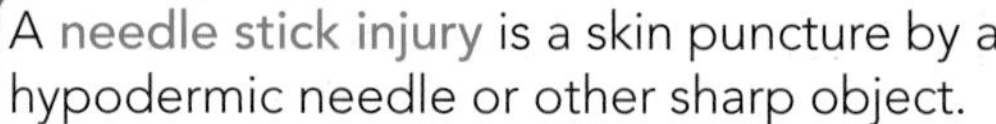

A needle stick injury is a skin puncture by a hypodermic needle or other sharp object.

A sudden illness can happen as the result of an underlying condition, for example diabetes or heart disease, or can happen completely out of the blue. A sudden illness could include minor illnesses, for example a head ache, ear ache, stomach upset, sore throat or indigestion; or it could lead to a major illness, for example a stroke, a heart attack or a diabetic coma. If professional help is not immediately available, emergency first aid will need to be administered promptly in order to prevent the condition worsening, aid recovery and preserve life.

## Evidence activity 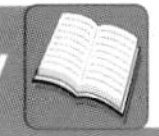

### 3.1 Describe different types of accidents and sudden illness that may occur in your own work setting

This activity enables you to demonstrate your knowledge of the different types of accidents and sudden illness that may occur where you work.

Talk with your colleagues, manager or employer, and look through your workplace accident record book and any care plans that are accessible to you, to find out what accidents and sudden illnesses are particular to where you work. Familiarise yourself with the potential source of accidents and with the signs and symptoms of each sudden illness. Use this information to make an awareness-raising poster for your workplace.

## 3.2 Procedures to be followed if an accident or sudden illness should occur

## Time to reflect 

### 3.2 Dealing with accidents and emergencies

Think about a time when you have witnessed or helped out at an accident or in an emergency situation. Was the situation dealt with effectively? If you had an accident or became suddenly ill, how would you like to be treated?

Your workplace must have procedures which must be followed in the event of an accident or sudden illness. Again, it is important that you only work within your sphere of competence and acknowledge that unless you are trained as a first aider, and your training is up to date, you should not administer any direct treatment to a casualty within the work setting. However, even if you are not directly dealing with the accident, you can play an important role in helping to manage the effects of the situation. You will also have a part to play in reporting and recording the accident in line with your organisation's policies. If you are the first person at the scene of an accident, you should summon help by finding a qualified first aider or calling an ambulance. You can also help by:

- assisting the person who is dealing with the emergency by responding to their instructions
- clearing the immediate area of people and other risks, for example broken glass
- offering support and reassurances to any witnesses who may be distressed.

The following is basic advice on first aid for use in the event of an accident and is no way intended as a substitute for effective training.

When approaching what looks like a serious accident, DR ABC may help you to remember what to do.

**D = Danger**

Never put yourself in danger, make the area safe, assess all casualties and get someone to call 999 for an ambulance. They should be prepared to describe what happened and where, the number of people affected and their condition.

**R = Response**

Gently shake the casualty's shoulders and ask loudly, 'Are you alright?'. If there is a response, reassure them that help is on its way. If there is no response:

- check that help is on its way
- open their airway
- check for normal breathing
- take appropriate action – cardiopulmonary resuscitation (CPR) if necessary.

**A = Airway**

To open the airway, place your hand on the casualty's forehead, gently tilt the head back and lift the chin with two fingertips. Remove any visible obstructions from the mouth and nose. Check that help is on its way.

**B = Breathing**

Look for chest movements that indicate breathing, listen at the casualty's mouth for breath sounds, and feel for air on your cheek. If the casualty *is* breathing normally, place them in the recovery position to keep the airway open. If the casualty is not breathing normally, start cardiopulmonary resuscitation (CPR). Check that help is on its way.

**C = Circulation**

CPR is a series of chest compressions and rescue breaths that maintain circulation. Do not carry out CPR unless you have been trained and have demonstrated competence. Check that help is on its way.

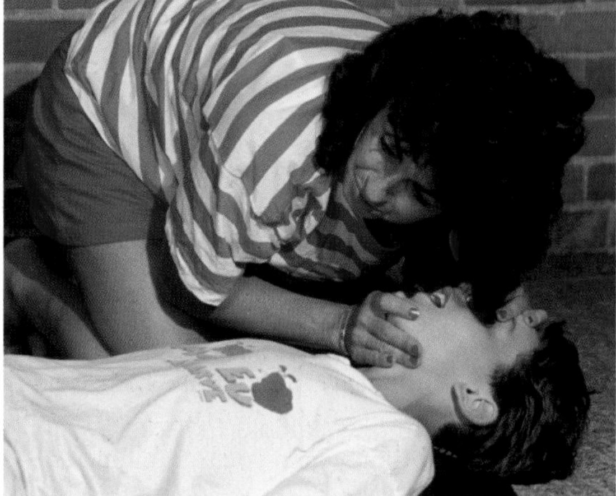

Figure 8.4 Dr ABC

## Severe bleeding

Apply direct pressure to the wound and raise and support the injured part (unless broken) to promote flow of blood back to the heart. Firmly apply a dressing and if bleeding seeps through, place an extra dressing on top. Call for help.

## Needle stick injury

Encourage bleeding by squeezing the affected site. Rinse under running water. If blood or body fluids have splashed into the eyes or mouth, wash with large amounts of cold water. Call for help.

## Broken bones and spinal injuries

If you suspect a broken bone or spinal injury do not move the casualty unless they are in immediate danger – get help immediately.

## Sprains and strains

Rest the injured area to promote healing and elevate if possible. Apply ice to reduce swelling and use a compression bandage and sling, if appropriate, to give support. Get help.

## Burns

Burns can be serious so if in doubt, seek medical help. Cool the affected part of the body with cold water until pain is relieved. Thorough cooling may take 10 minutes or more, but this must not delay taking the casualty to hospital.

Certain chemicals may seriously irritate or damage the skin. Avoid contaminating yourself with the chemical. Treat in the same way as for other burns but flood the affected area with water for 20 minutes. Continue treatment even on the way to hospital, if necessary. Remove any contaminated clothing which is not stuck to the skin.

## Epileptic seizures

A person who is having a seizure will not be able to maintain their own safety. It is therefore important that you ensure the person is safe and minimise the risk of injury throughout the seizure. If possible, loosen the person's clothing. Move any objects that could cause injury. If the seizure lasts for longer than five minutes, or this is the person's first seizure, you must call for an ambulance. Never attempt to restrain the person, or put anything in the person's mouth; and never attempt to move the person until he or she regains full consciousness, unless there is an immediate risk of injury.

## Dealing with violence

The risk of violence will depend on the environment in which you work, the type of people you work with and the type of service users you support. Workers who may be at risk should be trained in how to diffuse violence before there is a need for first aid; and in the event of exposure to violence, receive post-incident counselling and first aid as appropriate.

## Record keeping

Record keeping is important following all incidents involving injury or illness. The entry should be written as soon after the event as possible and should include the following information:

- The date of the entry.
- The date, time and place of the incident.
- Circumstances of the accident/illness.
- The name and address of the injured or ill person.
- Details of the injury/illness and any first aid given.
- What happened to the casualty immediately afterwards (went back to work, went to hospital).
- Your name and signature.

If the accident/illness is one which needs to be reported to the appropriate authorities, your manager should ensure this happens. This information can help identify accident trends and areas for improvement in the control of health and safety risks.

Basic advice on First Aid at Work, HSE 2008; www.nhs.uk

## Case Study

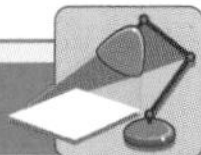

### 3.2 Responding to accidents and sudden illness

Aimee is a new support worker. She supports two young ladies (Ellie and Becky) who both have learning disabilities within their own home. On Saturday evening, Aimee is supporting Ellie to prepare some snacks as they are going to create a 'night in at the movies' and watch a DVD. Whilst preparing the snacks Ellie has an epileptic seizure and falls to the floor. There is a large table in the way and Ellie cuts her head as she falls. Aimee has received first aid training, but is frightened as she has never seen anyone have a seizure before. There is blood on the table and on the floor. Becky walks into the kitchen and is getting upset and distressed.

- How should Aimee deal with this situation?
- What are the issues within this scenario?
- Who should Aimee inform?
- What will Aimee need to record and how?

# LO4 Be able to reduce the spread of infection

## 4.1 Demonstrate the recommended method for hand washing

Hand hygiene is the single most effective method for preventing and controlling infection within the health and social care sector. Our hands normally have a resident population of **micro-organisms** that do us no harm, but transient micro-organisms picked up during everyday activities can cause infectious diseases, also known as healthcare associated infections. Hand washing with soap and warm water should remove transient organisms before they are spread, for example, to another person or a piece of equipment.

### Key term

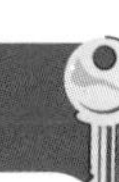

Micro-organisms are organisms such as bacteria, parasites and fungi that can only be seen using a microscope.

You should always wash your hands:

- when they are visibly soiled
- before preparing, eating or handling food
- after using the toilet, smoking, touching your body or hair and coughing or sneezing into your hands
- before an **aseptic** procedure, for example, changing dressings and giving injections

## Evidence activity

### 3.2 Explain procedures to be followed if an accident or sudden illness should occur

This activity enables you to demonstrate your understanding of the procedures to be followed if an accident or sudden illness should occur where you work.

Make a note of the types of accidents and sudden illnesses that have occurred, or may occur within your workplace.

For each scenario you have identified, make a memory card which details the first aid procedure for dealing with that situation. Your memory cards should include explanations for why these procedures should be followed.

- after a dirty procedure, for example disposing of body waste or soiled linen, even if you wore gloves
- after removing gloves
- after bed making
- before and after any situation which involves direct service user contact, for example bathing, toileting
- before starting work and before leaving work.

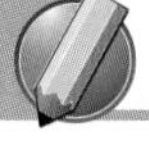

**Key term**

**Aseptic** means free of disease-causing micro-organisms.

For hand hygiene to be effective:

- fingernails should be kept short
- rings should *not* be worn
- watches, bangles and bracelets should *not* be worn
- sleeves should be rolled up to the elbow
- cuts and abrasions on the hands should be covered with a waterproof dressing.

## Hand washing technique

In most circumstances, washing hands with warm water and soap is usually sufficient to remove any transient micro-organisms. The Health Protection Agency describes a six point technique for effective hand washing as highlighted below.

Following the application of warm water and soap:

- Rub hands together, palm to palm to make a lather.
- Rub right palm over the back of the left hand, left palm over the back of the right hand.
- Rub palm to palm fingers interlaced.
- Rub backs of fingers to opposing palms with fingers interlocked.
- Rotational rubbing of right thumb clasped in left palm and vice versa.
- Rotational rubbing backwards and forwards with clasped fingers of right hand in left palm and vice versa.

See diagram opposite.

Don't forget to wash your wrists, rinse off the soap with warm running water and dry your hands thoroughly with a disposable paper towel and apply hand cream to help keep your skin in good condition. An effective hand washing technique should take around 15 seconds.

Washing with an alcohol rub is a useful alternative when your hands are not visibly dirty or when adequate hand washing facilities are not available. It also increases the removal of transient bacteria and should always be used prior to aseptic procedures. When using an alcohol rub, use enough to rub into all areas of the hands, paying attention to the thumbs, fingertips, between the fingers and the backs of the hands, until the hands feel dry.

**www.hpa.org.uk Hand Hygiene For Health Care and Social Care Staff Stop! Have You Washed Your Hands? HPA 2009**

**Practice activity**

**4.1 Demonstrate the recommended method for hand washing**

This activity enables you to demonstrate that you wash your hands effectively.

Practise washing your hands using the technique described above or the one recommended by your workplace. When you feel you are competent, ask your manager or employer to observe you.

## 4.2 Demonstrate ways to ensure that your own health and hygiene do not pose a risk to others at work

The very nature of working in a health or social care setting means that you must take great care to prevent the spread of infections.

If you work in a health or social care environment, it is essential that you are fit to perform your work safely and effectively without risk to your own or other people's

Evidence activity 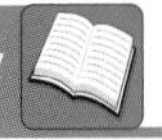

### 5.1 Identify legislation that relates to moving and handling

This activity gives you an opportunity to show your understanding of the legislation that relates to moving and handling.

Identify three pieces of legislation that specifically relate to moving and handling.

## 5.2 Principles for moving and handling equipment and other objects safely

There is a wide range of equipment available to support the needs of individuals who require assistance with moving and handling. Equipment basically falls into three categories:

1. Lifting equipment – hoists and slings which lift the full weight of the individual.
2. Moving and handling equipment – equipment designed to assist in a move, but does not lift the person, for example slide sheets, turning discs and transfer boards.
3. Equipment designed to promote independence – for example raised toilet seats, grab rails, walking sticks and zimmer frames.

Depending on where you work you may use a wide range of equipment, or you may rarely use equipment. Before you use any equipment it is essential that you have received training in its use and you have been assessed as competent in its use. Even if you receive general training, your employer must ensure you receive specific training on the equipment you are using. Every piece of equipment must have an instruction manual, and you should read this in order that you are aware of the instructions for use.

There is a wide range of possible moving and handling operations that may need to be undertaken within your workplace and it would be impossible to identify every scenario, however there are a few general principles that should be applied, depending on the activity you are undertaking. These principles must be outlined within your mandatory moving and handling training.

1. Avoid moving and handling where possible.
2. Ensure you are aware of the contents of associated risk assessments and work in line with them.
3. Always follow your workplace procedures and never undertake an activity for which you have not received training.
4. Always follow your workplace dress code.
5. If the load is a person, explain what you are going to do, reassure the person throughout the move and remind them to assist in the move as much as they can.
6. Ensure there is enough room to carry out the activity safely.
7. Maintain the natural curves of the spine, keeping the spine in line, create a stable base of support with your legs slightly apart, your knees slightly bent. Avoid stooping, bending at the waist and twisting.
8. If you are working with colleagues, identify a team leader who should give clear instructions, for example 'ready, steady, move'.
9. Use your large muscles in your legs to power the activity, keep the load as close to you as possible, and make sure you have a good grip. In the case of a person, check that the movement and your grip doesn't cause any discomfort.
10. Take your time and if for any reason you are not happy with the activity, get advice and report your concerns to your manager.
11. Know your limitations and do not exceed them.

Evidence activity 

### 5.2 Explain the principles for safe moving and handling

This activity gives you an opportunity to show your understanding of the principles for safe moving and handling.

Identify the factors that you take into account to ensure any moving and handling you undertake remains safe for:

- yourself
- the service user
- your colleagues.

## 5.3 Move and handle equipment and other objects safely

In recent years, and certainly since the introduction of the Manual Handling Operations Regulations, there has been a change in the techniques used for moving and handling. Over the years, some techniques have been classified as unsafe, and there has been a shift from teaching the various lifts and techniques to an emphasis on the avoidance of moving and handling activities.

This has led to an emphasis on the use of moving and handling equipment, aids and devices rather than care staff manually lifting service users and objects themselves. Even though the use of equipment can go a long way in reducing the risks associated with manual handling injuries, it is essential that this equipment is used safely in order that risks can be reduced further. Equipment used for moving and handling must always be operated correctly and maintained in a safe condition. Equipment used for moving and handling must:

- only be used following an appropriate level of instruction and training
- be inspected for defects prior to every use
- be maintained in accordance with the manufacturer's instructions
- be tested at the correct intervals (every six months for hoists and slings)
- be suitable for the task being performed
- be used only for the purpose for which it was designed
- be kept in a clean condition
- only be used within its safe working load.

**Practice activity** 

### 5.3 Safe moving and handling

This activity gives you an opportunity to practise moving and handling objects and equipment safely.

Identify any equipment you use for moving and handling within your place of work. Identify any practices you undertake to ensure the equipment is maintained and is safe to use. If you have been trained to use the equipment, undertake a moving and handling procedure, asking your manager to observe your practice. Ask for feedback and advice to assist in ensuring your practice remains safe.

# LO6 Be able to handle hazardous substances and materials

## 6.1 Hazardous substances and materials that may be found in the work setting

Hazardous substances can be found in many workplaces and include any substance that could cause ill health if a person comes into

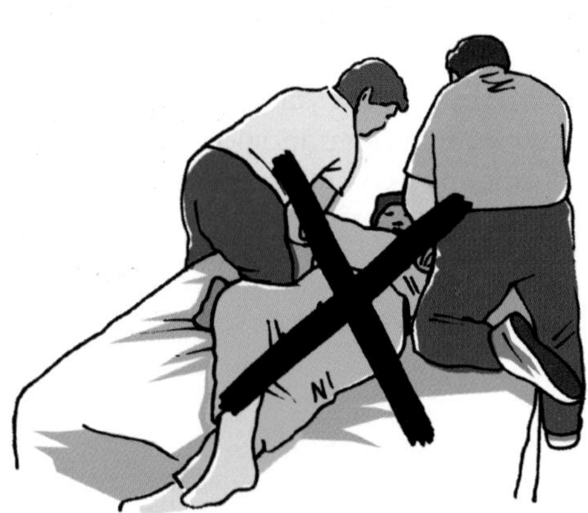

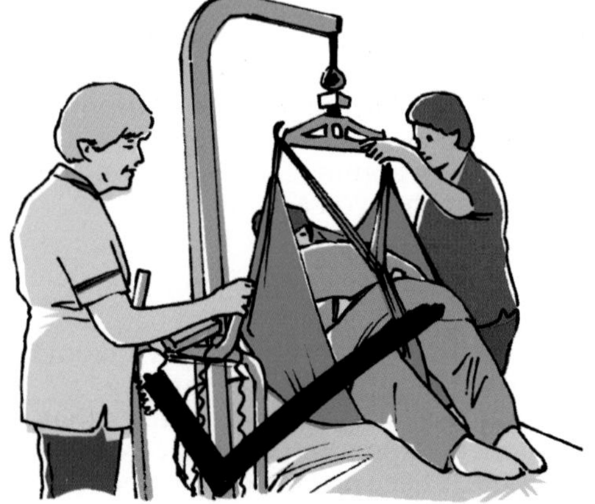

Figure 8.7 Changes in techniques

contact with it. There may be many reasons why a substance is classed as hazardous, for example it may be flammable, toxic, corrosive, cause disease or allergies.

Hazardous substances come in many forms including:

- liquids, for example cleaning chemicals
- solids, for example medication
- dust, for example any dust in substantial amounts
- fumes, for example from solvents
- gases, for example carbon monoxide
- biological organisms, for example micro-organisms and fungal spores.

## 6.2 Safe practices for storing, using and disposing of hazardous substances and materials

COSHH Regulations require that your employer has procedures in place for the safe storage, use and disposal of hazardous substances and materials. This will be identified within risk assessments. Manufacturer's instructions will also indicate safe storage, use and disposal. It is your responsibility to follow these procedures, as well as following instructions for the use of personal protective equipment, cleaning up spills and dealing with accidents.

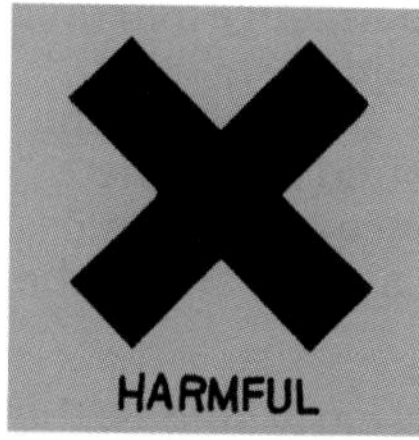

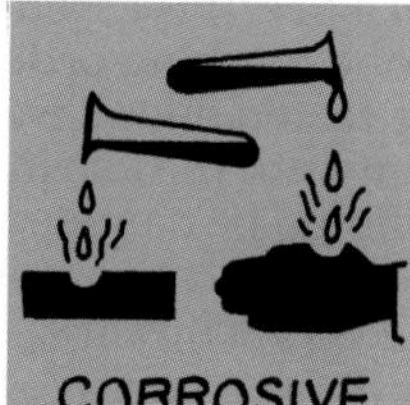

Figure 8.8 Examples of warning labels

### Evidence activity 

**6.1 Identify hazardous substances and materials that may be found in the work setting**

This activity gives you an opportunity to show that you know which of the substances you use at work are hazardous. Produce a poster for display in the staff room that identifies all the hazardous substances that you are exposed to at work.

### Evidence activity 

**6.2 Describe safe practices for storing, using and disposing of hazardous substances and materials**

This activity gives you an opportunity to show that you know how to safely store, use and dispose of hazardous substances and materials.

Go back to the hazardous substances you identified within Evidence activity 6.1 and using any resources available to you describe how each of these substances should be used, stored and disposed of.

# LO7 Be able to promote fire safety in the work setting

## 7.1 Describe practices that prevent fires from starting and spreading

The most effective way of dealing with a fire is to prevent it from spreading in the first place. In order for a fire to start, three things are needed. These are:

- Oxygen (in the air, but oxygen can also be given off by some chemicals).
- Fuel (this can be any combustible material and can be solid, liquid or gas).
- Heat (the cause of ignition, this could be from a cigarette, electric sparks, over heated equipment and so on).

Together, these three components make up the 'fire triangle'. Control of these three components or the removal of any one of them will prevent a fire from starting.

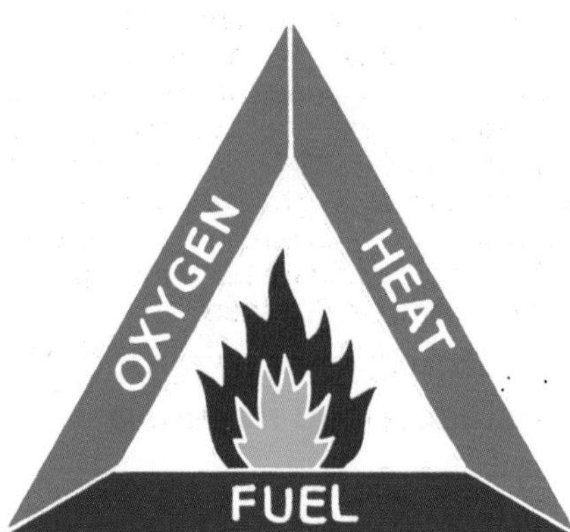


Figure 8.9 Combustion

The following steps can be taken to prevent fires from starting within your place of work.

- Containment – ensure any flammable materials are kept to a minimum and stored properly.
- Ignition – eliminate or control all sources of ignition.
- Exchange – try to use non-flammable substances.
- Separation – keep flammable items away from sources of ignition.
- Ventilation – ensure areas where flammables are stored are well ventilated as this will help to disperse any fumes.
- Use safe systems of work – sources of ignition should be well designed, maintained and controlled to ensure continued safety.

You must always follow your workplace policy and procedures in relation to fire safety. If you discover a fire in its very early stages you may be able to prevent it spreading. However, fire spreads very quickly and even a small, contained fire can produce smoke and fumes that can kill in seconds. If you are in any doubt, do not tackle a fire, no matter how small. If the fire is small, for example if it is in a frying pan or waste bin, you may be able to prevent it spreading by using a fire blanket.

Smoke alarms are important in preventing the spread of fire as they can alert people to the danger of a fire. It is essential that fire alarms are kept in good working order. Smoke alarms should be tested once a week, by pressing the test button until the alarm sounds; and the battery should be changed once a year (unless it's a ten-year alarm). Smoke alarms should be replaced every ten years.

Provided the fire is in its very early stages, the room is not filling with smoke and you are confident about your safety and have been appropriately trained, the spread of a fire could also be prevented by using the appropriate fire extinguisher. **You must always follow the advice you have been given within your fire training.** Ensuring that fire doors are closed could help to contain a fire until the fire services arrive.

### Evidence activity

#### 7.1 Describe practices that prevent fires from starting and spreading

This activity gives you an opportunity to show that you know how to prevent fires from starting and spreading.

Carry out a survey of your workplace to identify:

- Any potential fire risks. Make a note of how these risks could be minimised.
- Any measures aimed at preventing the spread of fire.

## 7.2 Emergency procedures to be followed in the event of a fire in the work setting

If you discover a fire within your workplace, it is important that you are aware of the procedures you must follow. Always ensure you adhere to your organisational policy and do not put yourself or anyone else at further risk.

1. DO NOT PANIC! Stay calm.
2. Immediately sound the fire alarm. If there is no alarm in the vicinity, shout 'FIRE' as loud as you can.
3. Only attempt to control a fire if it is small and contained, you can do so safely and you have been trained.
4. Dial 999 and ask for the fire brigade. Be prepared to give your name, address, the nature and exact location of the fire, how fast it seems to be spreading, the needs of people in the building and whether any are trapped or unable to escape.
5. Take able-bodied people out of the building or to the fire safe stairwell via the fire exit doors. Service users who are in bed should remain in their rooms with the door shut and await rescue by the fire brigade.
6. Close all doors behind you and proceed in a quiet and orderly manner. Walk, don't run. Don't stop to take any personal belongings with you.
7. Do not use the lifts.
8. If you encounter smoke or any blockage along an exit route, choose an alternative path.
9. When you leave the building, move well away from the doors to allow others behind you to emerge from the exits. Do not obstruct entrances or traffic routes.
10. Do not re-enter the building for any reason until the fire brigade gives the OK.

### Evidence activity

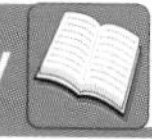

**7.2 Outline emergency procedures to be followed in the event of a fire in the work setting**

This activity gives you an opportunity to show that you know the procedures that should be followed in the event of a fire in your work setting.

Using any resources available to you, for example your workplace policy and your manager, make a poster to identify the emergency procedures that should be followed in the event of a fire within your workplace. Explain why these procedures must be followed.

## 7.3 Maintaining clear evacuation routes

Health and social care settings should have clearly designated fire escape routes, with signed fire exits and fire-proof doors that close automatically in the event of a fire. Fire escape routes should be well lit; fitted with fire alarms, smoke detectors and fire-fighting equipment, as well as adaptations such as handrails; and be wide enough to accommodate large groups of people and mobility aids, for example wheelchairs and walking fames. They also need to be free of obstructions at all times. Evacuation routes should also be clearly signposted.

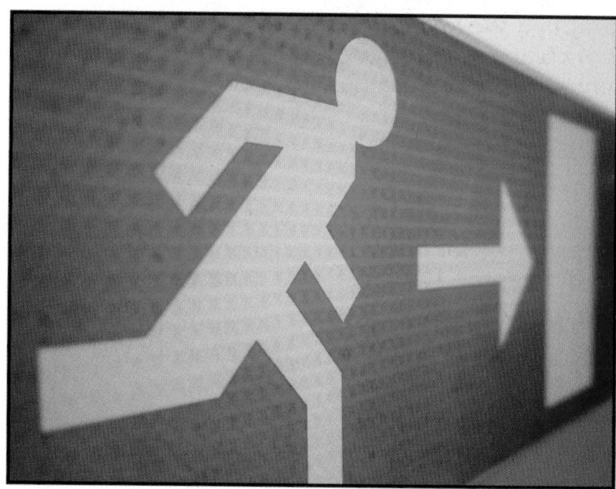

Figure 8.10 Clear evacuation routes

### Evidence activity 

#### 7.3 Explain the importance of maintaining clear evacuation routes at all times

This activity gives you an opportunity to show that you know why it is important to keep evacuation routes clear.

Familiarise yourself with the evacuation routes within your workplace and comment on whether there are any obstacles which could impede evacuation procedures in the event of a fire. What are the consequences of evacuation routes which are cluttered?

## LO8 Be able to implement security measures in the work setting

### 8.1 Use agreed procedures for checking the identity of anyone requesting access to premises and information

Not all visitors to your work settings may be genuine. It is important to be aware of the risks associated with bogus callers, claiming, for example, to be council employees, health workers, meter readers, repairmen, salesmen, even friends and relatives of the people you support. We all have a part to play in keeping the workplace safe and the people you work with have a right to feel safe and secure. It is therefore essential to check the ID of visitors and their right to enter before inviting them into your workplace.

Different organisations have different procedures for checking a caller's ID and their right to enter. However, as a general rule:

- Think before you open the door. Do you recognise the caller? Are they expected?
- Make use of any security measures that have been installed, for example an intercom system, chain lock and so on.
- Ask for proof of identity, for example an ID card.
- If an appointment has not been pre-arranged, politely ask them to wait outside while you confirm their visit with your manager.
- If you have any doubts or suspicions, do not let them in. Talk to your employer or manager, who may feel it necessary to call the police.

If after checking the person's ID you feel their visit is legitimate, ask them to complete the visitor's book on arrival and on exit. Ask the individual to wear a 'visitor's badge' as this will indicate to others that they have a right to be in the building. Anyone who is not known and who is not wearing a visitor's badge should arouse suspicion.

### Time to reflect

#### 8.1 Bogus callers

Think about a time when you have allowed someone access to your home or workplace without knowing for sure who they are or that they have a right of entry. What might have been the outcome? What checks should you have made before authorising access?

The overall aim of the Data Protection Act 1998 is to protect our right to privacy, particularly of personal information. You have a responsibility to ensure that information about the people you work with remains confidential and secure.

Personal information may only be disclosed to someone else with the service user's consent, in an extreme emergency, or if people need the information in order to support the individual. Therefore, if you are asked to disclose information about someone you work with, you must be satisfied that the person asking for the information has a right to know.

## Evidence activity 

### 8.1 Use agreed ways of working for checking the identity of anyone requesting access to premises and information

This activity gives you an opportunity to show that you know how to use procedures for checking the ID of anyone requesting access to your workplace and information about the people you work with.

Discuss the procedures your organisation has in place for checking visitors' and callers' ID with your manager. Write a short report to outline the key points discussed.

## 8.2 Implement measures to protect your own security and the security of others in your work setting

Health and social care organisations are accessible to the general public and therefore an easy target for individuals attempting to gain unauthorised access. Having identified the importance of checking the ID of people requesting access to premises and information, it is also important to consider other measures intended to promote security. These may include

- CRB checks – to identify the suitability of employees to work with vulnerable people.
- **CCTV** images, which help identify intruders, thieves, aggressive and dangerous encounters, abandoned packages that might contain explosives and so on.
- Keypad door locks –fitted to internal doors to prevent unauthorised people from accessing restricted areas, for example, where medicines or personal records are stored.
- Burglar alarms – to deter burglars and unwanted intruders.

**Key term**

CCTV means Closed Circuit Television.

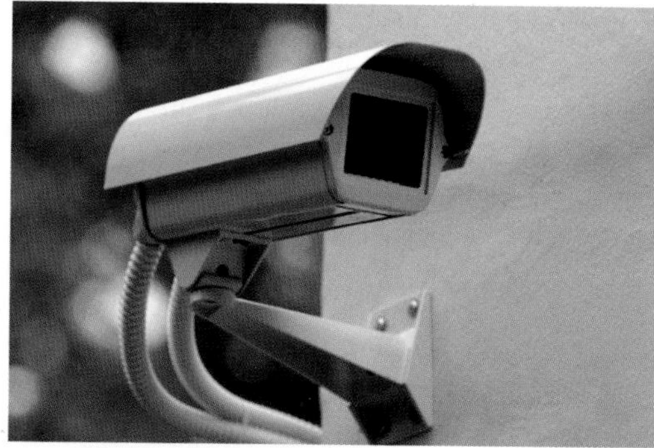

Figure 8.11 Security measures

Your workplace will have procedures detailing how you should:

- deal with potential breaches in security, including reporting, recording and support others following a breach
- deal with theft, bomb scares and missing persons
- use panic buttons, personal alarms, pagers, and mobile phones if you are in a compromised situation when working alone
- deal with challenging behaviour.

## Evidence activity 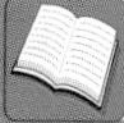

### 8.2 Implement measures to protect own security and the security of others in your work setting

This activity gives you an opportunity to show that you know how to protect yours and others security at work.

Identify security measures within your workplace. Under what circumstances are these security measures used?

## 8.3 Ensuring that others know your whereabouts

Many health and social care workers are employed as lone workers, for example some visit people in their own homes, collect and deliver prescriptions; and some use their car as a base.

Because of the nature of the job, lone working does carry some risks. Some examples include:

- care staff can suddenly become ill

- the office may not be available out of hours to answer queries
- risks associated with violence during darkness
- violence from people using the service or even their friends and relatives
- car accidents including breaking down
- accidents due to moving and handling .

## Case Study

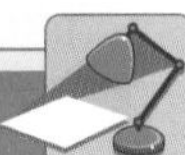

### 8.3 Suzy Lamplugh

In 1986, British estate agent Suzy Lamplugh vanished without trace. A major problem with the investigation of her disappearance was that no one realised she was missing until many hours after the incident happened. All her diary said was that she had an appointment to show a man around a house.

1. What do you think Suzy should have done before she went to her appointment?
2. How might Suzy have protected her security whilst she was out of the office?

Health and safety legislation requires employers to be able to trace lone workers and to have policies and procedures in place to ensure they are safe. This should include:

- Lone worker policy and procedures outlining how safety will be managed.
- Mobile phone policy and procedures explaining how and when mobile phones should be used.
- Communication policy and procedures detailing how you should check in and out of each visit and let the office know when you have reached home safely.
- Staff welfare policy and procedures ensuring you are equipped with a personal safety alarm.
- Staff learning and development policy and procedures requiring you to attend personal safety and awareness training.

Your main responsibility when working alone is to be aware of your surroundings and the possible threats to your personal safety. A disciplinary policy will set out procedures for disciplining you if you fail to follow measures set up to protect you.

**'We care because you care' Lone worker safety guide, Skills for Care 2010**

Suzy Lamplugh Trust www.suzylamplugh.org

## Evidence activity

### 8.3 Explain the importance of ensuring that others know your whereabouts

This activity gives you an opportunity to show you understand the importance of ensuring that others know your whereabouts.

Make a list of all the procedures you have to follow at work and the systems you use in your private life to let people know your whereabouts. Why is it necessary to follow these procedures and systems? What might happen if you didn't follow them?

# LO9 Know how to manage stress

## 9.1 Common signs and indicators of stress

We all experience pressure from time to time, and sometimes a bit of pressure can be motivating. It may be needed to complete a particular task. However, if the pressure builds up to the point that we can no longer cope, this can lead to stress. Some people thrive on stress and view it as a positive, energising emotion. But for most, it has negative consequences. According to the Health and Safety Executive, around 14 million working days and £4 billion are lost to work-related stress each year. There are some common signs, symptoms and indicators of stress.

- Cognitive symptoms – for example, memory problems, difficulty in concentrating, poor judgement, focusing on negative aspects, anxious or racing thoughts, constant worrying.
- Emotional symptoms – for example, moodiness, irritability or being short tempered, agitation, inability to relax, feeling

overwhelmed, a sense of loneliness and isolation and feelings of depression or general unhappiness.

- Physical symptoms – for example, aches and pains, diarrhea or constipation, nausea, dizziness, chest pain, rapid heartbeat, loss of sex drive and frequent colds.
- Behavioural symptoms – for example, eating more or less, sleeping too much or too little, not wanting to socialise with other people, postponing or neglecting responsibilities, using alcohol, cigarettes or drugs to relax, development of nervous habits, like nail biting.

**Evidence activity** 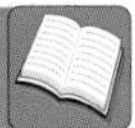

### 9.1 Identify common signs and indicators of stress

This activity gives you an opportunity to show that you know the signs of stress.

Think about a time when you have felt stressed. Which of the common signs and indicators can you relate to? Ask three of your colleagues what signs and indicators they experience when they feel stressed. Compare the answers.

## 9.2 Circumstances that trigger your own stress

The first step in managing stress is recognising the things that cause stress in your life. Every person's experience of stress is unique to them. There are many factors that can trigger stress. However, these triggers will very much depend on how you perceive stress. What is stressful for one person may not be stressful to another. Common stress triggers may include:

- money worries
- job issues
- relationships
- bereavement (loss of a loved one)
- family problems
- moving house.

Sometimes, there are no clear causes of stress. Some people naturally feel more frustrated, anxious or depressed than others, which can cause them to feel stressed more often.

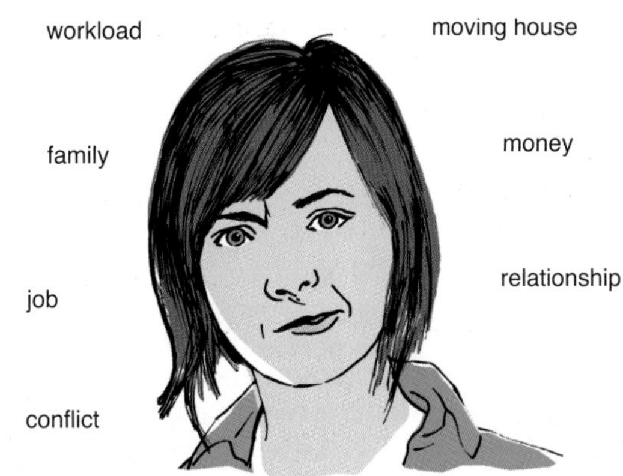


Figure 8.12 Triggers

**Evidence activity** 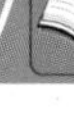

### 9.2 Identify circumstances that tend to trigger own stress

This activity gives you an opportunity to identify circumstances that tend to trigger your own stress.

Think about the things that make you feel stressed, for example certain work activities, being in a cramped space or having to make small talk with someone you don't know at a party. Now think about why they stress you. For example, why does one work activity stress you more than another? Is it because you don't like the people you are working with, because the activity is boring or you feel it could be done in a better way?

## 9.3 Managing stress

There are many strategies aimed at helping individuals to manage stress, and different people will find different ways of managing their own stress. If you can identify situations which lead to feelings of stress in yourself, you can then take steps to act upon the stressor before the feelings associated with stress get out of control. It is important to look at the ways in which you manage stress within your life in order to establish whether your coping mechanisms are beneficial, or whether they could be making your stress levels worse. Are they helpful or unproductive, healthy or unhealthy? Unfortunately, many people use mechanisms that could make their response to stress worse. Consider the following 'maladaptive' coping mechanisms.

- smoking
- drinking alcohol
- taking drugs
- over/under eating.

According to Professor Cary Cooper, an occupational health expert at the University of Lancaster, the keys to good stress management are building emotional strength, taking control of your situation, having a good social network and adopting a positive outlook. Professor Cooper suggests the following ways to managing stress.

1. Be active. Exercise will help you get rid of pent-up energy, calm your emotions and help you think more clearly.
2. Take control. Taking control is empowering and will help you find a solution that satisfies you, not someone else.
3. Connect with people. Talking things through with a friend will help you solve your problems. In addition, a good social support network will help you see things in a different way.
4. Have some 'me time'. Earmarking a couple of days a week for some quality 'me time' will help you achieve a healthy, stress-free work–life balance.
5. Challenge yourself. Setting yourself goals, such as learning something new, builds confidence and helps you take charge of your life.
6. Don't rely on alcohol, smoking and caffeine as your ways of coping. They might provide temporary relief but in the long term they don't solve problems, they just create new ones.
7. Do some voluntary work. Helping people in situations worse than yours will help you put your problems into perspective. And do someone a favour every day. Favours cost nothing and you'll feel better.
8. Work smarter, not harder. Good time management and concentrating on tasks that will make a real difference will help you feel more fulfilled.
9. Be positive. Try to be glass half full instead of glass half empty.
10. Accept the things you cannot change. Changing a difficult situation is not always possible. If you can't make any changes, accept things as they are and concentrate on everything that you do have control over.

www.nhs.uk; www.stress.org.uk

## Evidence activity

### 9.3 Describe ways to manage own stress

This activity gives you an opportunity to describe ways to manage your stress.

Think about the answers you gave within Evidence activity 9.2, where you have identified circumstances that trigger feelings of stress for you. Now describe the steps you take to manage those feelings of stress. Are the strategies you use healthy or unhealthy? What could you change to ensure your coping strategies are helpful to reducing your stress levels?

## Assessment summary

Your reading of this chapter and completion of the activities will have prepared you to demonstrate your learning and understanding of and competence in promoting and implementing health and safety in your workplace. To achieve the unit, your assessor will require you to:

| Learning Outcomes | Assessment Criteria |
|---|---|
| Learning outcome 1: Show you understand your responsibilities, and the responsibilities of others, relating to health and safety by: | 1.1 identifying legislation relating to health and safety in a health or social care work setting<br>See Evidence activity 1.1 p. 126. |
| | 1.2 describing the main points of health and safety policies and procedures as agreed with your employer<br>See Evidence activity 1.2 p. 127. |
| | 1.3 outlining the main health and safety responsibilities of yourself, your employer or manager and others in the work setting<br>See Evidence activity 1.3 p. 128. |
| | 1.4 identifying specific tasks relating to health and safety that should not be carried out without special training<br>See Evidence activity 1.4 p. 129. |
| | 1.5 explaining how to access additional support and information relating to health and safety<br>See Practice activity 1.5 p. 129. |
| Learning outcome 2: Understand the use of risk assessment in relation to health and safety by: | 2.1 explaining why it is important to assess health and safety hazards posed by the work setting or by particular activities<br>See Evidence activity 2.1 p.130. |
| | 2.2 explaining how and when to report potential health and safety risks that have been identified<br>See Evidence activity 2.2 p.130. |

| Learning Outcomes | Assessment Criteria |
|---|---|
| Learning outcome 2: Understand the use of risk assessment in relation to health and safety by: | 2.3 explaining how risk assessment can help address dilemmas between rights and health and safety concerns<br><br>See Evidence activity 2.3 p. 132. |
| Learning outcome 3: Understand procedures for responding to accidents and sudden illness by: | 3.1 describing different types of accidents and sudden illness that may occur in your work setting<br><br>See Evidence activity 3.1 p.133 |
| | 3.2 outlining procedures to be followed if an accident or sudden illness should occur<br><br>See Evidence activity 3.2, p.133 |
| Learning outcome 4: Be able to reduce the spread of infection by: | 4.1 demonstrating the recommended method for hand washing<br><br>See Practice activity 4.1 p.136. |
| | 4.2 demonstrating ways to ensure that your own health and hygiene do not pose a risk to an individual or to others at work.<br><br>See Practice activity 4.2 p.137. |
| Learning outcome 5: Be able to move and handle equipment and other objects safely by: | 5.1 identifying legislation that relates to moving and handling<br><br>See Evidence activity 5.1 p.139. |
| | 5.2 explaining the principles for moving and handling equipment and other objects safely<br><br>See Evidence activity 5.2 p.139. |
| | 5.3 moving and handling equipment and other objects safely<br><br>See Practice activity 5.3 p.140. |

| Learning Outcomes | Assessment Criteria |
| --- | --- |
| Learning outcome **6**: Know how to handle hazardous substances and materials by: | 6.1 identifying hazardous substances and materials that may be found in the work setting<br>See Evidence activity 6.1 p.141. |
| | 6.2 describing safe practices for storing, using and disposing of hazardous substances and materials<br>See Evidence activity 6.2 p.141. |
| Learning outcome **7**: Understand how to promote fire safety in the work setting by: | 7.1 describing practices that prevent fires from starting and spreading<br>See Evidence activity 7.1 p.142. |
| | 7.2 outlining emergency procedures to be followed in the event of a fire in the work setting<br>See Evidence activity 7.2 p.143. |
| | 7.3 explaining the importance of maintaining clear evacuation routes at all times<br>See Evidence activity 7.3 p.144. |
| Learning outcome **8**: Be able to implement security measures in the work setting by: | 8.1 using agreed ways of working for checking the identity of anyone requesting access to the premises and information<br>See Evidence activity 8.1 p.145. |
| | 8.2 implementing measures to protect your own security and that of others in the work setting<br>See Evidence activity 8.2 p.145. |
| | 8.3 explaining the importance of ensuring that others are aware of your whereabouts<br>See Evidence activity 8.3 p.146. |

| Learning Outcomes | Assessment Criteria |
|---|---|
| Learning outcome **9**: Know how to manage stress by: | 9.1 identifying common signs and indicators of stress<br>See Evidence activity 9.1, p.147 |
| | 9.2 identifying circumstances that tend to trigger your own stress<br>See Evidence activity 9.2, p.147 |
| | 9.3 describing ways to manage your own stress<br>See Evidence activity 9.3, p.148 |

Good luck!

## Weblinks

| | |
|---|---|
| Health and Safety Executive | www.hse.gov.uk |
| Health Protection Agency | www.hpa.org.uk |
| Infection Control services | www.infectioncontrolservices.co.uk |
| London Fire Brigade | www.london-fire.gov.uk |
| Fire Safety Advice Centre | www.firesafe.org.uk |
| Stress Management Society | www.stress.org.uk |
| Suzie Lamplugh Trust | www.suzylamplugh.org |

# 9 Handle information in health and social care settings

## For Unit HSC028

### What are you finding out?

We have all become more aware of identity theft and how easy it is to part with information innocently which is later abused. With the use of mobiles, texting and internet, information is now passed at a greater speed.

People in our care are not always aware of these dangers and are generally more vulnerable to types of abuse. Therefore this chapter will give you the information on protection we have available to support the people we look after.

People are frequently asked for personal and private information by various persons/organisations and with the development of technology available today, concerns regarding the safety and **confidentiality** of information have become paramount. With confidentiality people feel safe to part with vital information. To ensure that trust remains, certain laws and good practice codes are used within the healthcare setting. In 1996 the government commissioned a review of the transfer of patient-identifiable information from NHS organisations to other NHS and non-NHS organisations.

In December 1997 Dame Fiona Caldicott published the findings of this review, known as the Caldicott Report. The report highlighted 6 key principles and made 16 recommendations. Health and social care settings use these guidelines and legislation in making policies and procedures.

Legislation (laws) has been passed to promote the safety of individuals and it is important that you are aware of these and are able to enforce them. On applying for your role in a Health and Social Care setting, one of the forms you completed would be a CRB (Criminal Records Bureau) form. The CRB checks for any criminal activity. For a health and social care setting a POVA (Protection of Vulnerable Adults) check is also required, to ensure you are safe to work within this setting. These are only two of the laws that were put into effect to protect vulnerable people; we will go into more detail about these pieces of legislation later.

Within this chapter we will explore the legislation and your role in enforcing the law.

The reading and activities in this chapter will help you to:

- Understand the need for secure handling of information in health and social care settings
- Know how to access support for handling information
- Be able to handle information in accordance with agreed ways of working.

### Key term

**Confidentiality** is keeping a secret within a certain circle of persons.

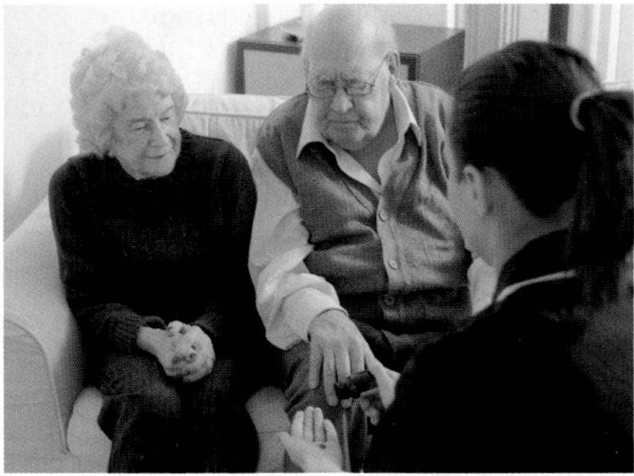

Figure 9.1 Health and social care setting

# LO1 Understand the need for secure handling of information in health and social care settings

## 1.1 Identify the legislation that relates to the recording, storage and sharing of information in health and social care settings

### Recording

Recording means a reproduction of information that is stored in a permanent manner. It needs to be accurate information, not a judgement but a true account of the situation. An example of this would be when completing an accident form, if we did not see someone fall, but found them on the floor; it would be inaccurate to state in the accident form that the person had fallen, as we would not have witnessed this. What we can report is the person was found on the floor: this is an accurate recording. The person may have just sat on the floor, not fallen. If we had inaccurately reported that the person had fallen, the doctor may request some medical test to identify why the person had fallen. This may cause distress for the person and would not benefit anyone.

It is very important that we do not put any of our own judgements into the report. An example of where this might occur would be if a person refused to go out for a walk and it was recorded in their notes that they did not enjoy going out of the home. From this report, fellow carers would possibly not encourage the individual to go out again. There may be several reasons the person did not want go out on this occasion, from something simple like it was too cold, to something more serious such as pains in their legs. Therefore, when recording, it is very important that we state the facts and not our thoughts. A more accurate account to be reported would be that this person refused to go out today, with no reason established as to why. Anyone reading the report would then be able to investigate the possible causes and include the person in other outings.

By recording events we are able to plan the best care for the individual. When you first started work you would not know if any of the persons you were looking after had any special needs or required a different type of approach due to not being able to hear, for example. Therefore everyone in care has an individualised care plan. The care plan needs to be accurate, honest and detailed so that everyone involved in their care knows how best to support the individual. The record must be precise and agreed with the person who is receiving the care. The care plan is a legal document; the individual has the right to see their records and should review these records frequently. When writing care plans it is important to keep in mind who has the right to read these records and the importance of factual recordings.

Everyone in a care home has a care plan; this is required to identify their needs and what assistance they required. Good practice says this should be written with the individual; they may not wish to share this information with their relatives and have this right due to the **Privacy Act 1974.** To access these records written consent is needed from the individual.

The **Equality Act 2010** identifies that anyone receiving care has the right to expect reasonable adjustments to providing access to goods, facilities, services and premises.

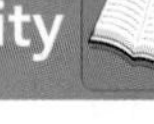

**Key terms**

The Privacy Act 1974 is legislation to protect your privacy.
The Equality Act 2010 is a legislation framework to protect the rights of individuals and advance equality of opportunity for all.

**Evidence activity**

**1.1 Identify the legislation that relates to the recording, storage and sharing of information in health and social care settings**

This activity will demonstrate that you can identify the legislation that relates to the sharing of information in health and social care settings.

Write a list of the legislation and acts of law that identify who can read an individual's health records/care plans

As you have identified there are many people who have rights to read the notes. Because of this, personal information is protected by legislation (law). The **Data Protection Act 1998** protects the individual from having their personal information shared; protection is also included in the **common law** of confidentiality and the **Human Rights Act 1998**.

## Key terms

Common law forms the basis of the legal system.

The Data Protection Act 1998 is legislation for the protection of an individual's information.

The Human Rights Act 1998 is legislation for the protection of an individual's fundamental rights.

The Data Protection Act has standards which must be met for obtaining, holding, using or disposing of personal data.

Common law states that information which has been obtained in confidence should only be disclosed when consent has been given, if there is sufficient robust public interest for justification or it is required by statute.

The Human Rights Act states that it has 'respect for individual private lives and prescribes the circumstances in which it is legitimate for a public authority to interfere with the enjoyment of this right'.

## Storage

To ensure we protect confidentiality we need to store records safely. As we use care plans frequently we may sometimes forget the importance of their security. It is very important that after reading or recording in the notes we place them back in a safe place. The reasons for this are to ensure no one else can read them that do not have authority to do so. Many different persons come into the homes for different reasons, such as delivery persons and relatives.

Principle 7 of the NHS code of practice states that records must be stored in an environmentally safe, protected area for current and archived records. To comply with this legislation in nursing homes most procedures state that personal information must be stored in a locked cabinet in a locked room; this complies with the Data Protection Act.

Records are required to be kept for an agreed period of time. Even after the person has died this information is still confidential and has to be kept for the recommended agreed times.

## Sharing

Confidentiality means we are only allowed to share the information the person has given us if they agree to the information being shared. People coming into care recognise we need to discuss this information with other medical professions and this should be talked about when taking the information.

In your placement there will be policies (principles or rules of what should occur in certain situations) and procedures (a series of actions or operations on how to do a task) on sharing of information, these policies and procedures are written following guidance given by the General Skills Council and the Care Standards Act 2000 (National Care Standards).

Sometimes we have to share information without consent, look at your procedures and policies and the NHS Code of Practice 2003 (Department of Health Guidelines) on confidentiality.

If someone has informed you they intend to harm themselves or others or if they have told you something that is unlawful you have a duty to disclose this information with the relevant bodies such as the police.

It is important to note that, when discussing something with the individual, if they inform you they wish to tell you something in confidence you can only keep this confidence if it does not break the law.

The sharing of information needs to be as secure as its storage. If a relative comes in and asks for information you need to do some checks first, to check they are a relative and that the person consents to them having the information.

When sharing information with other agencies you need to ensure the information you are sharing is factual and accurate, that the way you are sending the information is secure, that the individual consents to this information being shared and that delivery of the information is secure.

Evidence activity 

**1.1 Identify the legislation that relates to the recording, storage and sharing of information in health and social care settings**

This activity will demonstrate that you can identify the legislation that relates to the recording and storage of information in health and social care settings.

List the records you write in at your workplace and where you store these records.

## 1.2 Explain why it is important to have secure systems for recording and storing information in a health and social care setting

In this section it is important to look at the setting you are working in and think about the different forms of data (information) you use. When someone enters your work environment they will be asked to sign the signing in book, this is used for health and safety procedures, for example if a fire was to occur you would have a record of who was in the building. This type of data is publically shared with anyone else entering the building, and persons signing in are aware of the purpose of this information. Therefore consent is acknowledged.

For the persons you are looking after, generally vulnerable persons (a person over the age of 18 years; is or may be in need of Community Care Services by reason of mental or other disability, age or illness; and is or may be unable to take care of himself or herself and/or is unable to protect themselves against significant harm or exploitation) require protection from abuse.

When writing any personal details about the person you are caring for you need to ensure that this information is written in a secure environment, so persons not entitled to see the information cannot read what you are writing. When completed these records need to be stored, and only the persons with consent to see the records can do so. If we did not do this, think of what could occur.

Evidence activity 

**1.2 (a) Explain why it is important to have secure systems for recording and storing information in a health and social care setting**

This activity will help demonstrate that you understand why it is important to have secure systems for recording and storing information.

Write about a situation when you have recorded in the care plan. Where did you write them? Where did you put them when you finished? Could you have done anything differently to improve the confidentiality?

On starting a shift at work we sometimes make notes from the handover or care plans, what happens to these notes after we have finished work and how do we ensure the confidentiality of the individual?

Evidence activity 

**1.2 (b) Explain why it is important to have secure systems for recording and storing information in a health and social care setting**

This activity will help demonstrate that you understand why it is important to have secure systems for recording and storing information.

Write about the last time you made notes at a handover. How detailed were the notes? Was confidentiality maintained? What happened to the notes afterwards? Could you have done anything differently to improve confidentiality?

Most records are stored in metal cabinets to ensure that if a fire occurred the records would not be destroyed. When putting records onto a computer, staff are required to use a password/ code. This ensures that the records cannot be accessed by anyone else.

On entering a care setting personal records are taken, and one of the questions to be asked concerns the next of kin. When asking for the information, good practice is to check whether there is consent for that person to have personal information.

A 90-year-old was admitted to a care home: she had some mental health issues, her husband had died several years ago and she lived on her own. This lady had a solicitor who was looking after her financial situation. The 90-year-old lady continually stated she did not want the solicitor to be involved and therefore refused consent for her to have any information. As this lady was having memory problems it would have been easy to dismiss her refusal and give the information to the solicitor but, as the good practice guide informs us of correct procedure, the information was withheld. With further investigation it transpired the solicitor was abusing the person. She was selling all her personal effects and not putting the monies into the person's account. Fortunately this does not occur frequently.

Clear recording of information ensures we are able to deliver the best care; an example of this would be identifying clearly what the individual likes to eat, so that if they refuse a meal we can identify if this is due to foods they dislike. We need to record on a regular basis likes and dislikes to ensure the record is current. Sometimes individual's tastes buds can change and what they disliked at one time they may now like.

Everyone looking after the individual must know where the records are kept; again these must be in a secure place as they are not for public viewing. A record/personal data is a tool and we need to ensure that the care that is delivered is individual and personal. If correctly recorded and stored in a safe environment this tool enables us to deliver the care the person needs, wants and requires. It reinforces confidentiality and helps the individual trust the care they are receiving.

When working in a healthcare setting it is important to remain professional even when we have left work. In the past, carers have been dismissed due to breaches in confidentiality. Health and social care settings generally have an active social setting for staff, and after work you may go to the pub with your colleagues. These are the times that you must be extra sensitive about the personal information of the individual you look after, as a relative or friend may also be in the pub.

When writing an essay or work for a course, please beware of the need to hide the identity of the individual, this can be done by naming the person 'Mr/Mrs X'.

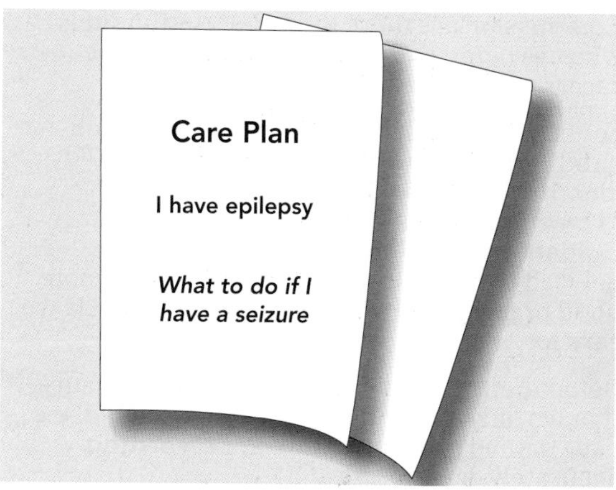


Figure 9.2 A care plan

# LO2 Know how to access support for handling information

## 2.1 Describe how to access guidance, information and advice about handling information

We have identified the various legislation regarding record keeping and storage. All care settings have policies and procedures for recording and storing information. When in the setting we can sometimes come across a situation not directly identified in these procedures.

In the healthcare setting you are working in, you will have a line manager to ask for some guidance; generally this would be the care supervisor or the registered nurse.

There may be times when asking someone does not seem practical, a scenario may be that a relative has come to the door demanding information. You need to remain calm and inform them that you will go and check. No one has the right of entry without consent, except for the police and fire services. Go and ask the person in charge.

When someone reports at the door always check their identity, even if they are in uniform, your role and duty is to protect the people you are looking after. Ensure every visitor signs in; this is a requirement for health and safety.

Healthcare settings have to be registered with the Care Quality Commission to enable them to be able to deliver care, the Care Quality Commission are there to support individuals who are being cared for and to support the carers who look after the individuals.

Legislation has clear guidelines to follow on handling of information; we have already identified the Confidentiality Act, Data Protection Act and General Social Skill's Guidance. These Codes of Practice were devised to help and support carers to promote good practice and safeguard the individuals we care for.

Before getting information, we need to ensure that we only take the information required, we have gained consent and we are recording accurately.

## Evidence activity 

### 2.1 Describe how to access guidance, information and advice about handling information

This activity will help demonstrate that you understand how to access information.

Identify a person you look after. What do you know about the person? Where can you find out their likes and dislikes? Who can you share the information with?

## Case Study 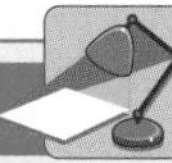

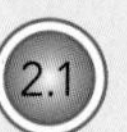

### 2.1 Mrs X

Mrs X has been admitted to the care home you are working in, when she is admitted you find £5,000 pounds on her personal belongings. Mrs X was not accompanied by any relatives and has a diagnosis of dementia. The next day a lady arrives claiming to be her daughter and asking if Mrs X has anything valuable to take away to be stored safely, claiming she has power of attorney (authorisation to act on behalf in legal and financial matters) for her aunt.

What would you do?

What checks would you need to complete?

Who would you ask for guidance?

## 2.2 Explain what actions to take when there are concerns over the recording, storing or sharing of information

Everyone employed in the healthcare setting is vetted before commencement of employment, they must be interviewed and at least two references must be obtained. A Criminal Record check is included and for those working with vulnerable adults a POVA (Protection of Vulnerable Adults) check is also completed.

As we have identified, various acts are available and in place to safeguard the people we look after. Part of your induction into the health and social care setting requires you to have training, part of this training identifies the need to correctly record, store and share information. This will be your first introduction to policies and procedures of your workplace.

Working in the health and social care setting requires you to adapt to the professional Code of Practice (General Skills for Care Council) and when you sign your contract, you will be signing to say that you agree to the responsibilities of a carer. Guidance for the role and responsibilities of a carer can be found at the General Skills for Care Council website and at the Skills for Care website:

www.gscc.org.uk

www.skillsforcareanddevelopment.org.uk.

Sometimes when working in a health and social care setting you may become concerned over the actions of another member of staff. If you see or hear anything that causes you concern you have a duty to report this. This reporting would follow the guidelines in your policy and procedures, generally speaking you would initially report to your line manager. If the matter was not resolved there, you would follow the next steps of the procedure. You are also able to go outside of the organisation to the Care Quality Commission. If you do not report any concerns you have, you will also be answerable to any enquiry.

### Evidence activity 

 2.2 **Explain what actions to take when there are concerns over the recording, storing or sharing of information**

This activity will help you demonstrate that you can explain what actions to take when there are concerns over sharing information.

You are reading Mrs X notes, which state that she is diabetic. You have found her today eating chocolate that is not diabetic chocolate, what would you do?

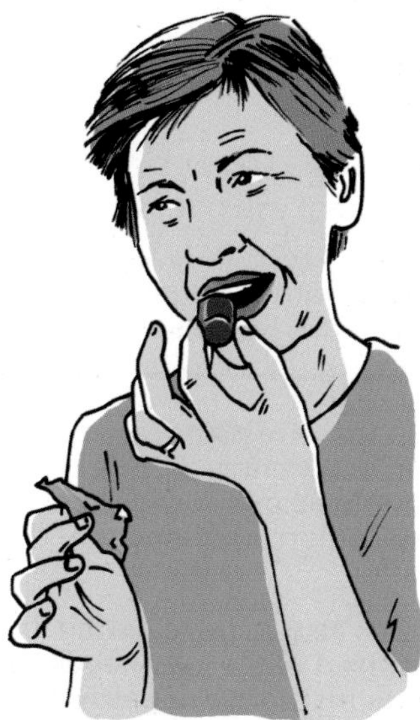

Figure 9.3

### Time to reflect 

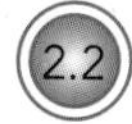 2.2 **Can you remember?**

Recall your introduction and the training you received on record keeping, storing and sharing information. What was the procedure in correcting an error written in the care plan, are you able to use corrective fluid, are you able to use pencil, and is the care plan a legal document?

Sometimes we need to transfer notes to a hospital when a person requires hospital treatment or attends outpatients. We need to ensure that sufficient information is being transferred and in a secure manner.

## LO3 Be able to handle information in accordance with agreed ways of working

### 3.1 Keep records that are up to date, complete, accurate and legible

As we have identified, keeping accurate records is required to help us look after people. Records are a legal document. In healthcare settings there are two forms of records: electronic and written.

Written records must be written so others can read them (those that are entitled to read them). They must be accurate and up to date. Care plan records should be written at least once a day. Care plans are a form of communication of care/personal needs. These records should be factual and non-judgemental. When starting work you should check the care plans to identify any changes to delivery of care.

## Case Study

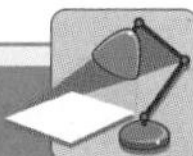

### Mrs X

Mrs X had arrived in the care home the night before. The carer, Mary, came on duty and went straight to Mrs X to assist her in getting dressed. Mary ran the bath and came to Mrs X and told her she was going to give her a bath. Mrs X began crying and screaming, Mary was aware that the more she tried to calm her down the more Mrs X was becoming frustrated. Mary left the room and went to the nurse in charge for advice.

The nurse in charge read the care plan and identified that Mrs X only likes showers and wears a hearing aid. Mrs X takes her hearing aid out night.

What should be the next action for the carer?

When writing care plans or passing information to relatives, doctors or social workers it is important that the information we give is an accurate (free from error) and true account of the situation. We cannot include our thoughts in the information.

When we send texts or emails, information can be easily misunderstood: this is partly due to the limited number of words used. Therefore we are not able to give emphasis to the importance of the message. In care plans we have to be very precise in our writing. An example of this would be:

- Mrs A did not like her tea.
- Mrs A appeared to not enjoy her tea and ate a very small amount.

The first statement informs us of very little, it does not tell us if she ate any of her tea, we don't know if she did not like all of her tea or just parts.

From the second statement we can identify that she had some food and there is a need to investigate why she did not enjoy her tea.

It is important that we add to this statement when we have identified why she did not enjoy her tea, to prevent it occurring again. It may be that Mrs A did not like gravy and that was put over her tea; if we had checked we could ensure it was noted in the care plan not to put gravy on the food next time.

Imagine the situation of someone having a broken leg. The care plan may initially state that no weight is to be put onto the leg. If we do not update the care plan and the person was on bed rest for a long period, further medical problems could occur such as muscle wastage, meaning they would be unable to put weight on the leg again, or sores due to lack of circulation.

Records must be updated on a regular basis, with accurate and readable information to ensure we give the best individual care for that person, with clearly defined problems and actions to resolve the problems. The individual needs to agree and understand the records. The individual has the right to read their notes. Records are a professional document to plan the individual's needs and actions to resolve their problems.

## Time to reflect

### Can you do better?

Think of the last entry you put into a person's care plan, how accurate was it and could others read it? Was it current?

## Evidence activity

### Keep records that are up to date, complete, accurate and legible

This activity helps demonstrate your ability to keep records that are up to date, accurate and legible.

Think of the last entry you put in a person's care plan, write what you put, what else you could have written, why it worked in communicating information and when it was reviewed.

When writing in the care plan we need to ensure we date and sign every entry. This is because it is a legal document that can be used in court. It also provides an audit trail of events of the care delivered.

Electronic records also require dating, but no signature is required as the user needs to sign into the account with the use of password/user name, this identifies the individual.

## 3.2 Follow agreed ways of working for recording information

If we notice that someone has lost weight, we have to record this information. It is not enough to just put in the care plan that Mrs X appears to have lost weight, the procedure we would follow is to first check if Mrs X has lost weight, we would do this by checking her last recorded weight and re-weighing and recording her new weight. We would then be able to say that Mrs X has lost so many kilos from last month and this needs investigating. This information would then be passed on to the nurse in charge who would then transfer this information to the doctor for further investigation.

This highlights the importance of regular weighing and recording of the information, as well as the importance of recording the information correctly and legibly for others to read and understand. The doctor can then confirm if the weight loss is a gradual loss or a sudden loss, and this enables a clearer diagnosis of the problem.

On identifying weight loss the next step would be to identify the eating pattern of Mrs X, for example has she been eating and are there any identified foods she prefers?

### Evidence activity

#### 3.2 Follow agreed ways of working for recording information

This activity will help you demonstrate that you can follow agreed ways of working for recording information.

Read this care plan entry and identify any errors:

'Joan Appleton was very slow in getting up today and angry. Joan did not wash herself properly and had thrown her clothes on the floor. Joan has put on weight and did not care what she was wearing and put her shoes on the wrong feet.'

It is alright to name the person in their own care plan as they have consented to this information being shared. 'Slow' is a word that has no measure; what you may think of as slow may be fast for someone else. 'Angry' is a very descriptive word, this statement does not clarify if the person has been asked if she was angry, it may be her facial expression and possibly not a true reflection of her mood. Joan may only have a quick wash in the morning and prefer a bath at the end of the day; a more accurate statement without being judgemental would be Joan washed around her face and top half of her body.

From this statement we don't know if the carer saw Joan throw the clothes on the floor or if the clothes had fallen on the floor. A better statement would be either: 'On entering the room I saw Joan's clothes on the floor' or 'Joan became cross and threw her clothes on the floor'.

Regarding the statement that Joan did not care what she was wearing, had Joan stated that or had the carer thought that?

The importance of recording actual and sufficient information to assist staff to deliver the best care to the individual as recommended in the Care Standards Act 2000.

## Follow agreed ways of working for storing information

We know electronic data is stored safely and is secure through the use of passwords and firewalls. If a fire or disaster occurs, as these records are stored electronically they are likely to be preserved. And we know that only persons with the correct passwords can read them; the Data Protection Act identifies the security and storage required.

Paper-based information needs to be stored in a secure container that cannot be destroyed by burning and is not accessible to the general public. All healthcare settings follow the guidelines for safe storage and record this information in their policies and procedures.

Records and data need to be stored even if the person that the records relate to is no longer living. They must be stored securely.

## Follow agreed ways of working for sharing information

When we are caring for people we need to be sure who we are allowed to share their information with. If the person we are caring for gives consent for a named person to see their records, then we can show them.

On entering care the individual will assist with the information for their care plan, they will be told that in order to help them this information sometimes needs to be shared with fellow medical staff. Good practice would be to inform the individual every time you are going to share the information. An example of this would be on a visit to the dentist, you should inform the individual that you are going to show the dentist the medication they are on so they know how best to treat you. For example, the dentist may need to prescribe some tablets that may not be effective with the medication the individual is taking.

On admission good practice would be to check if they have any relatives or friends that they would like you to share information with, and write this in the care plan, always advising the individual that the care plan can be changed if they so wish.

The main thing to remember when sharing information is that consent from the individual is paramount. Check the identity of the person you are sharing the information with, it is better to annoy someone and ask for extra identity then to give the information without consent.

When individuals are being cared for in a home it is easy to think that their relatives have the right to information, but remember that not all families are caring and looking out for the individual. If you have concerns or the individual appears anxious around a relative, you have the support of the advocacy agency. Always check your setting's policies and procedures, or with the nurse in charge.

## Assessment summary

Your reading of this chapter and completion of the activities will have prepared you to demonstrate your learning, understanding and competence of Handling Information in Health and Social Care settings. To achieve this unit your assessor will require you to:

| Learning Outcomes | Assessment Criteria |
|---|---|
| Learning outcome 1: Show you understand the need for secure handling of information in the health and social care setting by: | 1.1 explaining the legislation that relates to the recording, storage and sharing of information in the health and social care setting<br><br>Evidence activity 1.1, p.154 and p.156 |
| | 1.2 explaining why it is important to have secure systems for recording and storing information in a health and social care setting.<br><br>Evidence activity 1.2, p.156 |
| Learning outcome 2: Know how to access support for handling information by: | 2.1 describing how to access guidance, information and advice about handling information<br><br>Evidence activity 2.1, p.158 |

| Learning Outcomes | Assessment Criteria |
|---|---|
| Learning outcome 2: Know how to access support for handling information by: | 2.2 explaining what actions to take when there are concerns over the recording, storing or sharing of information.<br><br>Evidence activity 2.2, p.159 |
| Learning outcome 3: Be able to handle information in accordance with agreed ways of working by: | 3.1 keeping records that are up to date, complete, accurate and legible<br><br>Evidence activity 3.1, p.160 |
| | 3.2 following agreed ways of working for:<br>• recording information<br>• storing information<br>• sharing information<br><br>Evidence activity 3.2, p.161 |
| | Learning outcomes 1 and 2 can be assessed by reflective accounts (reflective accounts require an explanation of a situation, what happened, what you did, what you could have done differently and what you have learned). Reflective accounts are seen as good evidence as this will show your learning and development. They can also be assessed by oral or written questions. Professional discussion is a discussion on an agreed topic of the unit with your assessor. Professional discussion should be planned with sufficient time for you to read up on the topic and then discuss with the assessor. Witness or expert testimony is where someone in your workplace writes a statement stating that you have demonstrated the competence or knowledge for this unit. If you have evidence of prior learning in the subject, possibly a training day you have been on, this is classed as recognition of prior learning. Direct observation is required for most units; this is where your assessor will observe you in the workplace. |
| | Learning objective 3 needs to be observed by your assessor. |

Good Luck!

## Weblinks

| | |
|---|---|
| The Department of Health for Social Care | www.dh.gov.uk/en/SocialCare |
| The General Social Care Council | www.gscc.org.uk |
| Skills for Care and Development | http://www.skillsforcareanddevelopment.org.uk |
| The Care Quality Commission | http://www.cqc.org.uk |
| Public Services | http://www.direct.gov.uk |

# 10 Dementia awareness

# For Unit DEM201

## What are you finding out?

Dementia is the term used to describe the symptoms caused by certain diseases or conditions of the brain. There are many different types of dementia, some more common than others, and they are often named according to the condition that caused them.

Over 750,000 people in the UK are disabled in one way or another by dementia and 60,000 deaths a year are directly attributable to dementia. Because the **incidence** of dementia increases with age and more people are living longer, these numbers are expected to rise considerably.

Dementia is progressive and eventually severe, which means the symptoms gradually get worse, but how fast it progresses depends on the person concerned. Everyone is unique and experiences dementia in their own way.

The reading and activities in this chapter will help you to:

- Understand what dementia is
- Understand key features of the theoretical models of dementia
- Know the most common types of dementia and their causes
- Understand factors relating to an individual's experience of dementia.

**Key term**

Incidence means occurrence.

## LO1 Understand what dementia is

### 1.1 What is meant by the term 'dementia'?

The nervous system is a network of nerve cells that carry messages to all parts of the body. It works continuously to control the activities in the body. The brain is the most important organ in the nervous system. You will read about its structure and functions later. It is made up of billions of nerve cells, which are elongated living structures with many projections called dendrites. Dendrites connect nerve cells with each other and the point at which two cells connect is called a synapse.

Messages pass along nerve cells in the form of tiny electrical impulses. When an electrical impulse reaches the end of a dendrite, it triggers the release of a **neurotransmitter**. The neurotransmitter passes across the synapse to the dendrite of an adjoining cell, where it triggers an electrical impulse and the continuation of the message. This passage of messages is the basis for how the brain controls the body's activities, for example movement, cognitive abilities and physiological functions such as heart rate and breathing.

**Key term**

A neurotransmitter is a chemical that transmits messages between nerve cells.

If a disease or condition stops nerve cells from doing their job, for example, by starving them of oxygen or nutrients, or by isolating them from neighbouring cells, they will die. Dementia is caused by the death of nerve cells in the brain. Most dementias are progressive, which mean they gradually get worse. This is because when a nerve cell dies it cannot usually be replaced. As more and more nerve cells die the brain starts to shrink or atrophy. Brain atrophy can often be seen in the brain scan of a person with dementia.

Dementia is not a disease in its own right. It is also not a natural part of ageing – although the chances of developing dementia increase with age, people in their mid-life can be affected. As

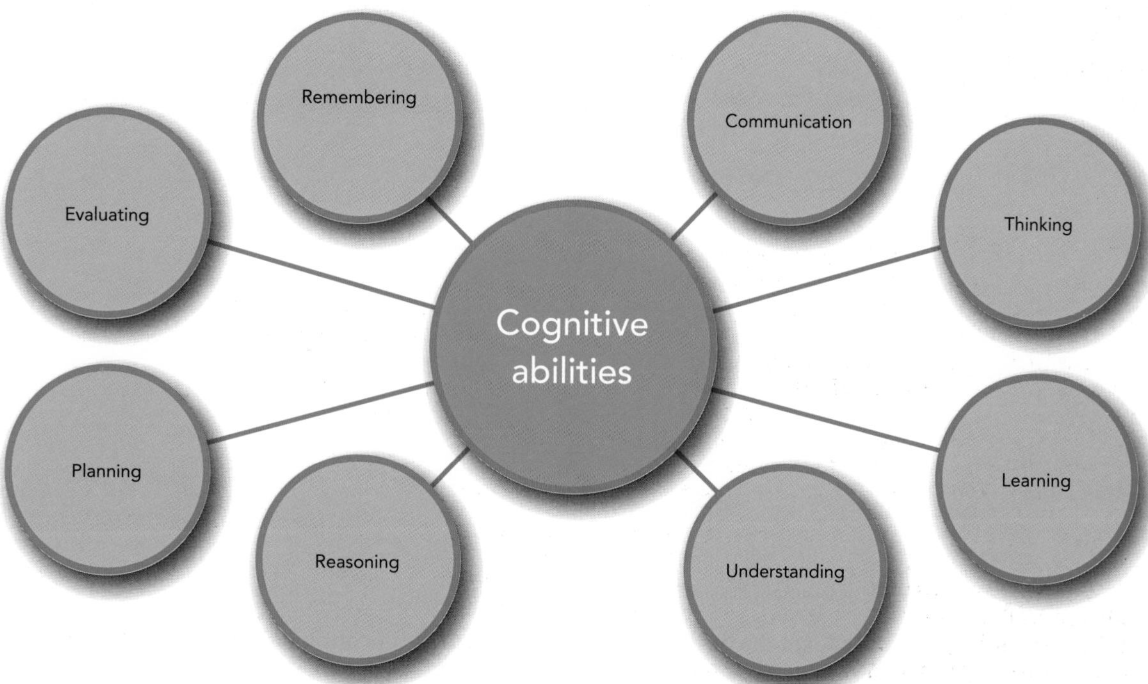


Figure 10.1 Cognitive abilities

you read above, it is the term used to describe the symptoms that are caused by diseases or conditions that affect the brain. Common symptoms include memory loss, impaired cognitive abilities and lack of physical coordination. However, the symptoms a person experiences depends on the area of the brain that is affected.

## Evidence activity 

### 1.1 Dementia

This activity allows you to demonstrate your understanding of the term 'dementia'.

Write a short quiz that finds out how much people know and understand about dementia. Include questions that ask about the incidence of dementia, the age of onset, why it develops, the **prognosis** for people with dementia and the symptoms they are likely to experience. Make sure you can give the correct answers!

### Key term

Prognosis is the prediction of the probable course and outcome of a disease.

## 1.2 Key functions of the brain that are affected by dementia

Common symptoms of dementia include **impaired** cognitive abilities; mood swings and depression; **disorientation**; problems processing (dealing with) nervous impulses, leading to disturbances such as **hallucinations**; and lack of physical coordination. However, as you read above, the symptoms a person experiences depends on the area of their brain that is affected.

The human brain is incredibly complex and is fed by a network of blood vessels that deliver oxygen and nutrients to the cells. It controls everything our body does, from coordinating our movements and our speech to keeping our heart beating and storing our memories. It can be divided into three main sections, the cerebral hemispheres, the cerebellum and the brain stem.

### Key terms

Disorientation is confusion due to the loss of spatial ability.
A hallucination is seeing and hearing things that don't exist.
Impaired means damaged.

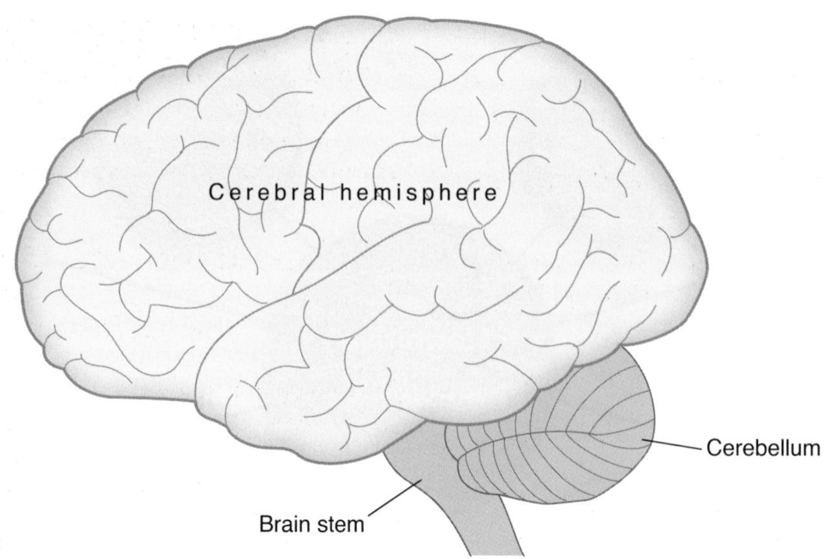


Figure 10.2 The brain

The cerebral hemispheres form the bulk of the brain.

- Their outermost layer is the cerebral cortex, which has a role in emotion, thought and planning.
- The left cerebral hemisphere is concerned with speech and language, mathematical ability and logic.
- The right cerebral hemisphere is concerned with **spatial ability**, face recognition, colour, shape, creativity and imagination.

## Key term

Spatial ability is the ability to understand the way our surroundings are laid out and to be aware of where we are within them.

Different areas of the cerebral hemispheres have different functions:

- The motor area has a role in controlling movement.
- The sensory area receives nervous impulses from sense organs in the skin and processes them so that we can feel the sensations of hot, cold, touch and pain.
- The visual area receives nervous impulses from the eyes and processes them into 'pictures' that we can see.
- The auditory area receives nervous impulses from the ears and processes them into 'sounds' that we can hear.

The cerebellum controls movement, posture and balance and the brain stem controls vital living functions such as breathing, heart beat and blood pressure.

At the centre of the brain is the limbic system, which contains the hippocampus. The hippocampus controls a number of functions but especially learning, memory and emotion.

Table 10.1 Key functions of the brain that are affected by dementia

| Area of the brain | Functions that are affected by dementia |
|---|---|
| Cerebral cortex. | Emotions and the ability to think and plan. |
| Cerebral hemispheres. | Communication, use of numbers, spatial awareness, creativity, the ability to recognise colours, shapes and faces, visual and auditory processing and movement. |
| Cerebellum. | Movement, posture and balance. |
| Hippocampus. | Emotions, memory and learning new things. |

www.alzheimers.org.uk, www.bbc.co.uk

## Evidence activity 

### 1.2 The key functions of the brain that are affected by dementia

This activity allows you to demonstrate your knowledge of how the functioning of the brain is affected by dementia.

Produce a labelled diagram of a section through the brain to show the position of the cerebral cortex, cerebral hemispheres, cerebellum and hippocampus. Briefly describe the function of each area and say how damage within each affects the way someone experiences dementia.

## 1.3 Why depression, delirium and age-related memory impairment may be mistaken for dementia

Delirium is caused by:

- prescribed and illegal drugs, such as anti-depressants and cannabis
- poisons, such as alcohol
- infections, such as pneumonia
- physiological disturbances and disorders, such as heart, kidney and liver failure
- a lack of oxygen to the brain
- mental health problems, such as depression, anxiety and dementia.

The symptoms of delirium are very similar to those of dementia. They include changes in attention, poor concentration, disorganised thinking and poor **short term memory (STM)**; a loss of awareness and disorientation; agitation and emotional and personality changes; hallucinations and rambling speech. But whilst delirium and dementia have many symptoms in common, and indeed delirium can be caused by dementia, delirium should not be mistaken for dementia as the treatment for each is different.

www.mentalhealth.org.uk

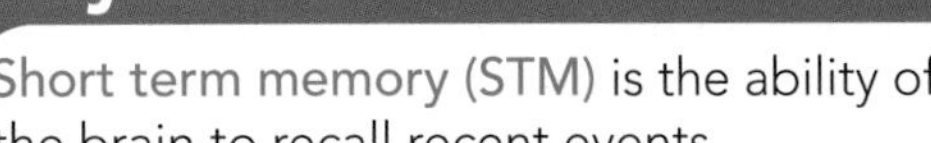

## Key term

Short term memory (STM) is the ability of the brain to recall recent events.

## Time to reflect

### 1.3 Think about this ...

Imagine that you come across someone in the street or in a shop who's obviously uncertain about where they are, very agitated and talking without making sense. What would be your first thoughts – that the person was the worse for drink, high on drugs, ill ... or experiencing the symptoms of dementia? What would you do?

Many people as they get older have trouble remembering names, what they did yesterday, what they just went upstairs for, where they've put their keys and so on. And it's not uncommon for these people to worry that they're developing dementia. However, in the majority of cases, age-related memory loss is just a normal part of the aging process and not a sign of dementia. Only when memory loss affects a person's ability to carry out daily activities should they seek treatment.

## Time to reflect

### 1.3 Going mad ... or just too much to remember?

What do you forget? Why do you forget these things? Does forgetting things impact on your day-to-day life? How can you help yourself to remember all the things you have to do?

In general, people with dementia are unaware of their forgetfulness – it's the people with memory loss that isn't caused by dementia who complain about it! 'Don't worry if you forget where you put your car keys. Only worry if you forget what they're used for!'

If the people you work with start to have difficulty remembering things, suggest they see their doctor but reassure any older people that age-related memory loss is quite normal. A doctor can treat memory loss if it is caused by, for example:

- the side effects of medication
- depression and anxiety
- sleep **apnoea**
- physiological disorders such as **hypertension** and diabetes
- **deficiency diseases** such as severe hypothyroidism (myxedema) and pernicious anaemia.

www.mentalhelp.net

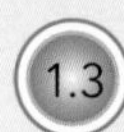

## Key terms

Apnoea means a pause in breathing.
Deficiency diseases are caused by a shortage of vitamins or minerals in the diet.
Hypertension means high blood pressure

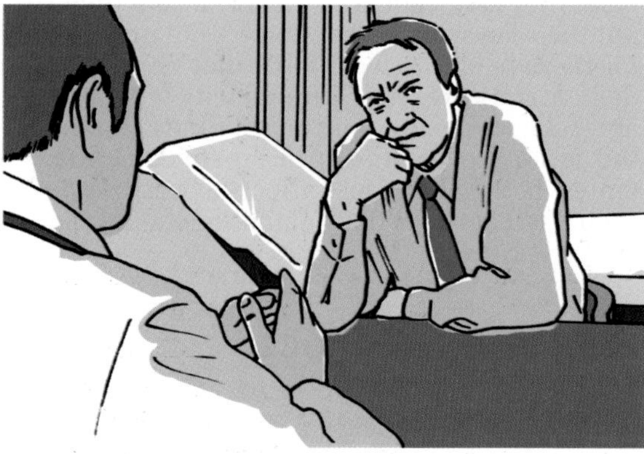

Figure 10.3 Getting help

You read earlier that the brain controls our emotions. Depression is a condition in which a number of emotions dominate a person's life and make it difficult for them to cope. It's a common symptom of dementia.

Symptoms of depression include:

- sadness, hopelessness, low self-esteem, guilt, thoughts of death and suicide
- anxiety, agitation, restlessness, irritability
- a loss of interest or pleasure in activities that were once enjoyed
- feelings of isolation and of being cut off from other people
- sleep disturbance
- problems with remembering, concentrating or making simple decisions
- weight loss or gain.

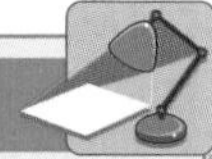

## Case Study

### 1.3 Jack

Jack lives on his own; in what some would call a hovel. He doesn't have any friends and no one has ever heard of any relatives. His immediate neighbours tell you that he has no conversation – he doesn't seem to be able to follow what they're saying, he has no contribution to make to conversation, and in fact he isn't interested in making conversation. He is becoming increasingly edgy, makes noises in the night, and people on the street are beginning to go out of their way to avoid him, especially children who have been led to believe that he is dangerous.

- What are your initial feelings about this situation? Poor Jack? Or would you too keep out of his way?
- What do you think could be the cause of his behaviour?
- What would you like to do to remedy the situation?

Similarities between dementia and depression mean that the two can be confused, and an older person with dementia may sometimes be wrongly thought to have depression, and vice versa. If the older people you work with start to behave in such a way that could indicate the onset of depression or of dementia, suggest they see their doctor as soon as possible so that an accurate diagnosis can be made and they can be treated.

www.alzheimers.org.uk

Evidence activity 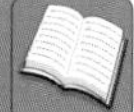

### 1.3 Why depression, delirium and age related memory loss can be mistaken for dementia

This activity allows you to demonstrate your understanding of why depression, delirium and age-related memory loss can be mistaken for dementia.

Complete the following table.

| Symptoms that are common to depression and dementia | Symptoms that are common to delirium and dementia | Symptoms that are common to age-related memory loss and dementia |
|---|---|---|
| | | |

## LO2 Theoretical models of dementia

In health and social care, a theoretical model is a framework for exploring health and social care needs, developing ideas for care and support and putting them into practice. This section looks at two important theoretical models of dementia, the medical model and the social model.

### 2.1 The medical model of dementia

The medical model is the traditional model in **Western societies** for understanding dementia. It dominated thinking among health and social care professionals until the early 1990s.

The medical model describes dementia as an **organic brain disorder** that causes impaired cognitive abilities about which nothing can be done. It promotes the view that the demented person is a problem. He or she can no longer function normally and needs to be cared for and controlled, by professional 'experts', away from the rest of us for whom the word 'demented' conjures up visions of madness, insanity and the horror of mental institutions.

### Key terms

An **organic brain disorder** is one where a person's behaviour changes because of damage to the brain.

**Western societies** are societies in the first or developed world, where medicine is based on science.

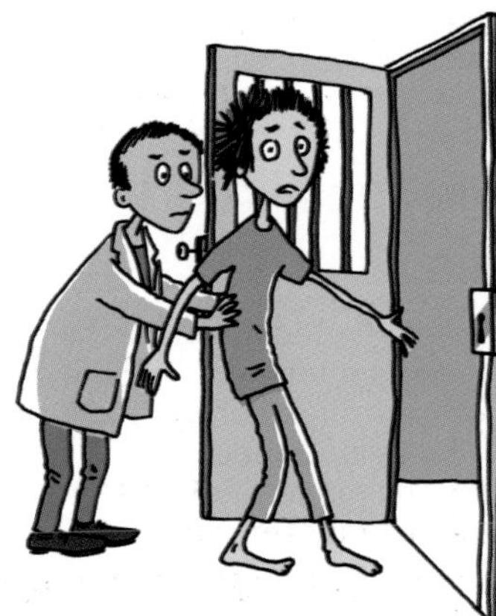

Figure 10.4 Mad or bad?

Even though medical professionals devised and continue to use the medical model of dementia, many of them have little knowledge and understanding of dementia, of how it progresses and how to make a diagnosis. They continue to dismiss the symptoms of dementia as depression, absent-mindedness or preoccupation. As a result, dementia is often only diagnosed during times of crisis.

> 'We had gone to him (the GP) for a lot of things and he was telling [the person with dementia] that it was in his mind, he hadn't got these problems, he needed to pull himself together.' (Carer)
>
> Living Well With Dementia: A National Dementia Strategy, DH, 2009

### Time to reflect

#### 2.1 How would you feel?

Imagine that you'd gone to see your doctor because you were losing your memory and worried you were developing dementia, and that he or she sent you away, telling you to 'pull yourself together'. How would you feel?

Because of this attitude and lack of knowledge, the **stigma** attached to having a mental health condition, and the understanding that nothing can be done to help, many people with worries about dementia avoid going to their GP. As a result they don't get diagnosed soon enough and help and support are often only put in place when there is a crisis.

**Key term**

Stigma means shame, disgrace.

## 2.2 The social model of dementia

Unlike the medical model, where the patient is the problem, the social model sees society as the problem. For example, the way society operates and the way it devalues people with mental health conditions makes it difficult for someone with dementia to lead a normal life. The social model involves understanding the experiences of living with dementia and providing care and support that meet an individual's physical, intellectual, emotional and social needs. It requires professionals to help people with dementia maintain a quality of life that is as comfortable as possible and of their own choosing.

### Research & investigate

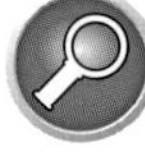

**2.2 Barriers that prevent people living a normal life**

Look around your neighbourhood, workplace, even your home, for barriers that prevent people with special needs from living as normal and comfortable a life as you. People with special needs include those with sensory impairments, physical disability, learning difficulty and mental health problems.

In the early stages of dementia, people are aware that their cognitive abilities are deteriorating. The medical model of dementia gives the professional making the diagnosis the authority to withhold information about the disease 'in the patient's best interest'. The social model says that the patient has a right to be told their diagnosis and what the future might hold as early as possible so that they can make choices about their future care. Professionals therefore need to know and be alert to the symptoms of dementia. They need to be able to make an accurate diagnosis as early as possible based on the person's strengths and skills, not on their impairments.

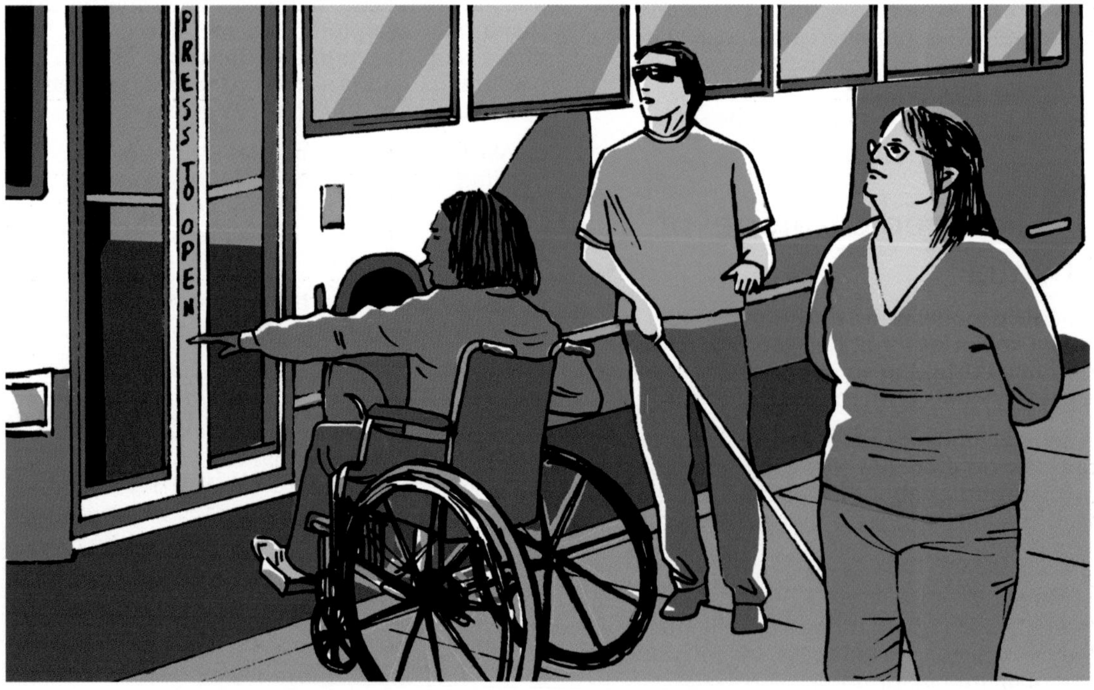


Figure 10.5 Barriers

## Time to reflect

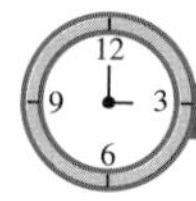

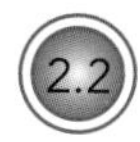

### To know or not to know … that is the question

Would you prefer to be told you have dementia or would you rather not know? If you would choose to remain ignorant, why? What do you think are the benefits of receiving a diagnosis of dementia early in its development?

The social model also requires that high-quality, **person-centred services** that enable people to adapt to and cope with their impairments should be available from the onset of dementia, throughout the illness until the end of life.

## Key term

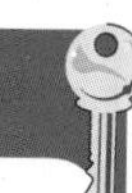

Person-centred services aim to improve a person's life by meeting their needs and involving them in the way the services are run.

## Evidence activity

### 2.1 and 2.2 The medical and social models of dementia

This activity allows you to demonstrate your knowledge of the medical and social models of dementia.

Complete the following table to show you know the main differences between the medical and social models of dementia.

| Aspects | The medical model | The social model |
|---|---|---|
| What are the health and social care needs of a person with dementia? | | |
| What is the treatment? | | |
| How should treatment be put into practice? | | |
| How does treatment impact on the person with dementia and their carers? | | |

## 2.3 Dementia as a disability

The medical model of disability sees disabled people as 'limited' by their disease or condition and treats them as inadequate. The social model of disability was developed by disabled people in response to the effect that the medical model had on their lives. For example, the **labels** 'disabled', 'limited' and 'inadequate' take no account of someone's skills and abilities; they refer only to what they can't do.

Being labelled 'disabled' and 'inadequate' also creates barriers to things that able-bodied people enjoy and take for granted, such as employment, education, housing, transport and so on. You looked at barriers earlier. In addition, it perpetuates **prejudice** and **discrimination**. Anti-discriminatory legislation is helping to remove barriers and shake off negative attitudes and discrimination but there is still a long way to go.

## Key terms

A **label** is a 'tag' that we use to describe someone and is usually based on their appearance and behavior.
A **prejudice** is an attitude or way of thinking based on an unfair pre-judgement of a person, rather than on a factual assessment.
**Discrimination** is the acting out of negative prejudices.

## Time to reflect

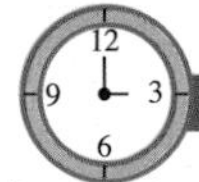

### 2.3 Do as you would be done by

- What labels and prejudices do you use and have with regard to people who have mental health problems such as dementia?
- Do you ever act out your negative prejudices? If so, what do you do?
- How would you feel if you were labelled and discriminated against because of a disease that affects your abilities and behaviour?

The social model of disability doesn't see disabled people as limited or inadequate; instead, it is the society they live and work in that limits or disables them. A simple example is that of wheelchair users. In an environment that has been adapted to their needs, for example where they can use public transport and gain access to buildings and services in the same way as an able-bodied person, they wouldn't be limited at all.

The social model of disability promotes the removal of labelling and barriers so that disabled people have the same opportunity as everyone else to decide how they live. Using the social model of disability to view people with dementia allows us to see them as individuals coping with their impairment and entitled to a quality of life and comfort of their own choosing.

www.nursingtimes.net; www.open.ac.uk

## Evidence activity

### 2.3 Dementia as a disability

This activity allows you to demonstrate your understanding of why the social model of disability should be used to view someone with dementia.

Consider the following common symptoms of dementia. Why is it good to view someone with these symptoms through the eyes of the social model of disability?

- Impaired cognitive skills, such as memory loss and an inability to communicate, think clearly, learn new things and understand.
- Depression.
- Delirium.
- Disorientation.
- Lack of physical coordination.

# LO3 The most common types of dementia and their causes

## 3.1 Common causes of dementia

As you know, dementia is a group of symptoms that are caused by certain diseases or conditions of the brain. There are over 100 different types of dementia, some of which are described below.

## Research & investigate

### 3.1 Did you know …?

Did you know that there are over 100 different types of dementia? Most people think of Alzheimer's disease when they hear the word dementia. How many people do you know – at work and in your personal life – who have Alzheimer's disease? And how many people do you know who have any other sort of dementia?

## Alzheimer's disease

This is the most common cause of dementia. It is a condition of the brain in which **plaques** and **tangles** develop, leading to the death of nerve cells. There is also a shortage of neurotransmitters. It is a progressive disease, which means that over time, more and more parts of the brain become damaged, resulting in symptoms getting more and more severe.

### Key term

Plaques are insoluble protein deposits that build up around nerve cells.
Tangles are insoluble twisted protein fibres that build up inside nerve cells.

## Vascular dementia

This is the second most common form of dementia and is triggered by blockages in the blood vessels in the brain. These blockages prevent enough blood and oxygen reaching the nerve cells, so they die. Areas of brain that have died in this way are called infarcts, so vascular dementia is also called multi-infarct dementia. It may be easier to think of vascular dementia as a series of strokes that result from other health problems, such as high blood pressure.

## Dementia with Lewy bodies (DLB)

This is a form of dementia that is similar to both Alzheimer's and Parkinson's diseases. Lewy bodies are tiny, spherical protein deposits in nerve cells. Their presence in the brain disrupts its normal functioning, including the passage of neurotransmitters. Lewy bodies are also found in the brains of people with Parkinson's disease, a progressive disease of the nervous system that affects movement. Some people who are initially diagnosed with Parkinson's disease go on to develop a dementia that closely resembles DLB.

## Fronto-temporal dementia

This covers a range of conditions, including **Pick's disease**, **frontal lobe** degeneration, and dementia associated with motor neurone disease. All are caused by damage to parts of the brain that are responsible for our behaviour, emotions and language.

### Key terms

Pick's Disease is a rare disorder that damages cells in the front part of the brain.
The frontal lobe is the front part of the brain.

## Korsakoff's syndrome

This is caused by a lack of vitamin B1 (thiamine), which damages the brain and nervous system, and is usually associated with heavy alcohol consumption over a long period of time. Alcohol can inflame the stomach lining, preventing the body from absorbing vitamin B1; and many heavy drinkers have poor eating habits, so fail to take in enough vitamin B1.

## Creutzfeldt-Jakob disease (CJD)

CJD is a type of prion disease. Prions are proteins that occur naturally on the surface of nerve cells in the brain but cause progressive brain damage if they become faulty.

## Mild cognitive impairment (MCI)

This is the term used to describe people who have some problems with cognitive abilities but whose symptoms don't yet affect their life. Identifying people with MCI is important because they can be prescribed medication to improve their symptoms and slow down the progression of dementia.

### Key term

Cognitive impairment means difficulty in carrying out cognitive abilities.

## Acquired Immune Deficiency Syndrome (AIDS)

People with AIDS sometimes develop cognitive impairment, particularly in the later stages of their illness. AIDS is caused by the presence of HIV (Human Immunodeficiency Virus) in the body. HIV attacks the body's immune system, making the person more susceptible to infection.

## Evidence activity 

###  3.1 The most common causes of dementia

This activity allows you to demonstrate your knowledge of the most common causes of dementia.

Produce a poster that identifies the most common causes of dementia. Using your experiences of people experiencing the different diseases (but remember to maintain confidentiality), illustrate your poster with brief, real life case studies of how they are affected.

##  3.2 Signs and symptoms of the most common causes of dementia

Table 10.2 Signs and symptoms of the most common causes of dementia

| Cause of dementia | Signs and symptoms |
|---|---|
| Alzheimer's disease | In the early stages, the person may be mildly forgetful, such as forgetting people's names and recent events; they may have problems finding the right words; be confused; lose interest in hobbies; have mood swings; and find it difficult to concentrate and make decisions.<br>As the disease progresses, memory loss and speech get worse; they may be confused by new surroundings and people; they may be aggressive, depressed and have trouble recognising family and friends. Day-to-day activities become difficult and they may lose their sense of time and place.<br>During the late stages, they become completely dependent on others; have difficulty eating and walking; become incontinent; and fail to recognise people and understand what's happening around and about. |
| Vascular dementia | People with vascular dementia have symptoms similar to other dementias but in particular they have problems concentrating and communicating; depression; the symptoms of a stroke, such as physical weakness or paralysis; memory problems; epileptic seizures; acute confusion; hallucinations and delusions; restlessness; wandering and getting lost; aggression; and incontinence. |
| DLB | People with DLB usually have some of the symptoms of Alzheimer's and Parkinson's diseases. They may have problems with attention and alertness, disorientation and difficulty thinking and planning ahead. They may also develop the symptoms of Parkinson's disease, for example slowness, muscle stiffness, trembling of the limbs, a shuffling walk, loss of facial expression and changes in the strength and tone of the voice.<br>Symptoms that are particular to DLB include hallucinations, sleepiness, restless, disturbed nights with confusion, nightmares and hallucinations; and a tendency to faint, fall, or have 'funny turns'. |

*Contd.*

| Cause of dementia | Signs and symptoms |
|---|---|
| Fronto-temporal dementia | Initially, people with fronto-temporal dementia experience personality and behaviour changes. For example, they start to lose the ability to empathise with others, which makes them appear selfish and unfeeling; become extrovert when they were previously introverted, or withdrawn when they were previously outgoing; behave inappropriately, for example, making tactless comments, joking at the 'wrong' moments, or being rude; lose their inhibitions, for example, sexual behaviour in public; become aggressive; and develop routines, for example, compulsive rituals. They may have language difficulties, such as finding the right words, starting conversations, using many words to describe something simple, or speak less and less. They may overeat or develop a liking for sweet foods.<br>In the later stages, symptoms become similar to Alzheimer's disease. |
| Korsakoff's syndrome | The main symptom is memory loss, particularly of things that happened after the onset of the condition. Other symptoms include difficulty in learning new information and skills; personality changes, from apathy through to talkative and repetitive behaviour; not realising that they have the condition; and **confabulation.** |
| CJD | Initially there are changes in personality, depression and loss of interest in life. As the condition progresses, there may be confusion, memory loss, anxiety, delusions, hallucinations, loss of coordination and balance, jerkiness, difficulty seeing or hearing, speech loss, paralysis and incontinence. Eventually, people with CJD go into a coma and are likely to die of an infection such as pneumonia. |
| MCI | People with MCI can manage their day-to-day activities. They have a good long-term memory but difficulty remembering recent events or new information. |
| AIDS | Symptoms of cognitive impairment resulting from AIDS include forgetfulness; problems with language and concentration; a 'drunken gait' – clumsiness and unsteadiness; jerky eye movements; personality changes; inappropriate emotional responses; mood swings; hallucinations; and loss of appetite. |

www.bupa.co.uk; www.alzheimers.org.uk

## Key term

**Confabulation** means inventing events to fill the gaps in memory.

## Evidence activity

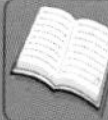

### 3.2 Signs and symptoms of the most common causes of dementia

This activity allows you to demonstrate your knowledge of the signs and symptoms of the most common causes of dementia.

Produce a set of memory cards to which your colleagues can refer if they are concerned that anyone they work with may be developing one of the dementias. Each card should state which type of dementia it refers to and describe the signs and symptoms most associated with the dementia concerned.

## Risk factors for dementia

### Time to reflect

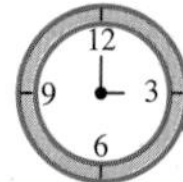

#### What do you know?

The media is awash with suggestions outlining what to do and what to avoid doing if you want to delay the onset of dementia. What do you remember of these suggestions? How do you think they might work?

### Evidence activity

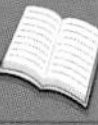

#### Risk factors for the most common causes of dementia

This activity allows you to demonstrate your knowledge of the risk factors for the most common causes of dementia.

Look at the case notes or personal histories of two or three people who you know have dementia. Find out whether they were – and continue to be – exposed to any of the risk factors in Figure 10.6. Present your findings to your colleagues, to raise their awareness of the factors that increase the risk of developing dementia.

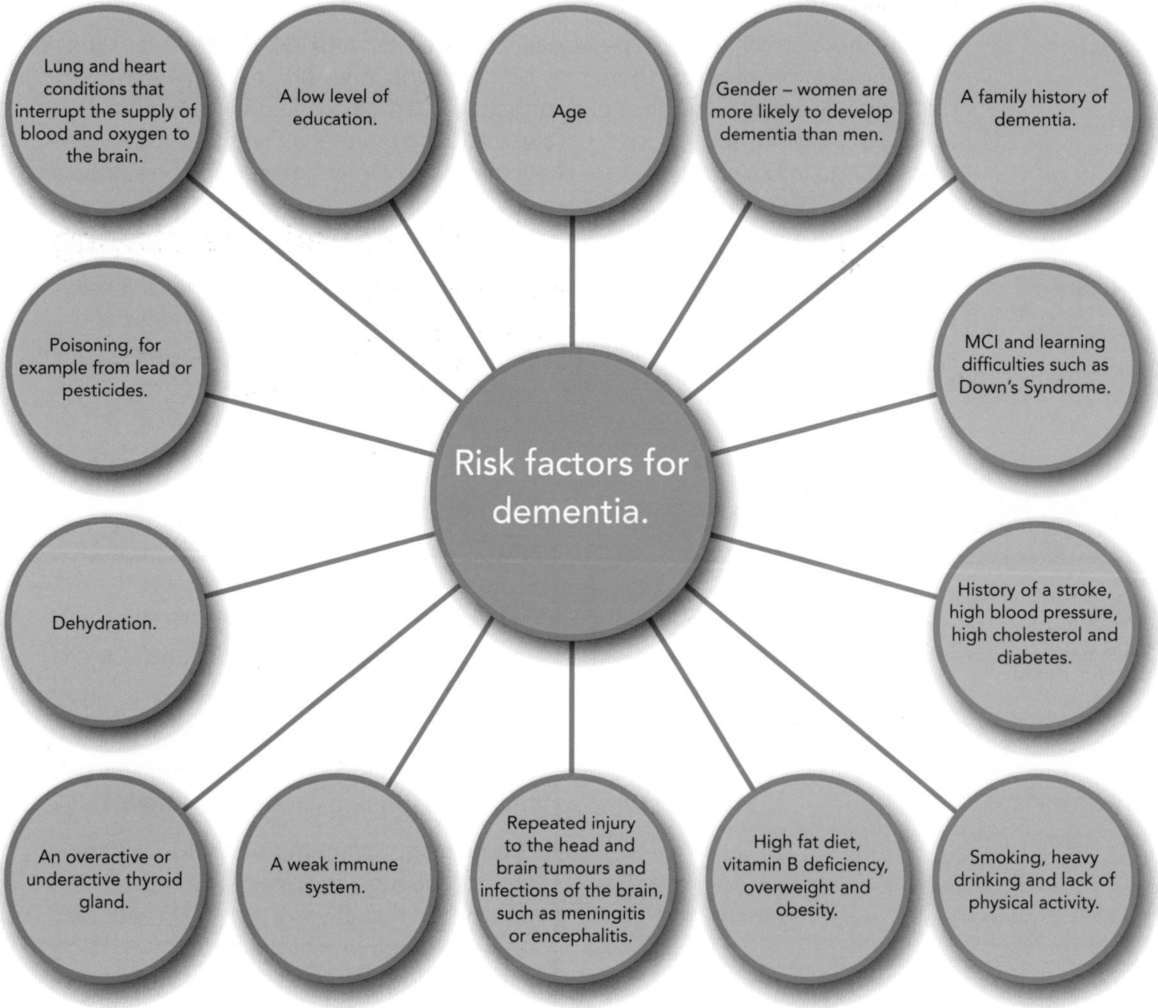

Risk factors for dementia.

- Lung and heart conditions that interrupt the supply of blood and oxygen to the brain.
- A low level of education.
- Age
- Gender – women are more likely to develop dementia than men.
- A family history of dementia.
- Poisoning, for example from lead or pesticides.
- MCI and learning difficulties such as Down's Syndrome.
- Dehydration.
- History of a stroke, high blood pressure, high cholesterol and diabetes.
- An overactive or underactive thyroid gland.
- A weak immune system.
- Repeated injury to the head and brain tumours and infections of the brain, such as meningitis or encephalitis.
- High fat diet, vitamin B deficiency, overweight and obesity.
- Smoking, heavy drinking and lack of physical activity.

Figure 10.6 Risk factors for dementia

www.nhs.uk

## 3.4 Prevalence rates for different types of dementia

There are currently 700,000 people with dementia in the UK.

- About 75 per cent of people with dementia have either Alzheimer's disease, vascular dementia or a combination of the two.
- 10 per cent of people with dementia have DLB.
- Approximately 2 per cent of people with dementia have Korsakoff's syndrome.
- During the period January to October 2010, 111 people were suspected of carrying CJD and 43 had died from the infection.
- Two thirds of people with dementia are women.
- There are over 11,500 people with dementia from black and minority ethnic groups in the UK.
- There are currently 15,000 younger people (under 65) with dementia in the UK.
- About 3 per cent of men and women between the ages of 65 and 74 have dementia.
- The proportion of people aged 85 and older with dementia is between 25 and 35 per cent.
- One third of people over 95 have dementia.
- There will be over a million people with dementia by 2025 and over 1.75 million by 2050.
- 60,000 deaths a year are directly attributable to dementia but delaying its onset by 5 years would reduce deaths directly attributable to dementia by 30,000 a year.
- The financial cost of dementia to the UK is over £17 billion a year but family carers of people with dementia save the UK over £6 billion a year.
- Two thirds of people with dementia live in the community, one third live in a care home and 64 per cent of people living in care homes have a form of dementia.

**http://alzheimers.org.uk; www.bgs.org.uk; www.alzheimers-research.org.uk; www.cjd.ed.ac.uk; www.hpa.org.uk; www.nhsdirect.wales.nhs.uk**

### Evidence activity 

#### 3.4 Prevalence rates for different types of dementia

This activity allows you to demonstrate your ability to identify the prevalence rate for different types of dementia.

Using an internet search engine such as Google, specialist journals, the press and reports produced by providers of health and social care services within your Local Authority, find out the prevalence rates for different types of dementia in the area covered by your Local Authority and for the UK as a whole.

# LO4 Factors relating to an individual's experience of dementia

## 4.1 The experience of living with dementia

The experience of living with dementia varies according to people's age, the type of dementia they have and their level of ability and disability.

> 'I have lost handling things like knives and forks.' (Person with dementia)
>
> 'I rely greatly on my wife and my carers … I'd be in terrible trouble without them.' (Person with dementia)
>
> 'He used to be an engineer and he was very precise in everything he did, and now when he gets problems doing things he gets very frustrated. Very frustrated. He gets angry and he'll shout at me, "I never used to be like this."' (Carer)
>
> **Living Well With Dementia: A National Dementia Strategy, Department of Health, 2009**

## Research & investigate 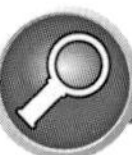

 Living with dementia

Think about the people you know who have been diagnosed with dementia. What skills and abilities do they still have? What skills and abilities have they lost?

As you know, the incidence of dementia increases with increasing age. Being diagnosed with dementia at any age is distressing, but particularly so for younger people who are still working, who have dependent family and financial commitments, such as a mortgage, and who value their relationships and physical and **intellectual fitness**. As you read above, there are currently 15,000 people under 65 with dementia in the UK. Their dementia is often referred to as 'early onset dementia', 'young onset dementia' or 'working age dementia'. Because most of us think of dementia as something that only affects older people, there is little public and professional awareness and understanding of early onset dementia and this can make it difficult for younger people with dementia to access appropriate support.

## Key term

Intellectual fitness means being open to new ideas, thinking critically, being creative and curious, and being motivated to learning new things.

Many dementia care services have a minimum age requirement of 65 and aren't available to younger people. Where services are open to younger users, they may not be appropriate to their needs. For example, younger people have different interests and abilities from older people and activities planned for older people are unlikely to meet the needs of a younger generation.

## Research & investigate 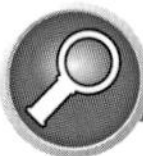

 Services for people with dementia

Check out the services provided within your local community for people with dementia.

What age groups do they cater for? What services and activities do they offer? Do they support carers of people with dementia? How do you think they could be improved?

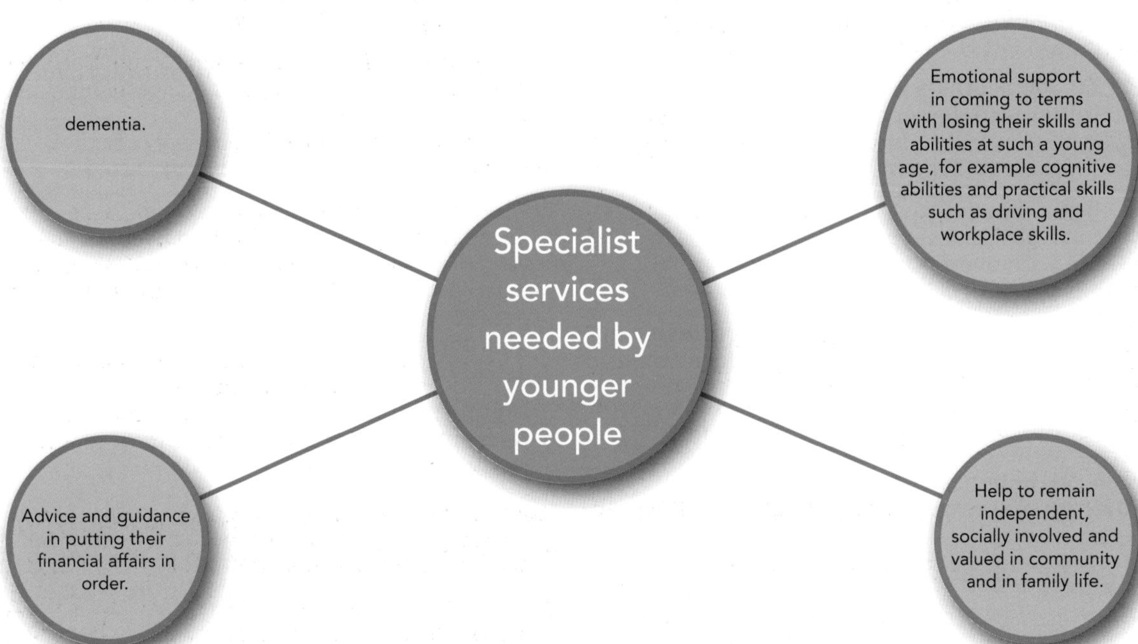


Figure 10.7 Specialist services needed by younger people with dementia

The lack of awareness and understanding of dementia, especially early onset dementia, can also make getting a diagnosis difficult. Medical professionals often misdiagnose younger people as being depressed or as suffering from the effects of stress. The author Terry Pratchett was 59 when he was diagnosed with Alzheimer's disease but prior to this he had been told by one specialist that he was too young to have Alzheimer's (www.dailymail.co.uk). This means that younger people with dementia receive very different levels of support from different doctors and professionals.

> 'We had an appointment with the local GP anyway, over a different matter, and while I was there I said, you know, I told him the symptoms and he pooh-poohed it.' (Person with dementia)
>
> **Living Well With dementia: A National Dementia Strategy, Department of Health, 2009**

Living with dementia at any age puts a strain on the relationship between the individual and their family. It can affect the sexual feelings and needs of both the person with dementia and their partner, and the person with dementia may lose their sexual inhibitions and behave in ways that are embarrassing to others and which confuse and distress themselves. Children and young people can be anxious and upset by their parent's changing behaviour, and caring for someone with dementia puts a strain on the carer's physical and emotional health. In addition, the impact of diagnosis can take the wind out of the family's sails, especially if they attach a stigma to the diagnosis. And it can devastate their quality of life, especially if the individual concerned is still the main breadwinner.

## Research & investigate

### 4.1 The impact of dementia on carers

Talk to two or three of the people you support who have dementia and their partners and children. Find out how dementia has impacted on each person, for example their lifestyle, relationships, health and career.

> 'I could cope with him in the day. I couldn't cope at night. Without sleep it was hopeless. I was on the verge. I said to the doctor, "If I don't kill him, I'll kill myself". That's how bad it was.' (Carer)

> 'My son is looking but he doesn't know me; my daughter ... never mentions it.' (Person with dementia)
>
> **Living Well With Dementia: A National Dementia Strategy, Department of Health, 2009**

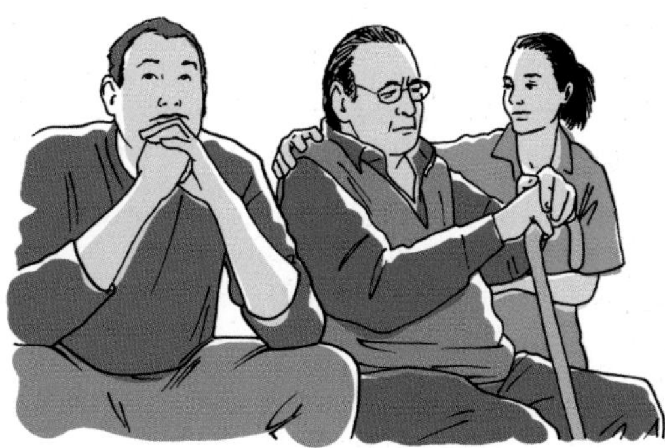

Figure 10.8 Living with dementia

The experience someone has of living with dementia depends on the area of their brain that is affected. For example, Alzheimer's disease can be caused by brain damage to the following:

- Front of the brain (frontal lobe). Damage here results in lethargy and a loss of motivation; an inability to plan and learn new things; **perseveration** such as picking at something or repeatedly folding a cloth; inappropriate behaviour, such as swearing and undressing in public; and so on. The front of the brain is also associated with personality, so damage to this area can alter personality, which is why someone with Alzheimer's disease is often not the person you used to know.
- Top area of the brain (parietal lobe). Damage here results in an inability to communicate, read and write, use numbers, perceive things normally, and recognise faces, surroundings and objects.
- Sides of the brain (temporal lobes). Damage to these areas affects the ability to take in new knowledge, hold on to it and retrieve it when we need it. The upshot is that we lose our short-term memory.
- Visual area (occipital lobe) at the back of the brain. Damage here can result in visual hallucinations and an inability to recognise objects. This explains why objects are not seen and understood correctly.

## Key term

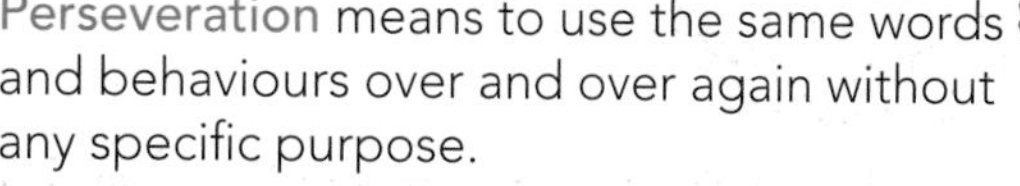

Perseveration means to use the same words and behaviours over and over again without any specific purpose.

DLB is caused when neurotransmitters fail to pass across synapses. The symptoms of DLB include those of Parkinson's disease – slowness, muscle stiffness, trembling of the limbs, a shuffling walk and loss of facial expression. You read earlier that DLB is characterised by the presence of Lewy bodies. These tiny spherical proteins are also found in the brain cells of people with Parkinson's disease and their presence disrupts the passage of the neurotransmitter called dopamine across synapses. Because dopamine is involved in the control of movement, its failure to pass between nerve cells results in the disabling symptoms of Parkinson's disease, which greatly affect the experience of someone living with DLB.

www.alzheimers.org.uk; www.parkinsonsawareness.eu.com; http://alzheimers.about.com

The experience someone has of living with dementia also depends on their level of ability and disability. People who have a learning disability are at greater risk of developing dementia as they get older. Whilst dementia affects them no differently from anyone else, there is a chance that the early stages may be missed because the individual concerned has difficulty communicating how their abilities have changed.

Studies have shown that all people with Down's syndrome develop the plaques and tangles associated with Alzheimer's disease. However, not all people with Down's syndrome develop the symptoms of Alzheimer's disease. The reason for this remains unexplained. People with other types of learning disability are also at risk of developing dementia and this is thought to be due to genetic factors or to brain damage.

Researchers in Sweden have discovered that education not only delays the early symptoms of dementia, it can also slow down its development. They found that educated people have less nerve damage during the early stages of dementia and tolerate more brain disease than less educated people. And according to British and French researchers, increasing education, eliminating depression and diabetes, and increasing fruit and vegetable consumption could lead to a huge reduction in new cases of dementia.

www.alzheimers.org.uk; www.alphagalileo.org; www.bbc.co.uk

## 4.2 The impact of attitudes and behaviours on people with dementia

You read earlier that there is often a stigma attached to dementia, as there is to other mental health conditions. For this reason, unless they are well supported, many people and their carers struggle socially and emotionally after a diagnosis. As Terry Pratchett said 'It is a strange life when you "come out". People get embarrassed, lower their voices, get lost for words.' And 'It seems that when you have cancer you are a brave battler against the disease, but when you have Alzheimer's you are an old fart. That's how people see you. It makes you feel quite alone.'

### Evidence activity

### 4.1 Factors that affect the experience of living with dementia

This activity allows you to demonstrate your knowledge of how different people experience living with dementia.

Complete the following table.

| Factor | How each factor can affect an individual's experience of living with dementia |
|---|---|
| Their age | |
| The type of dementia they have | |
| Their level of ability | |
| Their level of disability | |

## Research & investigate 

### 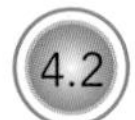 How did they feel?

Talk to people you know who have dementia. Find out how they felt when they were first diagnosed. How did their partners, family, friends feel?

'(The consultant) said it's dementia and I just burst into tears because I was so … I half expected it but it's still a terrible shock.' (Carer)

'You are just as likely of getting dementia as you are getting a haemotoma or lung cancer or whatever else. If there was that sort of attitude by society, then this would make the whole process … easier. So you know it is all part of the stigma, isn't it?' (Person with dementia)

**Living Well With Dementia: A National Dementia Strategy, Department of Health, 2009**

People who attach a stigma to dementia have a negative attitude to both the disease and the people who are living with it. They are prejudiced and their behaviour is often discriminatory.

## Time to reflect 

### 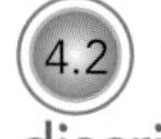 Dealing with prejudice and discrimination

You were asked to reflect on your prejudices and discriminatory behaviour earlier on. This time, think about how your friends, family and colleagues behave toward people with mental health conditions such as dementia. If they entertain negative attitudes or behave in discriminatory ways, why do you think this is? How could you help change their thinking and behaviour?

People are prejudiced against dementia because they don't know about the condition, don't understand the effects it has on the individuals concerned and are embarrassed or apprehensive. Misunderstandings and assumptions they have include that people with dementia are:

- dangerous
- unpredictable
- hard to talk with

Table 10.3 Prejudice and discrimination against dementia in society

| Where does prejudice and discrimination against dementia exist? | How is prejudice and discrimination against dementia shown? |
|---|---|
| The family | Family members are often embarrassed by or ashamed of their demented relative. |
| The community | The community is often superstitious of a person's unexpected, 'abnormal' behaviour and excludes them as a result. |
| The workplace | People in the workplace see an individual's declining abilities as 'inadequacies' that signal the need to remove them from employment. |
| Within public authorities and private organisations | Because people in public authorities and private organisations lack knowledge and understanding about the needs and abilities of people with dementia, they create barriers to their ability to access health and social care services, employment, education, housing, transport, leisure facilities, financial services and so on. |
| The media | The media, for example, TV, radio, newspapers and magazines, which continue to show people with dementia as inadequate and uncontrolled, ignoring the skills and abilities they retain. |

- have only themselves to blame for their condition
- will not improve with treatment
- could pull themselves together if they wanted.

And if people discriminate against a person with dementia, they treat them with suspicion and are intolerant of their behaviour.

Prejudice and discrimination, particularly in the early stages of the dementia, is emotionally destructive. It is cruel and humiliating, singles people out as being different and takes away any self-confidence and self-worth they have left. And unless support networks and appropriate services are in place, a further decline in memory and cognitive abilities causes people to withdraw and become socially isolated.

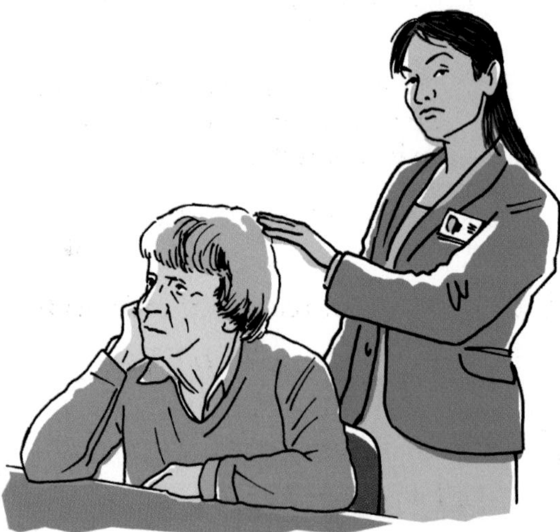

Figure 10.9 Discriminatory behaviour

You might be surprised to read that providers of health and social care services can also be guilty of prejudice and discriminatory behaviour. You read earlier that many medical professionals have little knowledge and understanding of dementia. They continue to dismiss the symptoms of dementia as depression, absent-mindedness or preoccupation, which has knock on effects on the provision of appropriate, high-quality, person-centred services.

> 'I consider that I didn't get a service from, not my doctor, my own GP. From my own GP I just got patted on the head.' (Person with dementia)
>
> **Living Well With Dementia: A National Dementia Strategy, Department of Health, 2009**

There is a wealth of health and social care workers supporting people with dementia. In addition to GPs, there are social workers and social care workers; nurses, including community, mental health and psychiatric nurses; psychologists and psychiatrists; pharmacists; physio, occupational and speech and language therapists; Dementia Care Advisors; advocates, support groups and, of course, carers – family, friends and so on. Good practice dictates that professionals and the general public become increasingly well-informed about dementia and the impact it has on the people living with it. Only when this is achieved can the fear, stigma and false beliefs associated with dementia be put to bed and people enabled to live well with their condition.

## Research & investigate 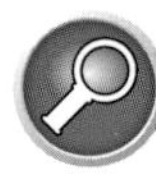

### 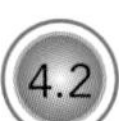 4.2 Workplace discrimination

Discrimination is illegal but will continue to take place until people shake off their negative attitudes. Find out how your workplace deals with discrimination against the people it helps and supports.

## Evidence activity 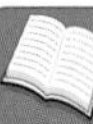

###  4.2 The impact of attitudes and behaviours on people who have dementia

This activity allows you to demonstrate your knowledge of the impact of attitudes and behaviours on people who have dementia.

Produce an information sheet for colleagues and visitors to your workplace that:

- lists the negative attitudes that people have about dementia and the discriminatory ways in which they behave as a result
- describes the impact that negative attitudes and discriminatory behaviour have on people who have dementia.

## Assessment summary

Your reading of this chapter and completion of the activities will have improved your knowledge and understanding of dementia.

To achieve the unit, your assessor will require you to:

| Learning Outcomes | Assessment Criteria |
|---|---|
| Learning outcome 1: Show you understand what dementia is by: | 1.1 explaining what is meant by the term 'dementia'<br>See Evidence activity 1.1, p.165 |
| | 1.2 describing the key functions of the brain that are affected by dementia<br>See Evidence activity 1.2, p.167 |
| | 1.3 explaining why depression, delirium and age related memory impairment may be mistaken for dementia.<br>See Evidence activity 1.3, p.169 |
| Learning outcome 2: Understand key features of the theoretical models of dementia by: | 2.1 outlining the medical model of dementia<br>See Evidence activity 2.1, p.171 |
| | 2.2 outlining the social model of dementia<br>See Evidence activity 2.2, p.171 |
| | 2.3 explaining why dementia should be viewed as a disability.<br>See Evidence activity 2.3, p.172 |
| Learning outcome 3: Know the most common types of dementia and their causes by: | 3.1 listing the most common causes of dementia<br>See Evidence activity 3.1, p.174 |
| | 3.2 describing the likely signs and symptoms of the most common causes of dementia<br>See Evidence activity 3.2, p.175 |
| | 3.3 outlining the risk factors for the most common causes of dementia<br>See Evidence activity 3.3, p.176 |

| Learning Outcomes | Assessment Criteria |
|---|---|
| Learning outcome 3: Know the most common types of dementia and their causes by: | 3.4 identifying prevalence rates for different types of dementia.<br>See Evidence activity 3.4, p.177 |
| Learning outcome 4: Understand factors relating to an individual's experience of dementia by: | 4.1 describing how different individuals may experience living with dementia depending on age, type of dementia, and level of ability and disability<br>See Evidence activity 4.1, p.180 |
| | 4.2 outlining the impact that the attitudes and behaviours of others may have on an individual with dementia.<br>See Evidence activity 4.2, p.182 |

Good luck!

## Weblinks

| | |
|---|---|
| The Alzheimer's Society | www.alzheimers.org.uk |
| BBC website | www.bbc.co.uk |
| Mental Health Foundation | www.mentalhealth.org.uk |
| Mental help website | www.mentalhelp.net |
| Nursing Times | www.nursingtimes.net |
| Open University | www.open.ac.uk |
| BUPA, Health information | www.bupa.co.uk |
| NHS website | www.nhs.uk |
| British Geriatrics Society | www.bgs.org.uk |
| Alzheimer's Research Trust | www.alzheimers-research.org.uk |
| The National Creutzfeldt-Jakob Disease Surveillance Unit | www.cjd.ed.ac.uk |
| Health Protection Agency | www.hpa.org.uk |
| NHS Direct, Wales | www.nhsdirect.wales.nhs.uk |
| European Parkinson's Awareness Association | www.parkinsonsawareness.eu.com |
| Alzheimer's Disease | http://alzheimers.about.com |
| Source of news about research | www.alphagalileo.org |

# 11 Understand the context of supporting individuals with learning disabilities

## For Unit LD201

### What are you finding out?

According to **mencap** there are around 1.5 million people who have a learning disability within the United Kingdom. Due to advances in health and social care and the fact that people are living longer, this figure is due to increase. One of the biggest problems for people who have learning disabilities is that other people generally don't understand what it means for someone to have a learning disability. A learning disability is not an illness or a disease, and it is not always possible to tell if a person has a learning disability. Having a learning disability does not mean a person has mental health problems, however some people who have a learning disability may develop mental health problems as a result of inadequate care and discrimination.

Learning disability is not what defines a person. It is merely a label used to diagnose people who have a learning disability. People with learning disabilities are all individuals with the right to the same life chances as other people. These people are individuals just like you and me.

The reading and activities in this chapter will help you to:

- Understand the legislation and policies that support the human rights and inclusion of individuals with learning disabilities
- Understand the nature and characteristics of learning disability
- Understand the historical context of learning disability
- Understand the basic principles and practice of advocacy, empowerment and active participation in relation to supporting individuals with learning disabilities and their families
- Understand how views and attitudes impact on the lives of individuals with learning disabilities and their family carers
- Know how to promote communication with individuals with learning disabilities

#### Key term

**Mencap** is the leading UK charity for people who have a learning disability and their families.

## LO1 Understand the legislation and policies that support the human rights and inclusion of individuals with learning disabilities

### 1.1 Identify legislation and policies that are designed to promote the human rights, inclusion, equal life chances and citizenship of individuals with learning disabilities

Most of the laws which concern people who have a learning disability also apply to other people. The main laws that are likely to make a difference to the lives of people who have learning disabilities are concerned with promoting:

- human rights
- anti-discriminatory behaviour
- equality
- inclusion citizenship.

## Key terms

**Citizenship** relates to being a citizen of a particular community with the duties, rights and privileges of this status.

**Equality** relates to being equal, especially of having the same political, social and economic rights.

**Inclusion** is a state of being free from exclusion.

Legislation aimed at promoting the human rights, inclusion, equal life chances and citizenship of individuals with learning disabilities include:

- The Human Rights Act 1998
- The Disability Discrimination Act 1995
- The Mental Capacity Act 2005
- The Equality Act 2010.

Valuing People Now is the UK Government's strategy for making the lives of people with learning disabilities and their families better by improving services. In particular, the strategy aims to make significant improvements in giving adults who have learning disabilities more choice and control over their lives through person-centred planning, advocacy and direct payments. You can find out more about Valuing People Now at www.valuingpeoplenow.dh.gov.uk.

## Key term

The **direct payments scheme** is a UK government initiative in the field of Social Services that gives service users money directly to pay for their own care, rather than through the traditional route of a Local Government Authority providing care for them.

**Person-centred planning** is a process of life planning for individuals, based around the principles of inclusion and the social model of disability.

Organisations that provide support for people who have learning disabilities should have policies in place which aim to reinforce this legislation. These policies set out the guidelines that all health and social care workers have to adhere to in order to ensure people who have learning disabilities are given the same opportunities as any other member of society.

## Evidence activity

### 1.1 Legislation and policies that are designed to promote the rights of individuals who have learning disabilities

This activity allows you to demonstrate your knowledge of the legislation and policies that are designed to promote the human rights, inclusion, equal life chances and citizenship of individuals who have learning disabilities.

Take a look at the policies within your place of work and make a note of any policies which promote human rights, inclusion, equal life chances and citizenship for the service users for whom you provide support.

How do the policies support these aspects of a person's life?

## 1.2 Explain how legislation and policies influence the day-to-day experiences of individuals with learning disabilities and their families

Policies are drawn up in line with current legislation. Policies can be drawn up nationally at governmental level and also locally at an organisational level. Policy makers can influence important decisions that affect people's everyday lives. We have already established that there are around 1.5 million people who have a learning disability in the UK, so all policies will affect these people in some way.

Policies should be based on the social model of disability, aimed at empowering people. People who have a learning disability are the experts in their own lives and their views are an essential part of any evidence base. Involving these people throughout the process of policy development will help identify gaps in knowledge and give an indication of whether the policy will work in the short and long term. Understanding the perspective, needs and priorities of people who have learning disabilities will help in the development of better policies and the delivery of effective services.

## Evidence activity 

### 1.2 How legislation and policies influence the day-to-day experiences of individuals who have learning disabilities and their families

This activity allows you to demonstrate your knowledge of the legislation and policies that influence the day-to-day experiences of individuals with learning disabilities and their families.

Think about the legislation and policies that are relevant to the people you support. How do legislation and associated policies influence the day-to-day experiences of these people and their families?

# LO2 Understand the nature and characteristics of learning disability

## 2.1 Explain what is meant by 'learning disability'

### Research & investigate 

#### 2.1 What is a learning disability

Think about the service users you support. How would you define their learning disability?

Defining the term 'learning disability' is not easy, because it does not have clear cut edges. No two people have the same level of 'ability' in the way they learn, and every person's experience of their learning disability will be individual to them.

In medical terms learning disabilities are known as **neurological disorders**. In simple terms, a learning disability may result when a person's brain development is affected, either before they are born, during their birth or in early childhood.

### Key term

**Neurological disorders** are disorders of the brain.

Learning disabilities are lifelong conditions that cannot be cured, and they can have a significant impact on the person's life. People with learning disabilities find it harder than other people to learn, understand and communicate. Some people with a mild learning disability may be able to communicate effectively and look after themselves, but may take a bit longer than usual to learn new skills. Others may not be able to communicate at all and may also have more than one disability. You may have heard a person's learning disability described as mild, moderate, severe or profound. If you hear these terms being used, it is important to remember that they are not separate compartments, they are simply stages along the scale of ability/disability.

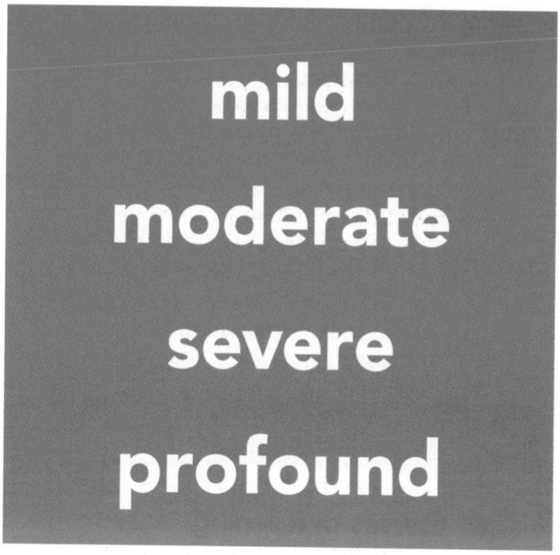

mild

moderate

severe

profound

Figure 11.1 Continuum of ability/disability

## Evidence activity 

### 2.1 Explain what is meant by 'learning disability'

This activity allows you to demonstrate your knowledge of what is meant by the term 'learning disability'.

How would you explain what the term 'learning disability' means to a new member of staff within your organisation?

## 2.2 Give examples of causes of learning disabilities

Learning disabilities are caused by the way the brain develops, either before, during or after birth. There are several factors that can affect the development of the brain.

### Before birth (pre-natal)

- Causes affecting the mother, for example rubella (German measles), excessive intake of alcohol, tobacco, recreational drugs and listeria (food poisoning).
- A child can also be born with a learning disability if certain genes are passed on by a parent. This is called an inherited learning disability. The two most common causes of inherited learning disability are Fragile X syndrome and Down's syndrome. Fragile X syndrome and Down's syndrome are not learning disabilities, but people who have either condition are likely to have a learning disability too. Fragile X syndrome is the most common cause of inherited learning disability, but not all people with Fragile X syndrome have a learning disability. All people who have Down's syndrome have some kind of learning disability.

### During birth (peri-natal)

- The most common cause includes problems during the birth that stop enough oxygen getting to the brain.

**Evidence activity** 

**Causes of learning disabilities**

This activity allows you to demonstrate your knowledge of the causes of learning disabilities.

Think about the service users you are supporting at the moment and, whilst respecting confidentiality, using any information that is available to you, identify the cause of their learning disabilities. Where on the continuum of learning disabilities do your service users sit?

### After birth (post-natal) or during childhood

- Illness, such as meningitis, or injury in early childhood.

Sometimes there is no known cause for a learning disability. There is a lot of information about particular syndromes and conditions. Check out the useful weblinks at the end of this chapter.

## 2.3 Describe the medical and social models of disability

**Time to reflect** 

**How do you feel about disability?**

It is important at this stage to examine how you feel about people who have a disability.

Think about the assumptions that are commonly made about people who have a disability in general. In a few words, what would you say are common assumptions often made about this section of the population? For example, would you say 'they need help?' or would you say you 'feel sorry for them?' or would you say 'people are disabled because of their environment?'.

Models of disability provide a framework for understanding the way in which people with impairments experience their disability. It is commonly accepted that there are two contrasting models of disability within our society. These are known as the 'medical model' and the 'social model'.

The medical model views the person who has a disability as the problem. This model holds the belief that the person who has a disability should adapt to fit in with society. If the person cannot fit in with society then it is their problem. The emphasis is on dependence which is backed up by the stereotypes of disability that lend themselves to pity, fear and patronising attitudes. The main focus is on the disability rather than the person.

The medical model highlights that people who are disabled cannot participate in society because their disability prevents them from doing so.

- You should not have relationships, you will never have a job, you are ill, you cannot do anything, you do not need an education, you can't walk properly, you need help
- You can't play sport, you need carers

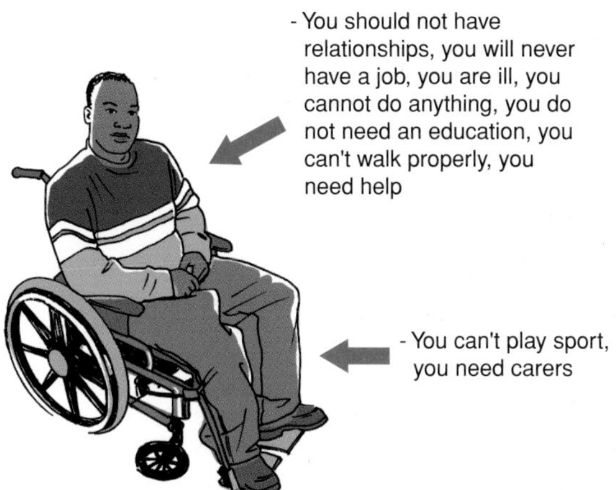

Figure 11.2 The medical model of disability

The social model of disability was developed with the input of people who have a disability. Instead of emphasising the disability, the social model centralises the person. It emphasises dignity, independence, choice and privacy.

This model makes an important distinction between impairment and disability.

Impairment is seen as something not working properly with part of the body, mind or senses, for example, a person may have a physical impairment, a sensory impairment or a learning impairment.

Disability occurs when a person is excluded by society, because of their impairment, from something that other people in society take for granted. That might be the chance to attend an event, access a service or get involved in an activity. The exclusion may affect a person's choices to live independently, to earn a living, to be kept informed, or just to make choices for themselves.

The social model of disability says that disabilities are created by barriers in society. These barriers generally fall into three categories, these are:

- The environment – including inaccessible buildings and services.
- Attitudes – including discrimination, prejudice and stereotyping.
- Organisations – including inflexible policies, practices and procedures.

Some people wrongly assume that the impairment causes the disability. However, the social model believes that it is the choices society makes that creates the disability. If things are organised differently, these people are suddenly enabled – though their impairment hasn't changed.

Everyone Welcome

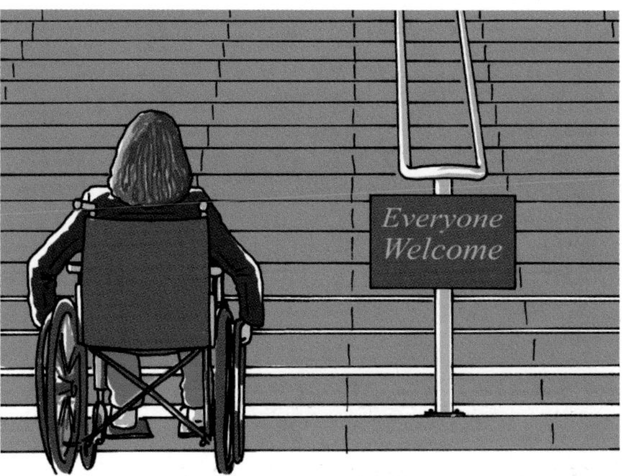

Figure 11.3 The social model of disability

**Evidence activity** 

**2.3 The medical and social models of disability**

This activity allows you to demonstrate your knowledge of the medical and social models of disability.

Look at the assumptions you made within the Time to reflect box. Would you say your beliefs support the medical model of disability or the social model of disability?

Take a look at the environment in which you work – are there any aspects of the environment that could disable a person? If so, what changes could be made to make the environment more enabling?

## 2.4 State the approximate proportion of individuals with a learning disability for whom the cause is 'not known'

There are a number of reasons for finding out the cause of a person's learning disability. Firstly, individuals and their families want to know and also have a right to know. There are also health factors as some forms of learning disability or syndromes can increase the likelihood of certain health problems occurring. Genetic counselling may also be required both for the family and for the person with the learning disability, especially where there is a wish to start a family.

We have identified some of the causes of learning disability within section 2.2, however, the British Institute of learning Disabilities (BILD) identifies that amongst people who have a mild learning disability, in about 50 per cent of cases no cause has been identified. In people who have severe or profound learning disabilities, cases which are of unknown cause are fewer, but still high at around 25 per cent.

**Evidence activity** 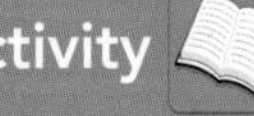

**2.4 The proportion of individuals with a learning disability for whom the cause is not known**

This activity allows you to demonstrate your knowledge of the approximate proportion of individuals who have a learning disability for whom the cause is not known.

Think about the service users you support. Do any of them have a learning disability for which the cause has never been identified?

How do your findings compare to those identified by BILD?

## 2.5 Describe the possible impact on a family of having a member with a learning disability

Over 60 per cent of people with learning disabilities live with family carers who often sacrifice their own lives in order to support the person.

Family members who provide care for those with a learning disability can suffer immense emotional and physical strain, and respite from their role can be made difficult by the adverse effects it can have on the person they are caring for.

While every family can have stresses and strains, these are very often exacerbated in families where a member of the family has a learning disability. Depending on the family members, the amount of support they receive, and the person who has the learning disability, this can impact on every aspect of the families needs, including economic needs, domestic needs, healthcare needs, relationship needs and self-identity needs. This can also impact on other aspects of family life leading to significant extra costs and complications.

A child who does not have a learning disability will usually mature and become more independent, eventually leaving the family home. A child with a learning disability, however, may not follow this pattern, and is more likely to remain within the family home into adulthood. This person may also require prolonged periods of intensive care. This could impact upon everyday occurrences such as family outings, which could become complicated or even impossible.

**Evidence activity** 

**2.5 The impact on a family of having a member with a learning disability**

This activity allows you to demonstrate your knowledge of the impact on a family of having a member with a learning disability.

Choose two service users for who you provide support and, whilst maintaining confidentiality, develop a case study for the two service users. For the two service users, identify the impact that their learning disability has had on other members of their family members, taking into account the:

- economic impact
- relationship impact
- domestic impact
- social impact
- self-identity impact
- healthcare implications.

# LO3 Understand the historical context of learning disability

## 3.1 Explain the types of services that have been provided for individuals with learning disabilities over time

Little is written about the lives of people with learning disabilities before the eighteenth century. There are however references to 'village idiots'. It is thought that these people represent a small minority of the people we would describe today as having a learning disability. Literacy skills were less in demand than labouring skills, so mild learning disabilities would easily go unnoticed.

The Poor Laws of 1834 led to the building of purpose built institutions called 'asylums' to house people described as 'mad' or 'mentally weak'. These were workhouses with harsh and rigid regimes, and contained many people who had learning disabilities. These people had little choice and were not valued as people. The asylums became overcrowded, and conditions worsened as attitudes changed and the people who were housed there began to be regarded as dangerous and a drain on society.

The development of institutions continued into the early 20th century, though the purpose of moving people to institutions changed. Laws were passed that encouraged the building of schools for 'mentally disabled' children, and in 1908 the Radner Commission stated that: 'Feeble-mindedness is largely inherited'. It was suggested that such people were genetically inferior and needed to be segregated from the rest of society.

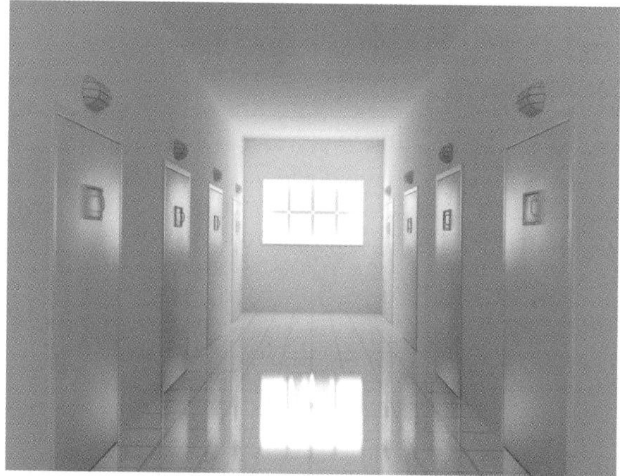

Figure 11.4 Institutionalisation

The 1913 Mental Deficiency Act stated that any person admitted to an institution had to be certified as 'mentally defective'. The institutions were now renamed 'colonies', and their purpose was to separate their residents from society. In 1929, the Wood Committee suggested that such people were a threat to society.

During the periods between the two World Wars, the numbers of people admitted to institutions increased. Laws were passed to further segregate all people who had learning disabilities and their families from the rest of society. Proposals were introduced to round up and separate all families of 'feeble minded people', including 'insane, epileptics and drunks', to name but a few.

It was suggested that such people would 'take over' and 'infect' others and that a 'racial disaster' would ensue. Cyril Birt was a member of the Eugenics' Society, a group that believed there was a problem of 'degeneracy' in society and that there was a need to separate those with learning disabilities, keeping men and women apart so they would not procreate. History shows that the theories of eugenics have justified many atrocities committed against people with a learning disability and the mentally ill, as well as the millions of victims of the Holocaust.

Fortunately, this country drew back from such unthinkable measures. However, this ideology continued to affect the huge numbers of people admitted to institutions right up until the late 1980s. In the 1930s, the IQ test was introduced – people scoring low on the test were categorised as 'mentally defective' and unable to learn.

The introduction of the National Health Service in 1946 and the development of the medical model of disability had an impact. The term 'mentally handicapped' came into use, and the 'institutions' turned overnight into hospitals, with the emphasis now on caring for their residents. Society had moved from seeing the 'mentally handicapped' as dangerous and degenerate to viewing them more sympathetically, as people in need of treatment, although still a drain on the public purse. People with a learning disability remained segregated and isolated, and the standard of care was extremely poor. This remained the case right up until the closure of the long-stay hospitals.

In 1959, the Mental Health Act began the idea that some people might not need to be cared for in a hospital. It was also the first time that people with a 'mental illness' were distinguished from those described as having a 'mental handicap'.

In 1967, national newspapers started to draw attention to the bad conditions in 'mental handicap' hospitals. In 1971, the Government published a paper, 'Better services for the

Mentally Handicapped', in response to continued reports about appalling conditions in the hospitals. This paper laid the foundations for 'Care in the Community', with the expectation that half of the people in hospitals should be living in the local community by 1990.

During the 1980s, the concept of 'normalisation' began to influence the delivery of care for people who had a learning disability. Normalisation theory emphasises the 'value of the individual', their right to choice and opportunity, and the right to any extra support they need to fulfil their potential. At this time there was also recognition that institutions were a major barrier to inclusion.

The idea that everyone in society has the right to a life with choice, opportunity and respect, with extra support according to their needs, helped to change the way services were planned and delivered. The National Health Service and Community Care Act 1990 recognised the right of disabled people to be an equal part of society, with access to the necessary support.

We might like to believe that the task of de-institutionalising the care of people with a learning disability is now complete. Nearly all the long-stay hospitals are now closed, and many rights are now law as detailed in the Disability Discrimination Act.

However, the reality is that many people are still denied the things that most people take for granted, such as a decent income, somewhere appropriate to live, the chance to work, leisure opportunities and choices in education.

### Evidence activity 

#### 3.1 The types of services that have been provided for individuals with learning disabilities over time

This activity allows you to demonstrate your knowledge of the types of services that have been provided for individuals with learning disabilities over time.

Find out about the history of your service users. Were any of them 'cared for' within an institution?

Make a note of the differences between the care that was provided within institutions and the support provided by your organisation.

Today's services aim to enable people and promote equal treatment and inclusion. This brings with it new challenges and responsibilities, the greatest of which is to change public attitudes towards people with a learning disability and raise understanding.

www.mencap.org.uk

## 3.2 Describe how past ways of working may affect present services

People who have worked in health and social care for some time may remember some of the institutions, and may have indeed worked in them. Some health and social care workers may therefore have adopted the medical model approach to disability. This will, without a shadow of a doubt, affect the care and support that these health and social care workers are delivering.

### Evidence activity 

#### 3.2 How past ways of working may affect present services

This activity allows you to demonstrate your knowledge of how past ways of working may affect present services.

How do you think past ways of working may affect present ways of working?

## 3.3 Identify some of the key changes in the lives of individuals who have learning disabilities

There have been major key changes in the lives of individuals who have a learning disability. We have already discussed the institutionalised medical model approach to care and support. Person-centred planning has generally led to positive changes for people who have learning disabilities. However, mencap report that people who have a learning disability are still treated differently.

## Where people live

There have been major changes in the living arrangements of people who have a learning disability. With a move away from an institutionalised approach to care, more people are being empowered to maintain their independence for as long as possible. Whilst over 60 per cent of people who have a learning disability live with their family, there are also a significant number of people who maintain their independence within their community through supported living.

## Daytime activities

With the introduction of self-directed support, service users are able to make choices about where they go and what they want to do during the day time. Self-directed support should enable service users to decide:

- how to live their lives
- where to live and who with
- what to do during the day
- how to spend their leisure time
- what to spend money on
- who they are friends with.

## Employment

Mencap report that only 1 in 10 people who have a learning disability are in employment. They are more excluded from the workplace than any other group of disabled people. Where they do work, it is often for low pay and part-time hours. Research shows that 65 per cent of people with a learning disability want to work, and that they make highly valued employees when given the right support.

### Research & investigate

**3.3 Why?**

Using any information that is available to you, take a look at why people who have a learning disability find it difficult to get paid work.

## Sexual relationships and parenthood

Discussions surrounding sexuality are uncomfortable for 'able bodied' people. This is a very private area of a person's life and one which we choose not to discuss openly. It is now recognised that people who have learning disabilities also have sexual feelings and may want to engage in close personal relationships. Some organisations run courses for people who have learning disabilities where they are taught about social and personal development. Because people with learning disabilities are a vulnerable group of people there are many aspects that need to be considered to ensure any relationship remains a safe and healthy relationship.

All too often support services start with the belief that people who have a learning disability won't make good parents and that their children should be taken away. Mencap also identify that this is backed up by research that shows that 40 per cent of parents who have a learning disability do not live with their children. Not all parents with a learning disability can look after their own children and the welfare of the child is essential. However, if parents who have a learning disability are provided with adequate support, they should be able to keep their children.

### Case Study

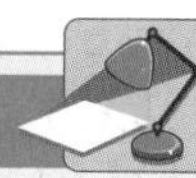

**3.3 Frank**

Frank is a young man who has learning disabilities. He confides in his support worker about the difficulties he is having with his girlfriend. Frank and his girlfriend (who also has learning disabilities) want to have sexual intercourse but they are unsure about 'safer sex'. The worker advises them of the different organisations that have up-to-date information in user friendly format that would provide them with some knowledge of 'safe sex'. The worker also advises them that these organisations can provide support and help in talking over the issues.

What responsibility does the support worker have at this stage?

What responsibility does the person with learning disabilities have?

Who else has responsibilities and what are they?

## Provision of healthcare

People who have a learning disability generally experience poorer health and poorer healthcare than other members of the public. However, as we are well aware, these people have just as much of a right to receive good healthcare. They will need healthcare in the same way that everyone else will, and some people with a learning disability will have additional health needs (for example, people with a learning disability are more likely to have epilepsy). Often, they need more support to understand information about their health, to communicate symptoms and concerns, and to manage their health.

### Evidence activity 

 3.3 Key changes in the lives of individuals who have learning disabilities

This activity allows you to demonstrate your knowledge of key changes in the lives of individuals who have learning disabilities.

Make a poster which identifies the key changes in the lives of people who have learning disabilities. The poster should take into account where people live, day time activities, employment, sexual relationships and parenthood and the provision of healthcare.

# LO4 Understand the basic principles and practice of advocacy, empowerment and active participation in relation to supporting individuals with learning disabilities and their families

## 4.1 Explain the meaning of the term 'social inclusion'

The term 'social inclusion' has come to replace older terminology, such as 'community development work'. In practical terms, social inclusion means working within the community to tackle and avoid circumstances and problems that lead to social exclusion, such as poverty, unemployment or low income, housing problems and becoming housebound and isolated due to illness.

Historically, people with learning disabilities have faced poor life chances, largely due to social exclusion. They have not been accepted by mainstream society, facing stigmatisation, prejudice and even fear, and this has led to these people becoming socially excluded within society.

Promoting social inclusion is closely linked to empowering the individual. This means giving people with learning disabilities a voice, allowing them to make choices for themselves about the direction of their own life based on their wishes and aspirations.

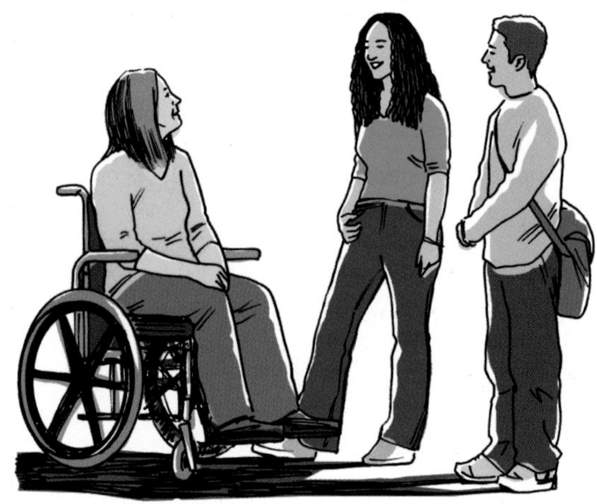

Figure 11.5 Social inclusion

### Evidence activity 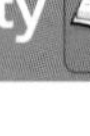

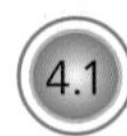 4.1 Social inclusion

This activity allows you to demonstrate your knowledge of 'social inclusion'.

Explain the steps you take to ensure social inclusion within your place of work.

## 4.2 Explain the meaning of the term 'advocacy'

The term 'advocacy' is concerned with 'speaking up for, or acting on behalf of, yourself or another person'. The other person is often receiving a service from a statutory or voluntary organisation. Some people require the assistance of an advocate because they are not clear about their rights as citizens, or have difficulty in fully understanding these rights. Other people may find it difficult to speak up for themselves. Advocacy can enable people to take more responsibility and control for the decisions which affect their lives.

Advocacy can help service users to:

- make their own views and wishes known
- express and present their views
- obtain independent advice and accurate information
- negotiate and resolve conflict.

**Evidence activity** 

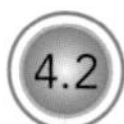

### 4.2 Advocacy

This activity allows you to demonstrate your knowledge of what is meant by the term 'advocacy'.

Think about a time when you have advocated the wishes of service users for whom you provide support. Explain the circumstances surrounding the episode. Why could the service user not speak out for him/herself?

What did you need to take into consideration prior to advocating the person's wishes?

## 4.3 Describe different types of advocacy

All people are very different from each other. Their needs for support are different, and may also change at different stages throughout their life. All advocacy types are of equal value. Which type of advocacy is used, and when, should depend on what is best suited to the person who seeks it. A single person may ask for different types of advocacy support at different times in their life.

What is essential to all types of advocacy is that it is the person who has a learning disability who is always at the centre of the advocacy process. Advocacy can therefore be described as a process which is person-centred. It is about the person's needs, what that person wants, and finding the best way of getting that across to the people who need to know.

Advocacy can be likened to a box of tools. Different types of advocacy can be used together or they can be used separately depending on the job that needs to be done.

### Professional advocacy

Professional advocacy is frequently described as the 'case-work' model. It is used for short to medium term involvement, which often supports people in finding a solution to a problem. Professional advocacy may be required where an individual requires support with issues requiring specific expertise, for example child protection, education, housing, employment and financial matters.

### Citizen advocacy

The advocate in this relationship is usually called the 'citizen advocate', and the person receiving the service is called the 'advocacy partner'. An advocacy partner is someone at risk of having choices, wishes and decisions ignored, and who needs help in making them known and making sure they are responded to. A citizen advocate is a person who volunteers to speak up for and support an advocacy partner and is not paid to do so. The citizen advocate is unpaid and independent of service providers and families and is a member of the local community. The advocacy relationship is based on trust and confidentiality.

### Crisis advocacy

Crisis advocacy provides support that aims to give the person a voice in a situation that requires a quick response. It is usually short term and aimed at helping the individual solve a problem.

### Peer advocacy

Peer advocacy is usually provided by a person who has experienced a similar situation. It is based on the fact that people who have experienced the same things feel they have a better understanding and can be more supportive. In the past, peer advocacy occurred when people with learning disabilities lived in isolated hospitals. They were often separated from others in their community and only had each other for company. There was no one else to speak up for them other than their fellow peers. As people with learning disabilities began to learn more about their rights and the obligations of citizenship, more of them began to speak up for each other. Peer advocacy is often of great support to an individual but is not recognised as being independent or unbiased.

## Self advocacy

Self advocacy is what most of us do most of the time. It is about speaking up for yourself. This type of advocacy should always be encouraged wherever possible. Many people who have learning disabilities have a good ability to speak up for themselves. However, they sometimes find it hard to get others to accept this or even to listen to them. Self advocacy groups are a good way to encourage this. Self advocacy groups are run by people who have learning disabilities. These are often groups of people who use services or have the same interests locally. They work together to make sure they have a say in how those services are run. Self advocacy groups are a very good way for people to support each other and they can help to build confidence so that people feel more able to speak up for themselves.

### Time to reflect

4.3 Self advocacy

How do you enable your service users to self advocate?

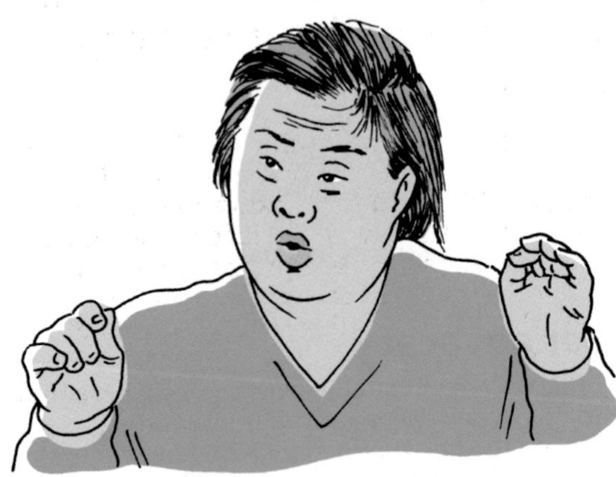

Figure 11.6 Self advocacy

## Legal advocacy

As the name suggests, legal advocacy is concerned with using the services of a lawyer or ombudsman to support an individual with specific legal issues.

### Evidence activity

4.3 Different types of advocacy

This activity allows you to demonstrate your knowledge of the different types of advocacy.

Give examples to demonstrate times that the different types of advocacy have been used within your organisation.

## 4.4 Describe ways to build empowerment and active participation into everyday support with individuals with learning disabilities

Empowerment is a word we hear a lot, and has become an important aspect of delivering health and social care services. Empowerment for people with learning disabilities is the process by which individuals develop increased skills to make decisions and take control over their lives. This helps individuals to achieve their goals and aspirations, thus maximising their quality of life.

A key feature in empowering people is giving them a voice and actively listening to what they have to say. Empowerment is, therefore, closely linked to the concept of person-centred care and various forms of advocacy.

For the person who has a learning disability, the subjective experience of empowerment is about rights, choice and control which can lead them to a more **autonomous** lifestyle. For the health and social care worker, it is about anti-oppressive practice, balancing rights and responsibilities and supporting choice and empowerment whilst maintaining safe and ethical practice.

### Key term

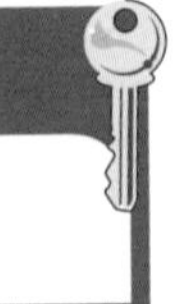

Autonomous means independent, not controlled by others.

Person-centred planning places the individual at the centre of all processes and uses techniques to ensure meaningful participation is key to empowering individuals in this way.

**Evidence activity** 

### 4.4 Building empowerment and active participation into everyday support

This activity allows you to demonstrate your knowledge of the ways to build empowerment and active participation into everyday support with individuals who have learning disabilities.

Explain the processes that are in place within your organisation to ensure the people you support are empowered and enabled to actively participate in decisions on a daily basis.

# LO5 Understand how views and attitudes impact on the lives of individuals with learning disabilities and their family carers

## 5.1 Explain how attitudes are changing in relation to individuals with learning disabilities

People who have a learning disability and their families have always been affected by the way they are viewed and treated by society. Sadly, the history of public and private attitudes to learning disability over time has been one of intolerance and lack of understanding.

**Evidence activity** 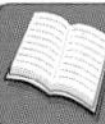

### 5.1 Changing attitudes in relation to individuals with learning disabilities

This activity allows you to demonstrate your knowledge of how attitudes are changing in relation to individuals with learning disabilities. We have already established that attitudes towards people who have learning disabilities have changed over time. With a move away from institutionalisation and an emphasis on inclusion, today's services aim to enable people who have learning disabilities, and promote equal treatment and inclusion.

Why do you think attitudes towards people who have a learning disability are changing?

## 5.2 Give examples of positive and negative aspects of being labelled as having a learning disability

The way people with learning disabilities have been portrayed has often been with a '**label**'. Terms like 'the mentally handicapped', 'the blind' and 'the mentally ill' place the person in a group which risks a stereotypical view. Being labelled as 'disabled' and 'inadequate' also creates barriers to things that 'able-bodied' people enjoy and take for granted, for example, relationships, employment, education, housing, transport and many more. In addition, it perpetuates **prejudice** and **discrimination**. Anti-discriminatory legislation is helping to remove barriers and shake off negative attitudes and discrimination, but there is still a long way to go.

In some respects, it is important to apply a 'label' to a certain condition as this will ensure the person who has a learning disability is given any support and care that is required to ensure they lead a good quality of life. It is the type of label that is applied that makes all the difference.

## Key terms

**Discrimination** is the acting out of negative prejudices.
A **label** is a 'tag' that we use to describe someone and is usually based on their appearance and behaviour.
A **prejudice** is an attitude or way of thinking based on an unfair pre-judgement of a person, rather than on a factual assessment.

The most important aspect to remember, with any label, is that the person is an individual with individual needs. This sometimes tends to be forgotten. If this view is not upheld, the more profound perception of the disability will result. Using the right positive language goes a long way to defining people with a learning disability as a person first.

### Evidence activity 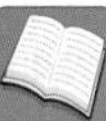

 **5.2 Positive and negative aspects of being labelled as having a learning disability**

This activity allows you to demonstrate your knowledge of the positive and negative aspects of being labelled as having a learning disability.

Identify any labels that you have heard applied to people who have a learning disability. Explain how these labels have affected individuals in a positive and negative way.

## 5.3 Describe steps that can be taken to promote positive attitudes towards individuals with learning disabilities and their family carers

It is now accepted that the way people are portrayed within the media can greatly influence public perception and attitude.

The recognition of the social model of disability has gone a long way in changing the attitudes of health and social care workers towards people who have learning disabilities and recognising that the person comes first.

Some employers undertake disability awareness training as part of their general staff training programmes, and this can go a long way in changing attitudes towards people who have learning disabilities.

More people who have learning disabilities are now using mainstream community facilities, such as colleges, hospitals, libraries and leisure centres. This sends out a clear message that segregation is no longer acceptable but more could be done to ensure that people are positively welcomed and included.

### Evidence activity 

 **5.3 Steps that can be taken to promote positive attitudes towards individuals who have a learning disability and their family carers**

This activity allows you to demonstrate your knowledge of the steps that can be taken to promote positive attitudes towards people who have a learning disability and their family carers.

What steps do you take to promote positive attitudes towards individuals who have a learning disability and their family carers?

## 5.4 Explain the roles of external agencies and others in changing attitudes, policy and practice

External agencies have an important role in facilitating changes in attitude, policy and practice. For example, support groups such as the Learning Disability Coalition, who are a group who represent 14 learning disability organisations and over 140 supporter organisations who have come together to form one group with one voice.

They believe that people with a learning disability have the right to live independent lives, with the support that they need. Their aim is to ensure the government provides enough money so that people with a learning disability have the same choices and chances as everyone else. They do this by:

- Providing a unified voice to government and other key decision-makers.
- Gathering evidence on cuts to services at local level.
- Raising awareness of the financial pressures on services for people with learning disabilities, and campaigning for better funding.
- Achieving an evidence-based assessment of the long-term resource requirements for people with learning disabilities.

www.learningdisabilitycoalition.org.uk

## Evidence activity

### 5.4 The roles of external agencies and others in changing attitudes, policy and practice

This activity allows you to demonstrate your knowledge of the roles of external agencies and others in changing attitudes, policy and practice.

Take a look at the Learning Disability Coalition website. Make a note of the agencies that have joined together to represent the voice of people who have learning disabilities. How do these groups work together to change attitudes and policy and how do they impact on changing your practice?

# LO6 Know how to promote communication with individuals with learning disabilities

## 6.1 Identify ways of adapting verbal and non-verbal communication when communicating with individuals who have learning disabilities

Communication is a two way process in which messages are sent, received and understood between people or groups of people. It is a basic human right upon which we build relationships, make friends and control our existence. It is the way we become independent and make choices. It is the way we learn and express our thoughts, feelings and emotions. The British Institute of Learning Disabilities (BILD) estimates that between 50 and 90 per cent of people who have learning difficulties also experience difficulties with communication. People who have learning disabilities do not have one recognised tool to help them communicate and every person is different. It is therefore essential that an assessment is undertaken to ensure effective methods of communication are identified for each individual person.

Generally, people in societies develop common languages in order that they can live together with a shared method of communication. In fact, communication is fundamental to being a part of society.

People who find it difficult to communicate, or are undervalued in their societies, will automatically feel excluded unless those around them are prepared to adapt their method of communication. Effective communication is therefore essential in order to promote the principles associated with independence, choice, rights and inclusion.

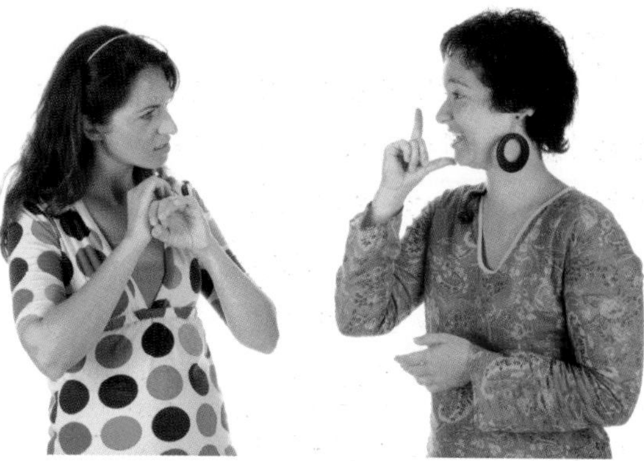

Figure 11.7 Accessible communication

Methods of communication vary and can either be verbal or non-verbal. A high percentage of communication is non-verbal.

- When communicating verbally it is important not to overestimate language skills. Equally it is important that the pace of communication is consistent with the person's level of understanding.
- Objects, pictures, signs and symbols are all powerful ways of communicating meaning.
- British sign language (BSL) has long been established as a language used by people who have a hearing impairment.
- Braille enables people who have a visual impairment to be able to read.
- People with more complex learning disabilities may not be able to use any recognised means of communication and will therefore be dependent on others to interpret their needs and choices through observation and response to their communicative behaviour.

**Evidence activity** 

### 6.1 Adapting verbal and non-verbal communication

This activity allows you to demonstrate your knowledge of adapting verbal and non-verbal communication when communicating with individuals who have learning disabilities.

Explain how the communication requirements of individuals are assessed within your organisation.

Think about the service users you support and identify ways in which the methods of verbal and non-verbal communication have been adapted to facilitate communication with these individuals.

## 6.2 Explain why it is important to use language that is both 'age appropriate' and 'ability appropriate' when communicating with individuals with learning disabilities

When communicating with people who have a learning disability, it is essential that the communication takes place at a pace and in a manner that the individual can process. This means that the information should be both 'age appropriate' and 'ability appropriate'. Communication must also take into account the person as a whole and sensitive consideration should be given to the person's cultural and religious beliefs.

**Evidence activity** 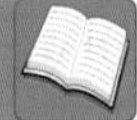

### 6.2 Age and ability appropriate language

This activity allows you to demonstrate your knowledge of the importance of using language that is both 'age and ability appropriate' when communicating with individuals who have learning disabilities.

Explain why it is important to use language that is both 'age appropriate' and 'ability appropriate'.

How do you ensure you take these factors into account when communicating with service users?

What could be a consequence of not taking these factors into consideration?

## 6.3 Describe ways of checking whether an individual has understood a communication, and how to address any misunderstandings

When communicating with a person who has a learning disability it is essential that the person understands what has been communicated. If the person has understood, this may be immediately obvious.

Within your role as a care worker you will want to help individuals communicate to the best of their ability and promote understanding of their needs and preferences whenever appropriate. However there will be times when you find that you are having difficulty with communication and you are unsure whether an individual has understood what you have communicated to them. Hopefully you will know your service users well, but it is also important to seek advice from a senior member of staff when misunderstandings occur. Individuals who are unable to successfully communicate with you, or understand what you are communicating to them, may become distressed.

The extent of the frustration and distress will vary from person to person but will be apparent through verbal communication, body language or facial expression.

## Evidence activity

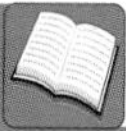

### 6.3 Checking understanding and addressing misunderstandings

This activity allows you to demonstrate your knowledge of the importance of checking whether an individual has understood communication and how you address any misunderstandings.

How do you check understanding when you are communicating with service users?

How do you address any misunderstandings as they arise?

## Assessment summary

Your reading of this chapter and completion of the activities will have prepared you to demonstrate your learning and understanding of supporting individuals who have a learning disability in your workplace. To achieve the unit, your assessor will require you to:

| Learning Outcomes | Assessment Criteria |
|---|---|
| Learning outcome 1: Understand the legislation and policies that support the human rights and inclusion of individuals with learning disabilities by: |  1.1 identifying legislation and policies that are designed to promote the human rights, inclusion, equal life chances and citizenship of individuals with learning disabilities<br>See Evidence activity 1.1 p. 186. |
| |  1.2 explaining how legislation and policies influence the day to day experiences of individuals with learning disabilities and their families.<br>See Evidence activity 1.2 p. 187. |
| Learning outcome 2: Understand the nature and characteristics of learning disability by: |  2.1 explaining what is meant by 'learning disability'<br>See Evidence activity 2.1 p. 187. |
| |  2.2 giving examples of causes of learning disabilities<br>See Evidence activity 2.2 p. 188. |

| Learning Outcomes | Assessment Criteria |
| --- | --- |
| Learning outcome 2: Understand the nature and characteristics of learning disability by: | 2.3 describing the medical and social models of disability<br><br>See Evidence activity 2.3 p. 189. |
| | 2.4 stating the approximate proportion of individuals with a learning disability for whom the cause is 'not known'<br><br>See Evidence activity 2.4 p. 190. |
| | 2.5 describing the possible impact on a family of having a member with a learning disability.<br><br>See Evidence activity 2.5 p. 190. |
| Learning outcome 3: Understand the historical context of learning disability by: | 3.1 explaining the types of services that have been provided for individuals with learning disabilities over time<br><br>See Evidence activity 3.1 p. 192. |
| | 3.2 describing how past ways of working may affect present services<br><br>See Evidence activity 3.2 p. 192. |
| | 3.3 identifying some of the key changes in the lives of individuals who have learning disabilities in:<br><br>a) where people live<br>b) daytime activities<br>c) employment<br>d) sexual relationships and parenthood<br>e) the provision of healthcare.<br><br>See Evidence activity 3.3 p. 194. |
| Learning outcome 4: Understand the basic principles and practice of advocacy, empowerment and active participation in relation to supporting individuals with learning disabilities and their families by: | 4.1 explaining the meaning of the term 'social inclusion'<br><br>See Evidence activity 4.1 p. 194. |
| | 4.2 explaining the meaning of the term 'advocacy'<br><br>See Evidence activity 4.2 p. 195. |

| Learning Outcomes | Assessment Criteria |
| --- | --- |
| Learning outcome 4: Understand the basic principles and practice of advocacy, empowerment and active participation in relation to supporting individuals with learning disabilities and their families by: | 4.3 describing different types of advocacy<br>See Evidence activity 4.3 p. 196. |
| | 4.4 describing ways to build empowerment and active participation into everyday support with individuals with learning disabilities.<br>See Evidence activity 4.4 p. 197. |
| Learning outcome 5: Understand how views and attitudes impact on the lives of individuals with learning disabilities and their family carers by: | 5.1 explaining how attitudes are changing in relation to individuals with learning disabilities<br>See Evidence activity 5.1 p. 197. |
| | 5.2 giving examples of positive and negative aspects of being labelled as having a learning disability<br>See Evidence activity 5.2 p. 198. |
| | 5.3 describing steps that can be taken to promote positive attitudes towards individuals with learning disabilities and their family carers<br>See Evidence activity 5. 3 p. 198. |
| | 5.4 explaining the roles of external agencies and others in changing attitudes, policy and practice.<br>See Evidence activity 5.4 p. 199. |
| Learning outcome 6: Know how to promote communication with individuals with learning disabilities by: | 6.1 identifying ways of adapting verbal and non-verbal communication when communicating with individuals who have learning disabilities<br>See Evidence activity 6.1 p. 200. |
| | 6.2 explaining why it is important to use language that is both 'age appropriate' and 'ability appropriate' when communicating with individuals with learning disabilities<br>See Evidence activity 6.2 p. 200. |

| Learning Outcomes | Assessment Criteria |
| --- | --- |
| Learning outcome **6**: Know how to promote communication with individuals with learning disabilities by: | 6.3 describing ways of checking whether an individual has understood a communication, and how to address any misunderstandings. See Evidence activity 6.3 p. 201. |

Good luck!

## Weblinks

| | |
| --- | --- |
| Office for Disability Issues | www.officefordisability.gov.uk |
| Understanding Individual Needs | www.understandingindividualneeds.com |
| About Learning Disabilities | www.aboutlearningdisabilities.co.uk |
| mencap | www.mencap.org.uk |
| Learning Disability Coalition | www.learningdisabilitycoalition.org.uk |
| The Foundation for People with Learning Difficulties | www.learningdisabilities.org.uk |
| Easyhealth | www.easyhealth.org.uk |

# 12 The principles of infection prevention and control

## For Unit IC01

### What are you finding out?

Infection is caused by **pathogens**. Not all infectious diseases are transmissible but some, such as influenza, MRSA, *C. difficile* and norovirus have the potential to spread from one person to another. Understanding how pathogens act and spread is crucial to their prevention and control.

Users of health and social care services are physically and emotionally vulnerable to infection. For example:

- Influenza vaccination is recommended for all elderly people in the UK aged 65 and over as well as people in at-risk groups, such as those suffering from conditions like asthma and COPD (chronic obstructive pulmonary disease).
- During the year to March 2010, just over half of reported cases of MRSA (meticillin-resistant *Staphylococcus aureus*) and *C. difficile* (*Clostridium difficile*) in England and Wales were contracted by patients whilst in hospital.
- In January 2010, norovirus, which thrives in schools, care homes and hospitals was claimed to have infected 500,000 victims per week, particularly elderly people and those with pre-existing health problems.

Infection prevention and control is therefore key to the work of health and social care employers and employees, who have a responsibility to comply with relevant legislation and regulatory and professional body standards. Health and social care employees also have a responsibility to understand the importance of infection control and risk assessment procedures, of Personal Protective Equipment (PPE) and of maintaining good personal hygiene.

www.rcn.org.uk; www.healthcarerepublic.com; www.hpa.org.uk; www.dailymail.co.uk

The reading and activities in this chapter will help you to:

- Understand roles and responsibilities in the prevention and control of infections
- Understand legislation and policies relating to prevention and control of infections
- Understand systems and procedures relating to the prevention and control of infections
- Understand the importance of risk assessment in relation to the prevention and control of infections
- Understand the importance of Personal Protective Equipment (PPE) in the prevention and control of infections
- Understand the importance of good personal hygiene in the prevention and control of infections.

#### Key term

A **pathogen** is a disease-producing bacterium, fungi, virus, infestation or prion.

## LO1 Roles and responsibilities in preventing and controlling infection

Many infectious diseases have the capacity to spread rapidly and have disastrous effects in health and social care settings. Infection is a major cause of illness and hospitalisation among people living in residential care homes; and healthcare-associated infections (HCAIs) can be life threatening. Many of these infections make underlying medical conditions worse and some HCAIs are resistant to antibiotics. For these reasons, everyone involved in providing health and social care has very clear roles and responsibilities in ensuring the prevention and control of infections.

## Research & investigate 

###  1.1 Superbugs

According to www.bbc.co.uk on 11 August 2010, a new superbug that is resistant to even the most powerful antibiotics has entered UK hospitals. Experts warn that it could produce dangerous infections that would spread rapidly from person to person and be almost impossible to treat.

Check out the press and the internet for other superbugs that have threatened health around the world recently. In what ways have they affected the people you support?

## 1.1 Your roles and responsibilities in preventing and controlling infection

As a health and social care worker you have roles and responsibilities in relation to infection prevention and control. You must:

- cooperate with your employer in preventing and controlling infection
- know and understand your organisation's infection prevention and control policies and procedures
- follow infection control procedures and apply standard infection control principles or precautions (you will read about these later) to all situations all of the time
- know how to get advice on the prevention and control of infection and stay up-to-date in your knowledge and understanding of the subject
- make your manager aware of any difficulties you have in following procedures
- report breaches in good practice and take corrective action as appropriate.

You also have a responsibility to be on your guard for potential outbreaks of infection and resistance to antibiotics and to inform your employer if you have any concerns.

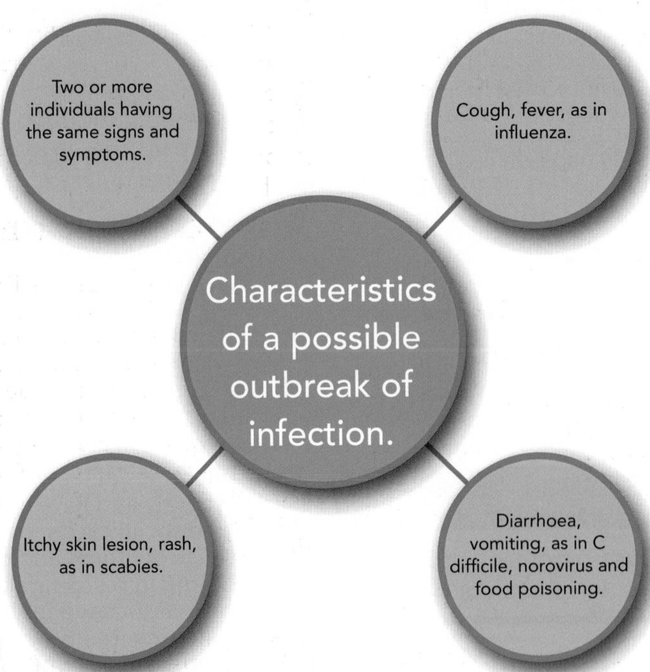


Figure 12.1 Characteristics of a possible outbreak of infection

Some job roles have an overall responsibility for infection prevention and control, such as Infection Control Champion, Infection Control Lead and Infection Control Link Person. Staff in these positions have a particular interest and up-to-date knowledge and expertise in infection prevention and control. Because of their experience, they are role models and a source of information and advice for colleagues, delivering training and promoting and maintaining safe practice. They work with patients, their relatives and friends, providing information on infection prevention and control. They liaise with health authorities, as appropriate. And their good communication skills enable them to influence and introduce any necessary changes in work practice.

### Evidence activity

#### 1.1 Your roles and responsibilities in preventing and controlling infection

This activity gives you the opportunity to demonstrate your understanding of your roles and responsibilities in relation to the prevention and control of infection.

What are your roles and responsibilities in relation to infection prevention and control? Why is it important that you act out your roles and responsibilities in your work?

## 1.2 Your employer's responsibilities in preventing and controlling infection

Policies set out the arrangements an organisation has for complying with legislation. In order to uphold the law, your employer should have written policies describing the arrangements at work to prevent and control infection.

Procedures describe the activities that need to be carried out for policies to be put into action. Infection prevention and control procedures should be **accessible** and your employer should have a system for ensuring that you understand them and follow them to the letter. Failure of your employer to minimise the risk of infection and protect everyone at your workplace against infectious disease constitutes neglect.

### Key term

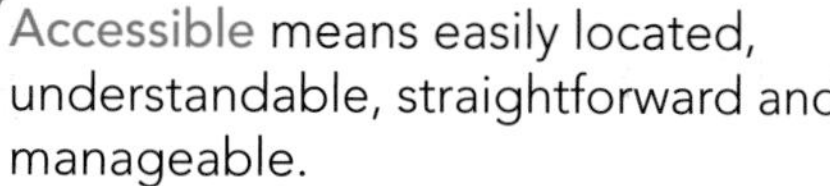

Accessible means easily located, understandable, straightforward and manageable.

Employers have a responsibility to regularly produce Infection Prevention and Control reports that describe:

- policies and procedures that are in place and how they are monitored
- any outbreaks of infection that have taken place and the action taken to rectify problems
- education and training that has taken place
- planned improvements to work practices.

The purpose of Infection Prevention and Control reports is to reduce infections and ensure improvements in infection prevention and control.

### Research & investigate

#### 1.2 Infection Prevention and Control reports

Have a look at the Infection Prevention and Control Report produced by your organisation. Maybe it is online, in which case use a search engine to find it; or perhaps it is hard copy (paper) only. What does the report tell you?

Employers have a responsibility to obtain and share with staff up-to-date advice and information about infection prevention and control. People qualified to offer advice and information include the specialist job roles you read about earlier, General Practitioners (GPs), Health Protection Nurses (HPNs), **Royal College of Nursing (RCN)** Nurse Advisers for Infection Prevention and Control, Community Infection Control Nurses (CICNs) and Environmental Health Practitioners (EHPs).

www.rcn.org.uk; www.cieh.org

### Key term

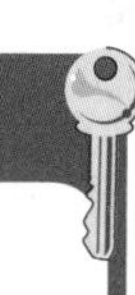

The Royal College of Nursing (RCN) represents nurses and nursing, promotes excellence in practice and shapes health policies.

Employers have a responsibility to report suspected outbreaks of infection, changes in resistance to antibiotics and notifiable diseases to the local **Health Protection Unit (HPU)**. Typical characteristics of a notifiable disease are:

- it is potentially life-threatening
- it spreads rapidly
- it cannot be easily treated or cured, for example, there is no vaccine or antibiotic available.

NB: At the time of writing (August 2010), the HPA, which has responsibility for dealing with public health issues such as infectious diseases, is to transfer its workload to the Secretary of State for Health.

www.hpa.org.uk

## Key term

Health Protection Units (HPUs) are local centres of the Health Protection Agency (HPA).

### Notifiable diseases

Acute encephalitis, acute poliomyelitis, anthrax, cholera, diphtheria, dysentery (amoebic or bacillary), food poisoning, leprosy, leptospirosis, malaria, measles, meningitis, meningococcal septicaemia (without meningitis), mumps, ophthalmia neonatorum, plague, paratyphoid fever, relapsing fever, rabies, rubella, smallpox, scarlet fever, typhus, tetanus, tuberculosis, typhoid fever, viral haemorrhagic fevers, viral hepatitis, whooping cough and yellow fever.

Employers have a responsibility to ensure that people with infectious disease are nursed in **isolation.**

## Key term

Isolation nursing is the physical separation of an infected patient from others.

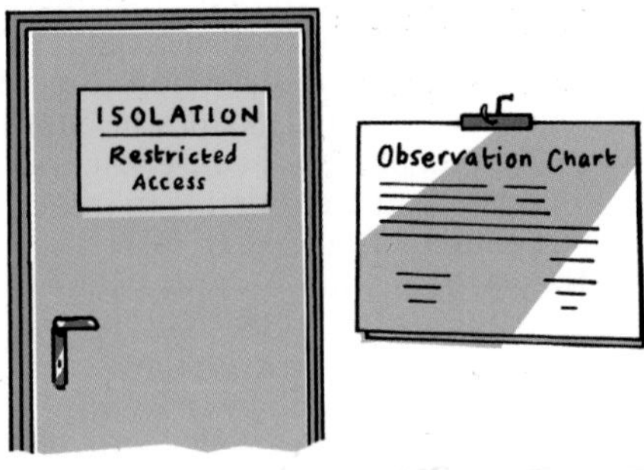


Figure 12.2 Isolation nursing

Employers also have a responsibility to ensure that staff:

- are immunised against infectious disease
- receive ongoing training in the prevention and control of infection
- have a personal development plan that shows what training they have completed and what they need to do.

Infection Control Guidance for Care Homes, DH, 2006

## Time to reflect

1.2 Immunisation

What diseases are you immunised against? Are your immunisations up to date? What could happen if you failed to be immunised properly?

## Evidence activity

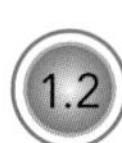

1.2 Your employer's roles and responsibilities in preventing and controlling infection

This activity gives you the opportunity to demonstrate your understanding of your employer's roles and responsibilities in relation to the prevention and control of infection.

What are your employer's responsibilities in relation to infection prevention and control? Why is it important that your employer fulfils these responsibilities?

## LO2 Legislation and policies relating to prevention and control of infections

### 2.1 Current legislation and regulatory body standards that relate to the prevention and control of infection

Table 12.1 Legislation relevant to infection prevention and control

| Legislation | Purpose of the legislation |
|---|---|
| Health and Safety at Work etc Act (HASWA) 1974. | Ensures the health and safety of everyone who may be affected by work activities. |
| Management of Health and Safety at Work Regulations (MHSWR) 1999. | Require employers and managers to carry out risk assessments to eliminate or minimise risks to health and safety, including from pathogens. |
| Personal Protective Equipment at Work Regulations (PPE) 1992. | Minimise the risks to health and safety associated with **cross-infection**. |
| The Health Act 2006. | Aims to prevent and control healthcare-associated infections (HCAIs) |
| The Health and Social Care Act 2008. | Aims to protect public health by preventing and controlling the spread of infectious diseases. |
| Reporting of Injuries, Diseases and Dangerous Occurrences Regulations (RIDDOR) 1995. | Require that certain work-related injuries, diseases and dangerous occurrences are reported to the Health and Safety Executive (HSE) or local authority. |
| Public Health (Control of Disease) Act 1984 and The Public Health (Infectious Diseases) Regulations 1988. | Require that outbreaks of infection, changes in resistance to antibiotics and notifiable diseases are reported to the HPU so that they can be managed to prevent their spread. |
| Food Safety Act 1990 and the Food Hygiene Regulations 2006. | Minimise the risks to health and safety associated with food handling. |
| Control of Substances Hazardous to Health Regulations (COSHH) 2002. | Minimise the risks to health and safety from the use of hazardous substances, including pathogens. |
| Hazardous Waste Regulations 2005. | Require that waste is dealt with so as to avoid putting health at risk. |
| Environmental Protection (Duty of Care) Regulations 1991. | Require that waste, including contaminated waste, is properly stored and adequately packaged whilst awaiting removal from the premises. |

**Key term**

Cross-infection is the spread of pathogens from one person, object, place or part of the body to another.

Regulatory bodies are organisations set up by the government to establish national standards for qualifications and best practice, and to ensure that the standards are consistently observed. They include:

- The Care Quality Commission in England, which regulates health and social care provided by the NHS, local authorities, private companies and voluntary organisations. Its standards of quality and care state that people can expect to be cared for in a clean environment where they are protected from infection.

www.cqc.org.uk

- The General Social Care Council in England, Care Council for Wales, Scottish Care Council and N Ireland Social Care Council. Their codes of practice dictate the standards of practice and conduct that social care workers and employers should meet, which includes protecting individuals from danger or harm.

www.gscc.org.uk; www.ccwales.org.uk; www.sssc.uk.com; www.niscc.info

- The GMC (General Medical Council), whose guides and strategies for improvement shape the role of healthcare professionals with regard to infection prevention and control.

http://www.gmc-uk.org

- The Nursing and Midwifery Council (NMC), whose code or 'Standards of conduct, performance and ethics for nurses and midwives' is a key tool in protecting and promoting health and well-being, requiring nurses and midwives to manage risks, including risk of infection.

www.nmc-uk.org

- The Health Professions Council (HPC), whose 'Standards of Conduct, Performance & Ethics' require **allied health professionals** to deal safely with risk of infection by taking precautions to protect everyone, including themselves, from cross-infection.

www.hpc-uk.org

- The Office for Standards in Education, Children's Services and Skills (OFSTED), which regulates and inspects care service provision for children and young people. For a care provider to meet OFSTED's standards and regulations, it has to demonstrate that children and young people are not at risk from cross-infection because of low standards of hygiene.

www.ofsted.gov.uk

**Key term**

Allied health professionals are clinical healthcare professionals as distinct from doctors, dentists and nurses, who work in a healthcare team to make the healthcare system function.

Some occupations are not covered by regulatory standards or codes of practice, for example healthcare assistants in England and Wales. Instead, National Occupational Standards (NOS) set out the **competences** that apply to their job roles and level of experience. NOS for workers in the health and social care sectors are written by the Children's Workforce Development Council (CWDC), Skills for Health and Skills for Care.

www.cwdcouncil.org.uk; www.skillsforhealth.org.uk; www.skillsforcare.org.uk

**Key term**

Competence is to do with having knowledge, understanding and capability.

**Evidence activity** 

**2.1 Current legislation and regulatory body standards that relate to the prevention and control of infection**

This activity gives you the opportunity to demonstrate your knowledge of current legislation and regulatory body standards which are relevant to the prevention and control of infection.

Summarise the Acts and Regulations, Regulatory Body Standards and National Occupational Standards that are relevant to your responsibilities in relation to infection prevention and control.

## 2.2 Local and organisational policies relevant to the prevention and control of infection

You read earlier that policies set out the arrangements an organisation has for complying with legislation. Infection prevention and control policies describe the measures that organisations take to comply with the legislation listed in Table 12.1.

Local authorities and health trusts produce **evidence-based policies** that guide health and social care settings within their districts and regions to comply with legislation whilst taking account of local needs. National initiatives and campaigns also help shape how local health and social care providers can minimise and prevent the spread of infection. For example the RCN 'Wipe it Out' campaign is aimed at reducing the **prevalence** of HCAIs, as are its booklets 'Good practice in infection prevention' and 'Guidance on Uniforms and Work Wear'.

### Key term

Evidence-based policies are policies that have been proved to work.
Prevalence means the proportion of individuals in a population having a disease.

The Department of Health has produced a number of documents addressing infection prevention and control at a local level, for example:

- Essential Steps to Safe Clean Care: Reducing Healthcare Associated Infections, which guides local health and social care providers in the use of best practice to prevent and manage the spread of infections.
- A Matron's Charter: An Action Plan for Cleaner Hospitals, which explains how staff, patients and visitors can make their local hospital a cleaner, safer place.
- Infection Control Guidance for Care Homes, which describes how everyone involved in providing residential care can protect residents and staff from acquiring infections.

Organisational policies relevant to infection prevention and control.
Hand hygiene.
Personal protective equipment (PPE).
Safe handling and disposal of sharps.
Safe handling and disposal of clinical waste.
Managing blood and bodily fluids and spills.
Cleaning and decontamination of equipment.
Achieving and maintaining a clean environment.
Training and education.

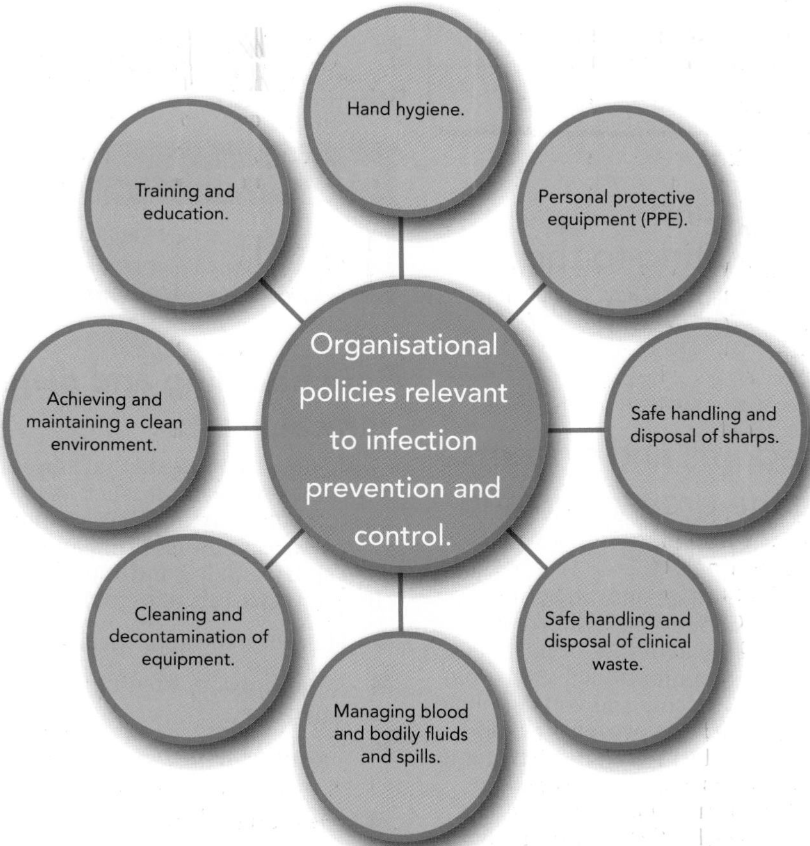

Figure 12.3 Organisational policies relevant to infection prevention and control

The Health Protection Agency provides support and advice to, for example, local authorities and health and emergency services. Its Guidance on Infection Control in Schools and Other Childcare Settings describes the importance of immunisation, personal hygiene and a clean environment.

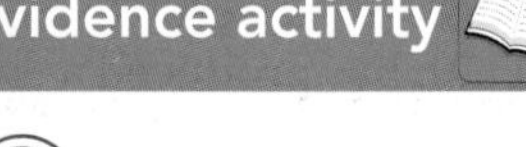

**Evidence activity**

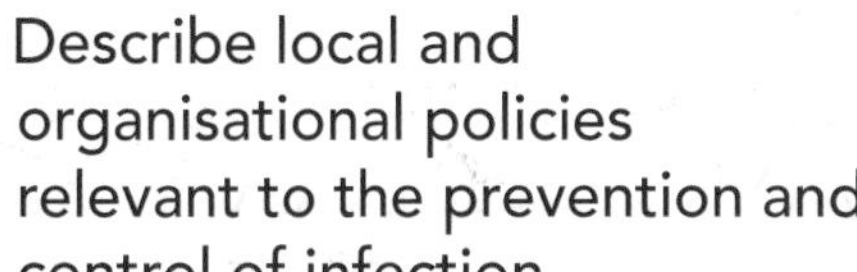

**2.2** Describe local and organisational policies relevant to the prevention and control of infection

This activity gives you the opportunity to demonstrate your knowledge of local and organisational policies relevant to the prevention and control of infection.

Describe infection prevention and control policies:

1. Written for your workplace. What is the purpose of each?
2. Written for health and social care organisations in your locality. Which organisations produced them? Why was it necessary for them to be produced?

# LO3 Systems and procedures relating to the prevention and control of infections

## 3.1 Procedures and systems relevant to the prevention and control of infection

Policies set out the arrangements an organisation has for complying with legislation. Procedures describe the activities or practices that need to be carried out for policies to be put into place. Figure 12.3 introduced you to policies that are relevant to infection prevention and control. You will read more about hand hygiene and PPE shortly but the following checklist summarises the practices or **standard precautions** that safeguard not only the individuals you work with but also you and your colleagues. Note that the checklist is not a substitute for your workplace's procedures.

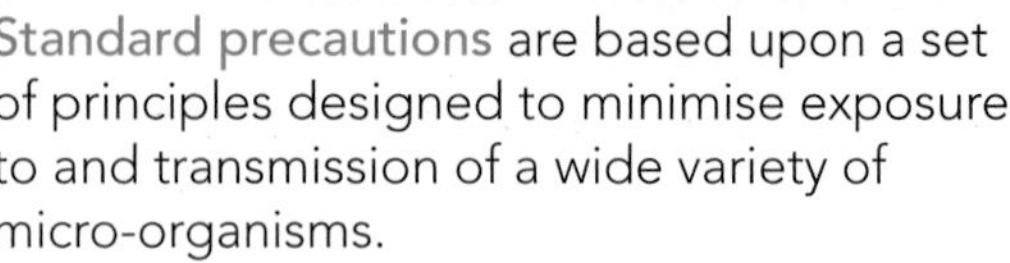

**Key term**

Standard precautions are based upon a set of principles designed to minimise exposure to and transmission of a wide variety of micro-organisms.

### Safe handling and disposal of *sharps*

- Don't attempt to use or dispose of sharps until you have had the appropriate training.
- Keep handling to a minimum and don't pass sharps directly from hand to hand.
- Never re-sheath needles and don't use bent or broken needles.
- Don't dismantle syringes or needles – dispose of them as a single unit.
- Dispose of sharps in the designated container at the point of use, that is where you are working.
- Store disposal containers in an area away from the public and don't fill them more than two-thirds full.

**Key term**

Sharps include needles, scalpels, stitch cutters and glass ampoules.

### Safe handling and disposal of clinical waste

Clinical waste is waste that can spread infection. It includes body fluids, such as blood; body waste, such as urine, faeces, vomit; soiled swabs, dressings, clothing and bed linen; and used sharps. Safe handling and disposal of clinical waste requires that you:

- Have had the appropriate training.
- Wear appropriate PPE and maintain good hand hygiene.
- Dispose of body fluids and waste down the sluice.
- Dispose of infected waste and used swabs and dressings in a yellow bag, for incineration.

- Dispose of soiled and infected clothing and linen in a clear alginate bag inside a red plastic bag, to be laundered.
- Report any dangerous handling and waste disposal to your manager.

## Managing blood and body fluids

Don't attempt to clean up spills or collect and handle specimens until you have had the appropriate training.

- Spills:
  - Wear appropriate PPE.
  - Clean up as soon as you can, using cleaning materials and disinfectants that are appropriate to the type of spill and the surface that has been spilled on.
- Collecting and handling specimens:
  - Wear appropriate PPE.
  - Make sure containers are suitable, sterile and leak-proof.
  - Label containers with relevant information and complete any accompanying forms.
  - Send specimens to the lab as soon as possible – never leave them lying around.
  - Enter test results into patient records as soon as you receive them, and report any abnormal results to the appropriate person.

## Decontamination of equipment

Don't attempt to use decontamination techniques and equipment until you have had the appropriate training. Always follow the manufacturer's instructions, and don't use decontamination equipment if you're not confident that it has been installed and maintained properly.

**Single-use equipment**, such as needles, should not be decontaminated and re-used. Dispose of it as appropriate.

### Key term

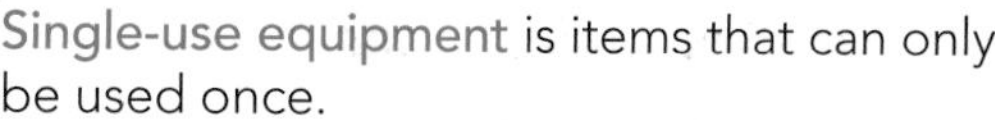

Single-use equipment is items that can only be used once.

Re-usable equipment, such as bed pans, must be decontaminated before re-use through a process of cleaning and disinfection or cleaning and sterilisation.

- Cleaning using detergent and hot water removes visible contamination but may not destroy pathogens. It is suitable for environmental cleaning.
- Disinfection uses chemicals or heat. It reduces the number of **viable** pathogens. Washer-disinfectors and ultrasonic baths use very high temperatures to disinfect equipment that would be damaged by chemicals; chemicals, such as formaldehyde and peroxide, are used when heat is insufficient.

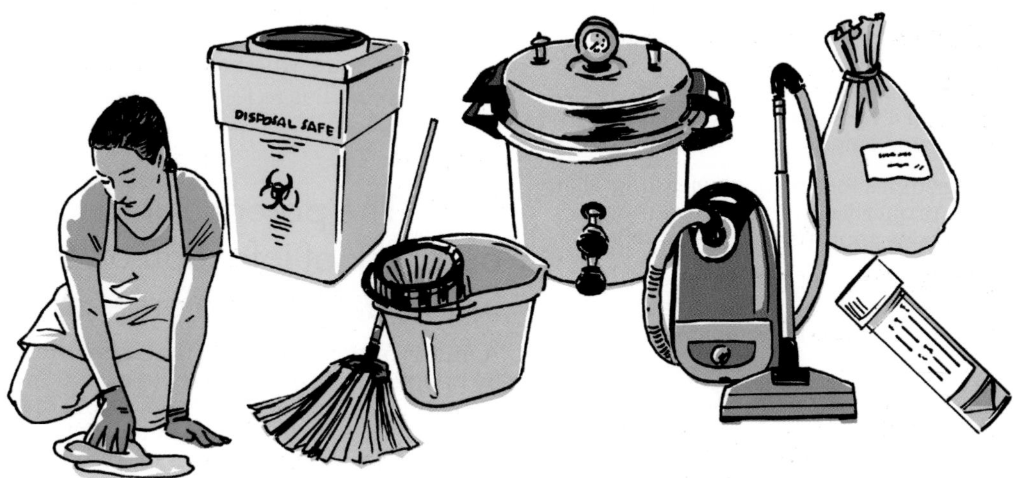


Figure 12.4 Standard precautions.

- Low risk equipment that does not touch broken skin or **mucous membranes** or is not in contact with patients, such as wheelchairs and bedframes, must be cleaned and/or disinfected after every use.
- Sterilisation ensures that an object is totally free from pathogens. You may have access to a sterile services department (SSD); or you could use a bench top vacuum steam steriliser.
- Medium risk equipment that touches intact skin or mucous membranes, for example a bed pan, doesn't need to be sterile when in use but must be cleaned and sterilised after every use.
- High risk equipment, such as equipment that touches broken skin or mucous membranes, penetrates the skin or enters the body, must be sterile when used and must be cleaned and sterilised after every use.

### Key terms

Mucous membranes are mucous-secreting membranes that line the body cavities and canals that connect with the external air, such as the alimentary canal and respiratory tract.

Viable means alive and able to reproduce.

## Achieving and maintaining a clean environment

A dirty environment carries a risk of infection. Dust and dirt, body fluids and waste, and household waste such as left-over food, provide conditions that support the growth and reproduction of a variety of pathogens. Health and social care settings should therefore have:

- fixed schedules for thorough cleaning of all areas, using properly maintained cleaning equipment that is appropriate to the surface being cleaned
- appropriate and clean facilities for the disposal of non-clinical, household waste.

### Time to reflect

Training

What training have you had in relation to infection prevention and control? How does training – or the lack of it – impact on your work?

## Training

All health and social care professionals should be trained in infection prevention and control, as part of their induction and on an ongoing basis to maintain and update their knowledge and skills. Training should cover the principles of infection prevention and control, including:

- relevant legislation
- policies and procedures, including standard precautions
- roles and responsibilities
- risk assessment
- use of PPE
- environmental and personal hygiene, including hand washing and skin care.

### Evidence activity

Procedures and systems relevant to the prevention and control of infection

This activity gives you the opportunity to demonstrate your knowledge of procedures and systems relevant to the prevention and control of infection.

Describe infection prevention and control procedures or standard precautions that:

1. you're required to follow in your work
2. a colleague, who has a different job role from you, has to follow in their work.

## 3.2 The potential impact of an outbreak of infection on the individual and the organisation

A minor outbreak of infection is characterised by people in close proximity to each other, such as in a ward or classroom or in adjacent rooms in a residential care home, developing similar signs and symptoms over a period of days or weeks. They are usually easily managed. A serious outbreak is characterised by 20 or more people throughout a health or social care setting developing signs and symptoms within 24 hours. Serious outbreaks are dealt with using serious outbreak procedures.

It's important to be able to recognise potential outbreaks so that prevention and control measures can be put in place as soon as possible. You read about the characteristics of a possible outbreak earlier. It's also important to report suspected or actual outbreaks without delay to the individual who has responsibility for managing infection control.

When a suspected outbreak has been reported, the individual or team responsible for managing infection will assess the situation and decide what action to take. This could include:

- isolating anyone who is infected
- ensuring that appropriate antibiotics are available
- restricting staff movement to limit exposure to the source of infection
- ensuring staff who are exposed to the infection use appropriate PPE and have a sufficient supply of alcohol gel
- employing additional staff, as cover for those who are sick or whose time is devoted to isolation nursing
- keeping relatives and friends informed, restricting visiting or closing the affected ward, department or setting
- informing the local HPU if the infection is a notifiable disease.

When the outbreak is under control, the environment and any equipment used during the outbreak should be thoroughly decontaminated. In addition a review should take place to check:

- the effectiveness of infection prevention and control procedures
- whether staff follow procedures to the letter
- whether there are any barriers to being able to follow procedures, for example time constraints, staff shortages and lack of resources
- the need for further training.

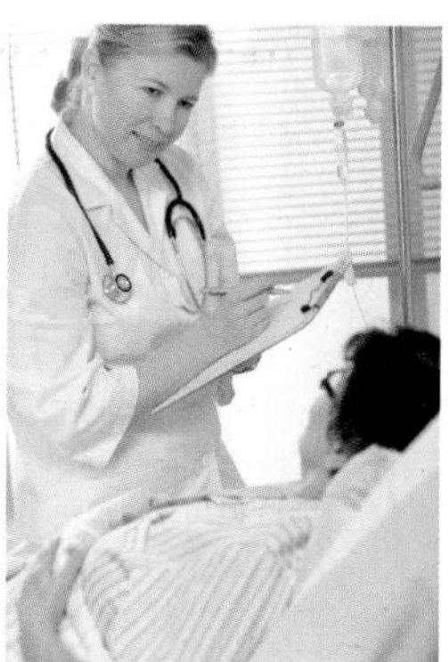

Figure 12.5 How do you feel?

It's also important to assess how patients feel that the situation was dealt with. Isolation nursing can create loneliness, depression and boredom; and disruption to routine can be stressful. The keen use of infection control measures can make people feel dirty or 'unclean' and worry that their disease will affect the attitude of staff towards them. And having a diagnosis sign on the door compromises their confidentiality.

Patients need to be encouraged to talk about their experiences of being in isolation so that strategies can be put into place for the future. And they and their relatives, who are understandably anxious, need to be helped to understand the need for the measures that are taken.

An outbreak of infection can also affect an organisation. For example:

- Healthcare-associated infections (HCAIs) infections such as *C. difficile* and MRSA are the focus of huge amounts of attention from the media, impacting on the reputation of the hospitals concerned and the morale of staff.
- Having to buy in additional resources, such as staff, impacts on finances.
- Lack of continuity of care due to use of agency staff affects the emotional well-being of patients.
- Additional work involved in dealing with an outbreak of infection is time consuming and can jeopardise job satisfaction and the day-to-day running of the organisation.

## Evidence activity

### 3.2 The potential impact of an outbreak of infection on the individual and the organisation

This activity gives you the opportunity to demonstrate your understanding of the potential impact of an outbreak of infection on the individual and the organisation.

Talk with your manager about an outbreak of infection at your workplace. How was the outbreak dealt with? How did it affect people and the organisation? Why did it have those effects? What steps were taken subsequent to the outbreak? Has there been a further outbreak of the same infection? If so, why?

# LO4 The importance of risk assessment in relation to the prevention and control of infections

## 4.1 What is meant by 'risk'?

A hazard is anything with the potential to cause harm, and a risk is the likelihood that a hazard will cause harm. For example, a broken paving stone is a hazard – it has the potential to cause someone to trip, fall and break a leg. But the likelihood or risk of this happening depends on factors such as age and ability. An able-bodied child is less likely to fall and break a bone then a frail older person or an adult with visual impairment.

The expression 'at risk group' is used to describe a group of people who have a higher-than-average risk of being harmed by hazards, for example because of their age, lifestyle, existing health status and genetic inheritance.

### Evidence activity

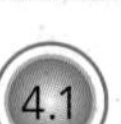

#### 4.1 Define the term risk

This activity gives you the opportunity to demonstrate your knowledge of the definition of 'risk'.

In your own words, what is meant by the term 'risk'?

### Case Study

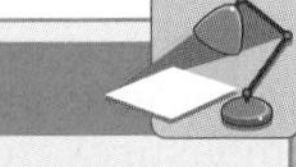

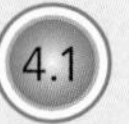

#### 4.1 Care in the community?

Cum-a-Cropper Community Centre is situated on a busy main road. It is an old house on three floors and the front door opens straight onto the pavement. Its ground floor kitchen/dining room, which is open plan and freely accessible, is much in need of a makeover, as are the two toilets, both on the second floor, neither of which has adequate disabled facilities. There is a lounge on the first floor and a TV and games room on the second floor. The garden is grassed.

The community centre is used by groups of children, young people, mothers and toddlers, elderly people, and people with learning and physical difficulties, including sensory impairments.

What hazards can you identify at Cum-a-Cropper Community Centre? How does the risk to health and safety vary within the different groups of people using the centre?

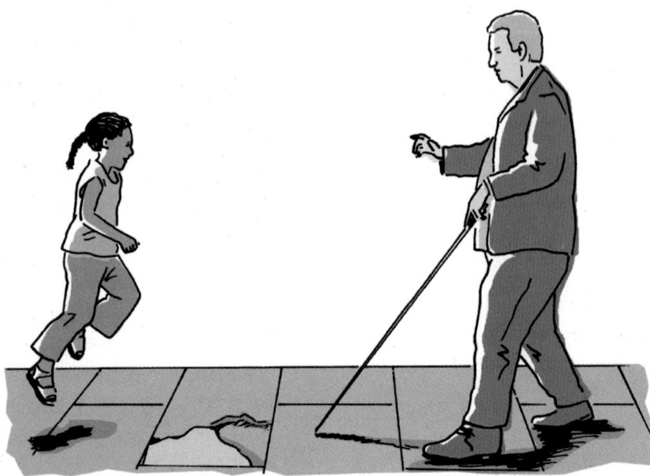

Figure 12.6 Hazards and degree of risk

## 4.2 Potential risks of infection within the workplace

Table 12.2 Potential risks of infection within the workplace

| Main route of spread of infection | Examples of pathogenic infections |
|---|---|
| Skin.<br>Direct contact is skin-to-skin contact between two people. Indirect contact is touching things that another person has used. | Bacterial infections such as MRSA and *C. difficile*; infestations such as lice; and fungal infections such as ringworm. |
| Airways (inhalation). | Bacterial and viral infections such as influenza, pneumonia, bronchitis and tetanus. |
| Digestive tract (eating and drinking). | Bacterial and viral infections such as *E. coli*, Salmonella, rotavirus and norovirus. |
| Use of healthcare instruments, such as sharps. | Viral infections such as HIV AIDS and Hepatitis B. |

Infection can occur anywhere where pathogens are present. Failure to prevent pathogens being brought into health and social care settings by patients, staff and visitors, and failure to control outbreaks of infection once they have established, can have dire effects on vulnerable, at risk groups.

HCAIs are infections acquired in hospital or brought into hospital by people already infected. They include:

- MRSA (Meticillin-resistant *Staphylococcus aureus*), a bacterium that is resistant to the antibiotic meticillin. Many of us carry *Staph. aureus* (SA) on our skin without developing an infection, but if it enters the body, it can cause blood poisoning and infections such as boils, abscesses and impetigo. It is spread by direct contact with infected patients and also indirectly, by touching contaminated sheets, towels, clothes and dressings. At risk groups include people who take frequent courses of antibiotics, are already in poor health, have an open wound or skin condition such as psoriasis, or have an in-dwelling device such as a **catheter** or a drip.
- *Clostridium difficile* (*C. difficile*), a bacterium that is present in the large bowel but that doesn't cause problems in healthy people. It is spread in the same way as MRSA but contaminated surfaces are more likely to be bedpans and toilets. Symptoms include stomach ache, diarrhoea, bleeding of the bowel, blood poisoning and fever. It can also be fatal. At risk groups include elderly people and people already in poor health.

### Key term

A **catheter** is a plastic tube inserted into the body to drain fluid.

The head louse is a tiny, wingless parasitic insect that lives among human hairs and feeds on blood from the scalp. They are very common and their bites cause the scalp to itch, which, if scratched, can become infected. Whilst head lice can't fly or jump, they have claws that allow them to cling firmly to hair. They spread mainly through head-to-head contact, but also indirectly when clothing and hair equipment is shared. At risk groups are people who have close contact, especially children.

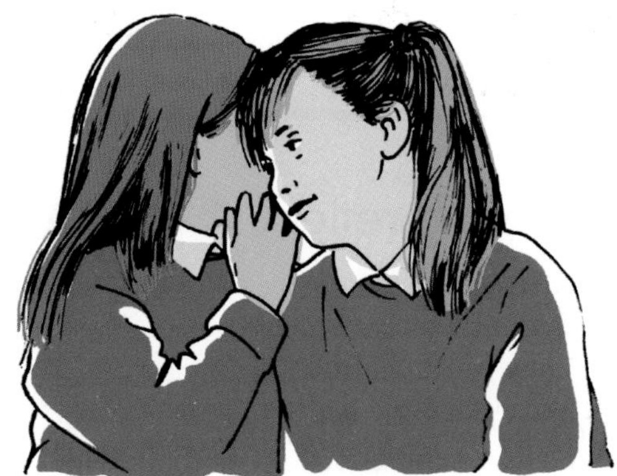

Figure 12.7 Spreading head lice

Ringworm is caused by a fungus that lives on dead skin, hair and nails. When it affects the skin between the toes, it's known as athlete's foot, and appears as red, scaly patches. Ringworm of the scalp starts as a small sore that becomes scaly, causing hair to fall out or break into stubble. Ringworm of the nails causes them to become thick, discoloured and brittle. It is spread directly and indirectly, for example from damp clothing and wet surfaces. At risk groups include people who use swimming pools and changing rooms and people in hospitals and residential care who share bathrooms.

Influenza is a highly infectious illness caused by a flu virus. It infects the respiratory system, causing fever, aches and pains, a dry cough, nausea and loss of appetite. Like the common cold, it is spread by inhaling small droplets of saliva that contain the virus and which are coughed or sneezed into the air by an infected person. It is also spread by indirect contact, for example when an infected person touches surfaces such as door handles with unwashed hands. At risk groups include elderly people and people with weak immune systems, such as cancer and AIDS patients.

Pneumonia is a bacterial or viral infection of the lung tissue and bronchitis is a bacterial infection of the **bronchi**. They are spread in the same way as influenza and can occur together as broncho-pneumonia. Symptoms include aches and pains, fever, chest pain, cough, breathlessness, and yellow/green, sometimes bloodstained sputum. At risk groups include people who are frail and elderly and already in poor health, for example with a chest disease. Pneumonia is a common cause of death in people in the late or terminal stages of a cancer.

### Key term

Bronchi are the large airways that carry air into the lungs.

## Time to reflect

### 4.2 Infections

Think about the infections you have had from time to time. What caused them? Why do you think you caught them? How did they affect you? How could you avoid catching them again?

Tetanus is caused by the bacterium *Clostridium tetani*, which is found in soil and animal manure. If the bacterial **spores** get into a wound they release a toxin that attacks the nervous system and causes problems such as muscle spasm, as in lockjaw. At risk groups include people who work with soil and animal manure, children playing outdoors, and people in health and social care settings where cleanliness is not maintained.

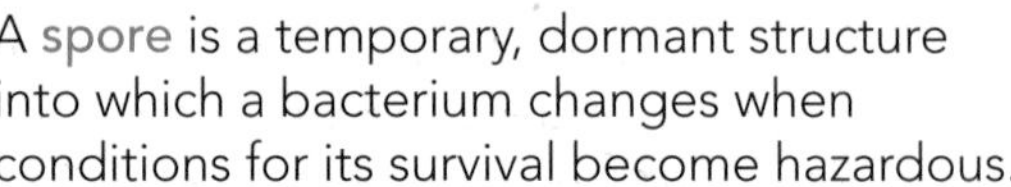

### Key term

A spore is a temporary, dormant structure into which a bacterium changes when conditions for its survival become hazardous.

Food poisoning is caused by poor standards of personal hygiene, poor hygiene in food storage, preparation and eating areas, and incorrect storage and cooking temperatures. Food poisoning bacteria include *Escherichia coli* (E. coli) and Salmonella; and viruses such as rotavirus and norovirus. In addition to growing and reproducing in food, they are carried by people on their bodies and clothes; by animals in their urine and faeces; and on kitchen surfaces and equipment. Signs and symptoms include nausea, stomach ache, diarrhoea and vomiting, and at risk groups include babies, children, elderly people and people with pre-existing health problems.

Hepatitis B is a highly infectious virus that damages the liver. It is 50 to 100 times more infectious than HIV (Human Immunodeficiency Virus) but like HIV is carried in body fluids such as blood, saliva, semen and vaginal fluid. At risk groups are drug users who use contaminated needles, patients exposed to contaminated equipment and blood, for example during transfusions, and people who have unprotected sex. Hep B is also an important complication of accidental **needle stick injuries** and therefore a risk factor for unvaccinated healthcare and body art workers.

www.patient.co.uk; www.nhs.uk; http://kidshealth.org; http://hcd2.bupa.co.uk; www.bbc.co.uk

### Key term

A needle stick injury is a skin puncture by a hypodermic needle or other sharp object.

## Evidence activity 

### 4.2 The potential risks of infection within the workplace

This activity gives you the opportunity to demonstrate your knowledge of the potential risks of infection within your workplace.

Bearing in mind the type of setting in which you work, the care that is provided and the characteristics of the people you support, for example their age, lifestyle and existing health status, outline potential risks of infection within your workplace.

## 4.3 Carrying out a risk assessment

The Management of Health and Safety at Work Regulations (MHSWR) 1999 require your employer to carry out risk assessments to eliminate or minimise any risks associated with infection. And because you have a responsibility to cooperate with your employer or manager's efforts to improve health and safety, you should be thinking 'risk assessment' as you carry out each and every activity.

## Time to reflect 

### 4.3 Risk assess or risk averse?

Do you think 'risk assessment' as you carry out your activities? Or are you blind to things that could go wrong? Can you see the benefit of being on the alert for potential hazards and associated risks?

According to the HSE, there are five steps to a risk assessment. In relation to the prevention and control of infections:

**Step 1**: Identify hazards.

- Inspect the cleanliness and hygiene of people, equipment and the working environment.
- Check that facilities for maintaining cleanliness and hygiene are in good repair.
- Check that infection prevention and control procedures are understood and followed to the letter.
- Check that systems are in place for monitoring the use of procedures, educating everyone concerned about the importance of following procedures and supervising them to ensure that they put their learning into practice.
- Review records relating to infectious outbreaks to check that they are appropriately dealt with.

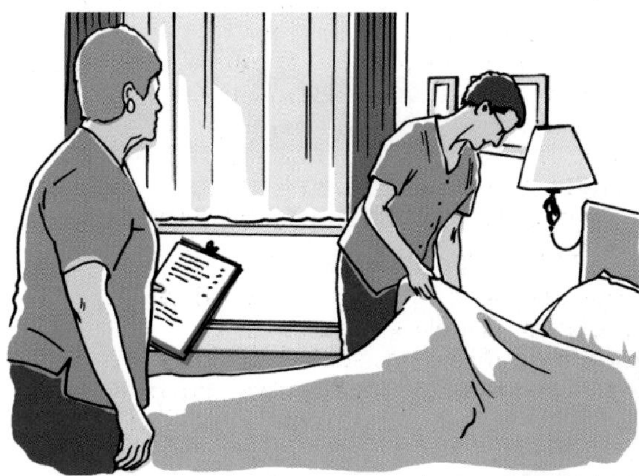

Figure 12.8 Identifying hazards

**Step 2:** Decide who might be harmed and how.

The people who could be harmed include those you support, yourself, your colleagues and any visitors; and harm would result from exposure to infection.

**Step 3**: Assess the risks arising from the hazards and decide whether existing precautions are adequate or if more should be done. If something needs to be done, take steps to eliminate or control the risks.

The risk that a hazard will cause harm depends on factors such as age, ability, health status and so on. The people you support are particularly at risk. Are existing precautions adequate to safeguard them? Can you eliminate the hazards?

If not, can you control risks arising from the hazards?

**Step 4**: Record the findings and say how the risks can be controlled to prevent harm. Inform everyone about the outcome of the risk assessment as everyone will be involved in controlling the risk.

It's very important to let everyone know the upshot of your risk assessment. Risks will remain unless you let people know how they must adapt their work practices.

**Step 5**: Review the assessment from time to time and revise it if necessary.

Review is very important. Unless you review the effect of changes to work practices you won't know if the changes are effective! Also, you may have been asked to use new equipment, materials and procedures, which could lead to new hazards. So don't be afraid to suggest further changes if necessary. Whilst you don't want to continually re-invent the wheel, there is an argument for never standing still, that things can only get better!

www.hse.gov.uk

### Evidence activity 

#### 4.3 The process of carrying out a risk assessment

This activity gives you the opportunity to demonstrate your knowledge of the process of carrying out a risk assessment.

1. Identify an infection hazard, for example, that colleagues aren't washing their hands as often as they should.
2. Who might be harmed and how?
3. What are the risks to health of the hazard? What can be done to eliminate or control these risks?
4. How could you make people aware of changes that need to be made to eliminate or control the risks?
5. When do you think you should review the effectiveness of the changes?

## 4.4 The importance of carrying out a risk assessment

As you know, all organisations have a legal obligation to carry out risk assessments. Failure of your employer to fulfil their legal obligations puts their reputation and financial standing at risk. This in turn could affect your employment status.

Risk assessment helps prevent and control the risk of infection. It helps maintain your health and that of everyone you work with, including members of the public. Because ill health harms lives, you have a moral obligation to think 'risk assessment' as you carry out each and every activity. By doing so, you will alert yourself to the standard of your work practice.

www.hse.gov.uk

### Evidence activity 

#### 4.4 The importance of carrying out a risk assessment

This activity gives you the opportunity to demonstrate your understanding of the importance of carrying out a risk assessment.

Identify a couple of activities that you carry out and which have been risk assessed, for example preparing food and helping someone use the toilet. Why do you think these activities have been risk assessed? Why is it important that you follow procedures for these activities to the letter?

# LO5 The importance of using personal protective equipment (PPE) in the prevention and control of infections

## 5.1 Demonstrate correct use of PPE

Personal protective equipment (PPE) is equipment that is used to protect against risks to health or safety. It must be used where there are risks that cannot be adequately controlled in other ways; it must have instructions on how to use it safely; and people who use it must be trained in its use and supervised to make sure they use it correctly.

Section 5.7 describes the correct practice in putting PPE on and taking it off; and Section 5.8 the correct procedure for its disposal. Read those sections before attempting the following activity.

Practice activity 

### 5.1 Demonstrate correct use of PPE

This activity gives you the opportunity to practise using PPE correctly.

Ask an experienced colleague to observe you using PPE, including:

- putting it on
- taking it off
- disposing of it.

Are you both confident that you use it correctly?

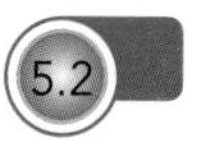

## 5.2 Different types of PPE

See page 222 for Evidence Activity 5.2.

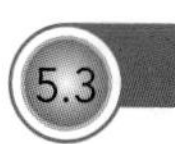

## 5.3 The reasons for using PPE

There are different types of PPE, each helping prevent the spread of pathogens from one person, object, place or part of the body to another.

Research & investigate 

### 5.3 PPE used at your workplace

Look around your workplace. What PPE do your colleagues use? When do they use it? Why do you think they use it?

### Body protection

Some procedures involve contact with blood and body fluids and waste. If an activity involves a risk of extensive splashing to your skin and clothing, wear a full-body fluid-repellent gown. If splashing would be restricted to your trunk area or you are carrying out procedures that involve contact with mucous membranes or breaks in the skin, wear a disposable, single use apron.

You should also wear a disposable apron if you are handling food, cleaning, making beds, disposing of waste and decontaminating equipment. Don't wear an apron all the time, 'just in case'; but do wear one where there is a possibility of risk, not just to protect you against infection but also to protect others against any pathogens you may be harbouring in your clothes.

### Face protection

Some cleaning materials cause breathing problems, such as asthma. Dirt and dust may contain bacterial spores, which can be inhaled during cleaning. And some infections are caught by inhaling the small droplets coughed or sneezed into the air by an infected person. To protect your airways and lungs against inhalation hazards, use PPE that covers your nose and mouth, such as a face mask.

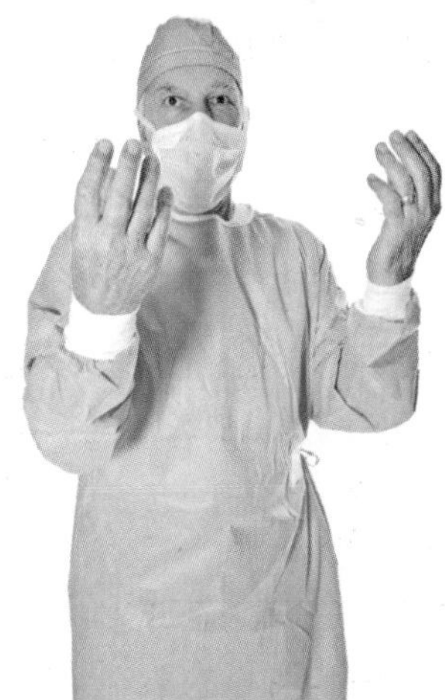

Figure 12.9 PPE

### Eye protection

Activities that require you to work with chemicals and body fluids and waste are 'splash hazards'. Wear PPE, such as visors and safety goggles, to protect your eyes against splashes.

### Gloves

Single-use disposable gloves are absolutely vital for protecting you and the people you work with against infection. You should use them for all procedures that involve contact with:

- people suspected or known to have an infection
- anything that may have been touched or used by someone who has an infection
- body fluids and waste, including soiled linen and clothing
- breaks in the skin and mucous membranes
- sterile instruments
- hazardous chemicals.

Evidence activity 

###  5.2 & 5.3 Different types of PPE and the reasons for their use

This activity gives you the opportunity to demonstrate your knowledge and understanding of types and use of PPE.

Complete the following table to show you know when to use PPE, what PPE to use and why you should use it.

| Items of PPE | When I wear it | Why I must wear it |
|---|---|---|
| | | |
| | | |
| | | |
| | | |
| | | |

## 5.4 Current regulations and legislation relevant to PPE

See page 223 for Evidence Activity 5.4.

## 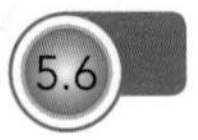 5.6 Your employer's responsibilities regarding the use of PPE

Table 12.3 Current legislation and regulations and your employer's responsibilities

| Relevant legislation and regulations | Responsibilities of your employer |
|---|---|
| Personal Protective Equipment at Work Regulations (PPE) 1992 | To provide you with PPE that:<br>• is appropriate and suitable<br>• is maintained and stored properly<br>• has instructions on how to use it safely<br>• you can use correctly. |
| Health and Safety at Work, etc Act (HASWA) 1974 | To write health and safety policies and procedures regarding the use of PPE and make you aware of them. |
| Management of Health and Safety at Work Regulations 1999 | To carry out risk assessments to eliminate or reduce risks to health and safety, including using PPE, and provide you with clear information, supervision and training in how to use PPE. |
| Provision and Use of Work Equipment Regulations (PUWER) 1998 | To make sure suitable replacement PPE is always readily available and that it is well looked after and properly stored when not being used. |
| Control of Substances Hazardous to Health Regulations (COSHH) 2002 | To carry out risk assessments on activities that involve exposure to hazardous substances and write procedures for their correct and safe use, including using PPE. |

*Contd.*

| Relevant legislation and regulations | Responsibilities of your employer |
|---|---|
| Health and Social Care Act (2008) | To make sure PPE is clean and fit for purpose, to minimise the risk of HCAIs. |
| Department of Health (2004) Standards for better health (England only) | To maintain safety of patients, staff and visitors by having systems that reduce the risk of infection, including using PPE. |
| Food Safety Act 1990 and the Food Hygiene Regulations 2006. | To make sure that food safety hazards are controlled, including using PPE. |
| Hazardous Waste Regulations 2005. | To make sure that hazardous waste, including used PPE, is dealt with so as to avoid putting health at risk. |
| Environmental Protection (Duty of Care) Regulations 1991. | To make sure that waste, including used PPE, is properly stored and adequately packaged whilst awaiting removal from the premises. |

**Evidence activity** 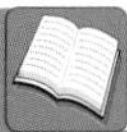

 & 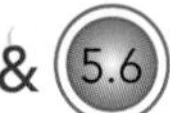

### Current regulations and legislation relevant to PPE and your employers' responsibilities regarding the use of PPE

This activity gives you the opportunity to demonstrate your knowledge of current regulations and legislation relevant to PPE and your employers' responsibilities regarding the use of PPE.

- List the Regulations and Acts of Parliament that are relevant to your work with regard to infection prevention and control.
- Describe how this legislation affects your employer's responsibilities regarding the use of PPE.

## 5.5 Your responsibilities regarding the use of PPE

The Health and Safety at Work Act 1974 states that it is your duty while at work to take reasonable care of yourself and anyone else who may be affected by your actions. In relation to prevention and control of infection, this means knowing:

- what PPE to use, when and how to use it and why
- the correct procedures for putting it on and taking it off
- appropriate decontamination and disposal methods.

You also have a responsibility to cooperate with your employer in relation to health and safety issues. This means you must:

- Follow procedures and comply with requests to use PPE. In some jobs, failure to use PPE properly can be grounds for disciplinary action, even dismissal. However, you can refuse to wear PPE if it puts your safety at risk, for example if it's the wrong size or you might be at risk because of poor fit.
- Make sure you are properly trained in how to use PPE.
- Report any concerns you have that PPE isn't being used appropriately.
- Suggest changes in the use of PPE that you think would be beneficial.

**www.direct.gov.uk**

A short guide to the Personal Protective Equipment at Work Regulations 1992, HSE 2005

**Research & investigate** 

 **Responsibilities**

Find out what could happen if you failed to:

- comply with requests to wear PPE
- attend training in the use of PPE
- raise concerns that PPE wasn't being used appropriately.

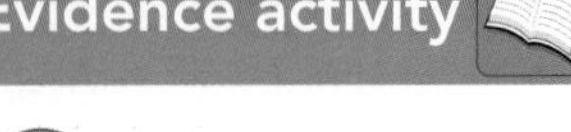

### Your responsibilities regarding the use of PPE

This activity gives you the opportunity to demonstrate your knowledge of your responsibilities regarding the use of PPE.

Describe your responsibilities with regard to the use of PPE.

## 5.7 The application and removal of PPE

It is important that you know the correct procedure for putting on and taking off a range of PPE.

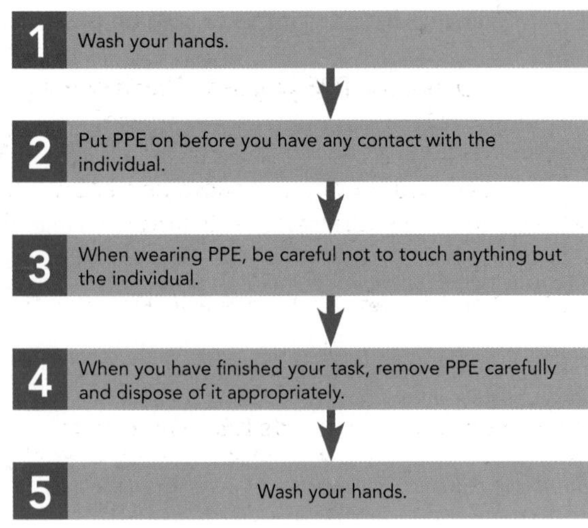


Figure 12.10 Five key points about the use of PPE

### Putting PPE on

1. If you need to wear a gown put that on first. Choose the appropriate gown for the task and the right size for you. The opening should be at the back and it should be secured at the neck and waist.
2. Face protection goes on next. Some masks are fastened with ties, others with elastic. If yours has ties, place it over your mouth, nose and chin and tie the upper set at the back of your head and the lower set at the base of your neck. If it has elastic head bands, separate the two bands, hold the mask over your nose, mouth and chin, then stretch the upper band over the upper back of your head and the lower at the base of the neck. Adjust to fit.
3. Eye protection is third to go on. Position goggles or visor over your eyes and secure them to your head using the ear pieces or head band. Adjust to fit.
4. Gloves are last to go on. Choose the type needed for the task and in the size that fits you best. Insert your hands and adjust for comfort and so that you don't feel restricted. If you are wearing a gown, tuck the cuffs under each glove to provide a continuous barrier protection for your skin.

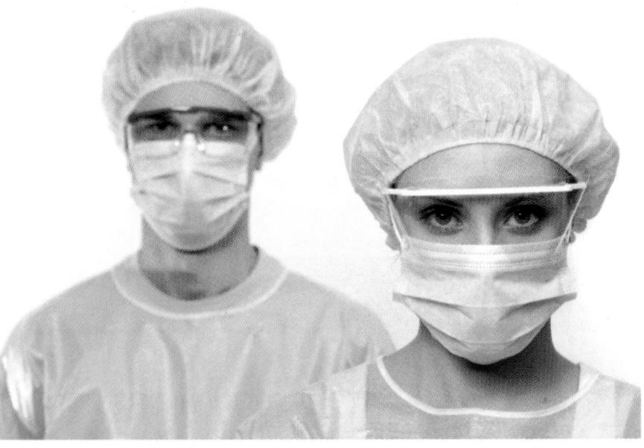

Figure 12.11 Face and eye protection

When wearing PPE, safe practice dictates that you:

- don't touch or adjust it while working
- don't touch anything with contaminated gloves
- take your gloves off if they get torn and wash your hands before putting on a new pair.

### Taking PPE off

At the end of an activity, the outside of anything on your front and arms is considered to be contaminated. Clean areas are inside the gloves and gown, the back of the gown and apron, and the ties and elastic of face and eye protection.

1. As gloves are the most contaminated items of PPE, they are taken off first. Using a gloved hand, grasp the outside of the opposite glove near the wrist and peel the glove away from the hand so that it is inside-out. Hold the removed glove in the other, gloved hand, slide one or two fingers of the ungloved hand under the wrist of the remaining glove and peel it off from the inside, creating a bag for both gloves. Dispose of as appropriate.
2. Eye protection comes off next. Grasp the 'clean' ear or head pieces and lift away from face. Dispose of as appropriate
3. Body protection is third to come off. Untie your apron, roll up so only the 'clean' part is

visible and dispose of appropriately. Remove a gown by:

- slipping your hands inside at the neck and shoulder and peeling away from the shoulders
- slipping the fingers of one hand under the cuff of the opposite arm and pulling your hand into the sleeve, grasping the gown from inside
- pushing the sleeve off the opposite arm.

Fold or roll into a bundle with only the 'clean' part visible and drop into the appropriate container.

4. Finally but most importantly, wash your hands. You will read about good hand washing technique shortly.

www.cdc.gov

**Evidence activity** 

### 5.7 Correct practice in the application and removal of PPE

This activity gives you the opportunity to demonstrate your knowledge of how to apply and remove PPE.

Produce a poster to be displayed in your staff room that tells colleagues how they should put PPE on and take it off. Check out websites and PPE catalogues for diagrams to illustrate your poster.

## 5.8 The correct procedure for disposal of used PPE

Clinical waste includes all items contaminated by body fluids and waste that are or could be infectious.

Single-use PPE, for example white or clear plastic aprons and disposable gloves, masks and eye protection, should be used for just one procedure or **episode of care**. If it gets contaminated by body fluids and waste, it must be disposed of as clinical waste in a yellow bag or container for collection and incineration by trained personnel. If it is not contaminated it should be double bagged and disposed of as domestic waste.

**Key term**

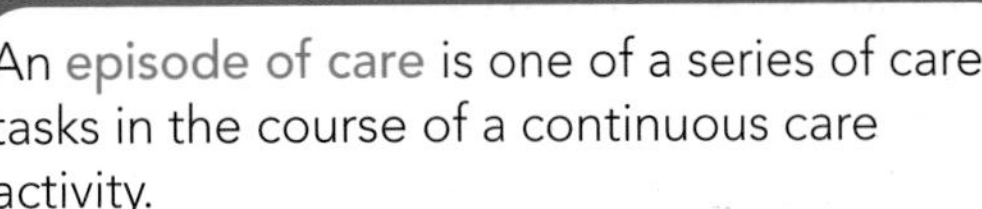

An episode of care is one of a series of care tasks in the course of a continuous care activity.

Re-usable PPE should be decontaminated according to the manufacturer's instructions.

Blue disposable plastic aprons should be used for food handling only and disposed of in domestic waste bins. Domestic household gloves should be washed with detergent and hot water and left to dry after each use to remove visible soiling. If they are worn frequently, are torn or becoming stained, they should be disposed of in domestic waste bins and replaced.

**Time to reflect** 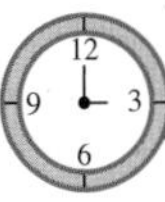

### 5.8 Disposal of PPE

Think about the PPE you use. Which of it is disposable and which can you re-use? How do you dispose of single-use items? What do you do with re-usable items? Do you need to make changes to your methods of disposal?

Waste bins should be lidded, foot-operated and kept clean, and the bags in them should never be filled more than two thirds full. Waste bags awaiting collection must be secured to prevent leakage and labelled to show the place of origin. They should be stored in a designated area that is kept clean and locked, to prevent access by the public, animals and vermin.

**Evidence activity** 

### 5.8 The correct procedure for disposal of used PPE

This activity gives you the opportunity to demonstrate your knowledge of the correct procedure for disposal of used PPE.

Produce a set of coloured, illustrated memory cards to remind your colleagues how they should dispose of used PPE.

# LO6 The importance of good personal hygiene in the prevention and control of infections

## 6.1 The key principles of good personal hygiene

Infection prevention and control is based on the use of practices and procedures that reduce the likelihood that infection is spread from one person, object, place or part of the body to another. High standards of personal hygiene are key to infection prevention and control, not least because much of health and social care requires being in very close proximity with vulnerable individuals.

Ten Top Tips for maintaining good personal hygiene.

1. Keep your hands clean. This is top of the list in controlling the spread of infections that cause diarrhoea and vomiting and respiratory diseases. You will read about good hand washing technique in the next section.
2. Shower or bath daily. Perspiration and dirt provide the perfect environment for many bacteria, fungi and viruses to live and reproduce; and stale sweat is not pleasant to smell. Use a good quality, unperfumed anti-perspirant.
3. Keep your hair clean and tidy and cover or tie it back if it is longer than collar length, especially when handling and serving food and drink. By paying regular attention to your hair, you will look and smell fresh and also be aware of any infestations.
4. Keep your nails short and clean. Bitten nails look revolting and dirt under nails harbours a range of **micro-organisms**. False nails are also a health and safety hazard and shouldn't be worn at work.
5. Keep your feet clean and covered. Dirty, sweaty feet also look revolting and are a **reservoir** for micro-organisms.
6. Keep your clothes clean. Parasites such as fleas and pubic lice can live in clothing, and dirty clothing smells, particularly if you smoke. Don't wear sleeves that go below your elbows at work, so that you can wash your hands and forearms effectively.
7. Keep your teeth clean. Nothing looks worse than dirty, stained teeth. And an unclean mouth provides living conditions for the bacteria that cause bad breath.
8. Don't wear jewellery or body piercings, apart from a plain ring, metal ear studs and a fob watch. Jewellery can carry micro-organisms, and piercings can be infected, especially when new.
9. Cover wounds. Cover any wounds with a coloured plaster and check out what you can and can't do while wearing the plaster, especially if you work with food.
10. Either shave regularly or keep facial hair clean and tidy. Your organisation may have requirements with regard to beards and moustaches.

### Key terms

**Micro-organisms** are organisms such as bacteria, parasites and fungi that can only be seen using a microscope.

A **reservoir** is an environment in which a micro-organism can live and reproduce.

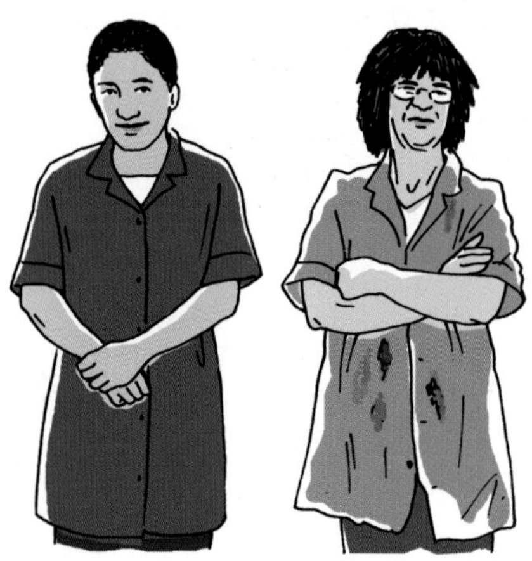

Figure 12.12 Personal hygiene

### Evidence activity

#### 6.1 The key principles of good personal hygiene

This activity gives you the opportunity to demonstrate your knowledge of the key principles of good personal hygiene.

How do you maintain good personal hygiene? In what ways could you improve your personal hygiene? Why is it so important for a health or social care worker to maintain good personal hygiene?

Practice activity 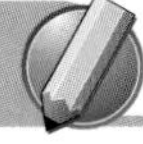

### 6.2 Demonstrate good hand washing technique

This activity gives you the opportunity to develop a good hand washing technique.

Using the information above, practise washing your hands so that you can be confident that they are completely free from contamination. Ask a more experienced colleague to observe you and act on any feedback they give you.

## 6.2 Good hand washing technique

See page 228 for Practice Activity 6.2.

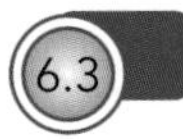

## 6.3 Correct sequence for hand washing

Hand hygiene involves washing your hands with soap and water to ensure that they are thoroughly decontaminated. It is a standard precaution against the spread of infection and you should do it before any activity with an individual whether your hands are visibly dirty or not.

1 Wet your hands and forearms and apply soap.

2 Rub palm to palm.

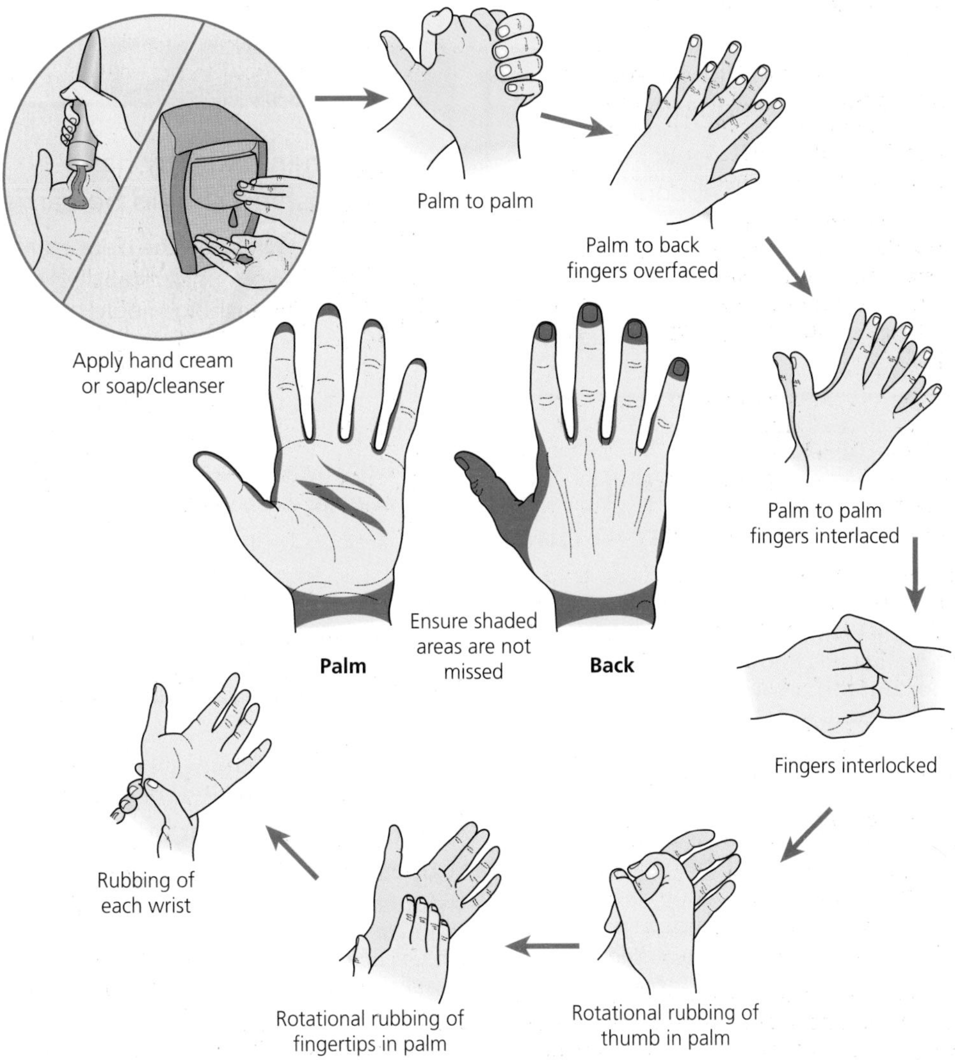

Apply hand cream or soap/cleanser
Palm to palm
Palm to back fingers overfaced
Palm to palm fingers interlaced
Fingers interlocked
Rotational rubbing of thumb in palm
Rotational rubbing of fingertips in palm
Rubbing of each wrist
Palm
Ensure shaded areas are not missed
Back

Figure 12.13 Effective hand washing

3 Rub with your fingers interlaced.

4 Massage between fingers, right palm over back of your left hand, left palm over back of your right hand.

5 Scrub with your fingers locked, including finger tips.

6 Rub rotationally with your thumbs locked.

7 Rinse thoroughly.

8 Dry the palms and backs of your hands using a paper towel.

9 Work the towel between your fingers.

10 Dry around and under your nails.

**Good practice in infection prevention and control, RCN, 2005, 2010**

NB Use the same technique when using alcohol gel.

**Evidence activity** 

### 6.3 The correct sequence for hand washing

This activity gives you the opportunity to demonstrate your knowledge of the correct sequence for hand washing.

Produce an illustrated poster for your staff room that describes the correct sequence for effective hand washing.

## 6.4 When and why hand washing should be carried out

Hands are top of the list when it comes to spread of infection and hand hygiene contributes significantly to reducing the risks of cross-infection. In fact it is known to be the single most important thing we can do to reduce the spread of disease.

**Time to reflect** 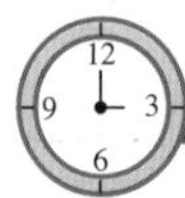

### 6.4 Now wash your hands

When do you wash your hands at work? Do you think you wash them sufficiently often? If not, what prevents you from washing them? Shortage of time? The condition of your skin? The soap isn't very nice? There are never enough towels?

Hand washing should be carried out before:

- having direct contact with the people you support, such as when giving personal care and carrying out first aid or healthcare procedures, for example catheter care, PEG feeding and collecting specimens
- administering medication
- using PPE
- handling food.

Hand washing should be carried out after:

- having direct contact with a patient, as above
- removing PPE, including gloves
- using the toilet, coughing, sneezing and touching your clothing, hair and so on
- domestic activities such as handling raw and waste food, cleaning and making beds.

**Evidence activity** 

### 6.4 When and why hand washing should be carried out

This activity gives you the opportunity to demonstrate your understanding of when and why hand washing should be carried out.

Think of five or six activities that you carry out in your day-to-day work.

- For which of these activities would you need to wash your hands?
- When would you wash them – before the activity, after, or before and after?
- Why do you need to wash your hands as you have described?

## 6.5 Products that should be used for hand washing

You have a duty of care to the people you work with, their family and friends, your colleagues and yourself to help prevent cross-infection. For this reason, you should raise the alarm if hand washing facilities and products aren't available for everyone to use.

Products that should be used for hand washing.
Soap or soap substitutes, which are milder than soap and less likely to dry the skin.
A supply of hot water from elbow or wrist lever operated mixer taps.
Wall mounted dispensers containing non-abrasive paper towels.
Foot-operated waste bins
Pump-action alcohol hand gel at point of care for use when the hands aren't visibly dirty and providing soap and water facilities would not be practical.
Pump-action antiseptic hand wash, which is used to disinfect the hands before surgery, prior to the insertion of an indwelling device and if there is an outbreak of infection.
Pump-action skin moisturiser, to soften the skin and prevent it from irritation or drying due to repeated hand-washing.
Information and advice about what to do in the event of, for example, a skin disorder such as dermatitis or eczema.

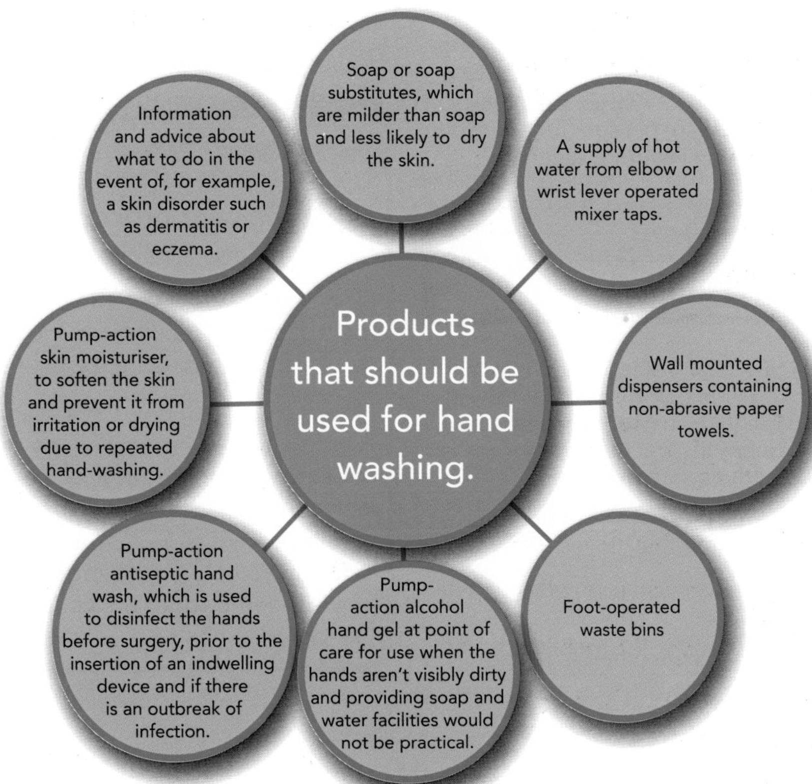

Figure 12.14 Products that should be used for hand washing

## Key terms

An indwelling device is a device that is inserted into the body, like a catheter.
Point of care is the location where care is given.

## Evidence activity 

### 6.5 Products that should be used for hand washing

This activity gives you the opportunity to demonstrate your knowledge of the types of products that should be used for hand washing.

Survey your workplace for hand washing products and facilities. Does it score well? Or are there any shortfalls in provision? Who should you report shortfalls to? Why is it important that hand washing products and facilities are in good supply?

## 6.6 Correct procedures that relate to skin care

Healthy, intact skin provides an effective barrier against cross-infection. Cover any breaks in your skin with a waterproof dressing and check the dressing regularly, replacing it if necessary. And keep your hands in good condition by using a good quality **barrier hand cream**.

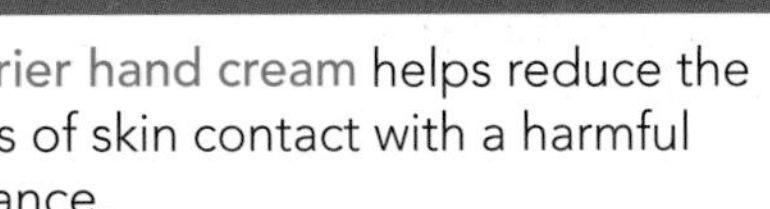

## Key term

A barrier hand cream helps reduce the effects of skin contact with a harmful substance.

Occupational skin diseases are caused by irritants and allergies. Soap, water and alcohol gel used for hand hygiene can cause irritation, for example, irritant contact dermatitis; and latex rubber gloves can cause allergies, for example, allergic contact dermatitis. Signs of occupational skin disease include dryness, redness, itching, inflammation, **vesicles**, cracking, scales and thickening. Some skin disorders, for example eczema, are made worse by frequent hand washing. If, as a result of wearing gloves and washing your hands, you develop signs of an occupational skin disease or your existing condition gets worse, seek medical advice from an appropriate person, for example your GP or Occupational Health Officer.

## Key term

A **vesicle** is a blister.

Gloves protect against risk of infection but they can cause skin problems if, for example, they are inappropriate to the task, are too large or small, or are damaged. Sensible precautionary measures help to reduce skin problems:

- Never wear gloves for more than one hour at a time, particularly single-use gloves.
- Never use lubricants such as powder to help put them on.
- Never use barrier cream when wearing them.
- After taking them off, wash and dry your hands, using a mild soap and a non-abrasive paper towel, and apply a quality moisturiser to return lost oils to the skin.

Hand protection and skin care management, MRC, 2006

## Evidence activity

### 6.6 Correct procedures that relate to skin care

This activity gives you the opportunity to demonstrate your knowledge of the correct procedures that relate to skin care.

Keep a record of how you care for your hands at work. Are you happy that you are looking after them sufficiently well? How can you improve your skin care regime? Why is it important to look after them as well as you can? Who can you speak to if you have any concerns about the condition of your hands?

## Assessment summary

Your reading of this chapter and completion of the activities will have prepared you to demonstrate your learning and understanding of the role of the health and social care. To achieve the unit, your assessor will require you to:

| Learning Outcomes | Assessment Criteria |
|---|---|
| Learning outcome 1: Understand roles and responsibilities in the prevention and control of infections by: | 1.1 explaining employees' roles and responsibilities in relation to the prevention and control of infection<br>See Evidence activity 1.1 p. 207. |
| | 1.2 explaining employers' responsibilities in relation to the prevention and control of infection.<br>See Evidence activity 1.2 p. 208. |
| Learning outcome 2: Understand legislation and policies relating to prevention and control of infections by: | 2.1 outlining current legislation and regulatory body standards which are relevant to the prevention and control of infection<br>See Evidence activity 2.1 p. 210. |

| Learning Outcomes | Assessment Criteria |
|---|---|
| Learning outcome 2: Understand legislation and policies relating to prevention and control of infections by: | 2.2 describing local and organisational policies relevant to the prevention and control of infection.<br>See Evidence activity 2.2 p. 212. |
| Learning outcome 3: Understand systems and procedures relating to the prevention and control of infections by: | 3.1 describing procedures and systems relevant to the prevention and control of infection<br>See Evidence activity 3.1 p. 214. |
| | 3.2 explaining the potential impact of an outbreak of infection on the individual and the organisation.<br>See Evidence activity 3.2 p. 215. |
| Learning outcome 4: Understand the importance of risk assessment in relation to the prevention and control of infections by: | 4.1 defining the term risk<br>See Evidence activity 4.1 p. 216. |
| | 4.2 outlining potential risks of infection within the workplace<br>See Evidence activity 4.2 p. 219. |
| | 4.3 describing the process of carrying out a risk assessment<br>See Evidence activity 4.3 p. 220. |
| | 4.4 explaining the importance of carrying out a risk assessment.<br>See Evidence activity 4.4 p. 220. |
| Learning outcome 5: Understand the importance of using personal protective equipment (PPE) in the prevention and control of infections by: | 5.1 demonstrating correct use of PPE<br>See Practice activity 5.1 p. 221. |
| | 5.2 describing different types of PPE<br>See Evidence activity 5.2 p. 222. |
| | 5.3 explaining the reasons for use of PPE<br>See Evidence activity 5.3 p. 222. |

| Learning Outcomes | Assessment Criteria |
|---|---|
| Learning outcome **5**: Understand the importance of using personal protective equipment (PPE) in the prevention and control of infections by: | 5.4 stating current relevant regulations and legislation relating to PPE<br>See Evidence activity 5.4 p. 223. |
| | 5.5 describing employees' responsibilities regarding the use of PPE<br>See Evidence activity 5.5 p. 224. |
| | 5.6 describing employers' responsibilities regarding the use of PPE<br>See Evidence activity 5.6 p. 223. |
| | 5.7 describing the correct practice in the application and removal of PPE<br>See Evidence activity 5.7 p. 225. |
| | 5.8 describing the correct procedure for disposal of used PPE.<br>See Evidence activity 5.8 p. 225. |
| Learning outcome **6**: Understand the importance of good personal hygiene in the prevention and control of infections by: | 6.1 describing the key principles of good personal hygiene<br>See Evidence activity 6.1 p. 226. |
| | 6.2 demonstrating good hand washing technique<br>See Practice activity 6.2 p. 228. |
| | 6.3 describing the correct sequence for hand washing<br>See Evidence activity 6.3 p. 228. |
| | 6.4 explaining when and why hand washing should be carried out<br>See Evidence activity 6.4 p. 228. |
| | 6.5 describing the types of products that should be used for hand washing<br>See Evidence activity 6.5 p. 229. |

| Learning Outcomes | Assessment Criteria |
|---|---|
| Learning outcome 6: Understand the importance of good personal hygiene in the prevention and control of infections by: | 6.6 describing correct procedures that relate to skin care.<br>See Evidence activity 6.6 p. 230. |

Good luck!

## Weblinks

| | |
|---|---|
| Royal College of Nursing | www.rcn.org.uk |
| Healthcare Republic, a website for healthcare professionals | www.healthcarerepublic.com |
| Health Protection Agency | www.hpa.org.uk |
| Daily Mail newspaper | www.dailymail.co.uk |
| Chartered Institute of Environmental Health | www.cieh.org |
| Care Quality Commission | www.cqc.org.uk |
| General Social Care Council in England, | www.gscc.org.uk |
| Care Council for Wales | www.ccwales.org.uk |
| Scottish Care Council | www.sssc.uk.com |
| N Ireland Social Care Council | www.niscc.info |
| General Medical Council | http://www.gmc-uk.org |
| Nursing and Midwifery Council (NMC) | www.nmc-uk.org |
| Health Professions Council (HPC) | www.hpc-uk.org |
| Office for Standards in Education, Children's Services and Skills (OFSTED) | www.ofsted.gov.uk |
| Children's Workforce Development Council (CWDC) | www.cwdcouncil.org.uk |
| Skills for Health | www.skillsforhealth.org.uk |
| Skills for Care | www.skillsforcare.org.uk |
| Health information for patients | www.patient.co.uk |
| NHS website | www.nhs.uk |
| Children's health information | http://kidshealth.org; |
| Health information from BUPA | www.bupa.co.uk |
| BBC website | www.bbc.co.uk |
| Government website about public services | www.direct.gov.uk |
| Centre for Disease Prevention and Control | www.cdc.gov |

# 13 Move and position individuals in accordance with their plan of care

## For Unit HSC2028

### What are you finding out?

For a number of reasons many people who use health and social care services need help and support to move and change position. Incorrect moving and handling techniques, whether **manual** or with the help of equipment, can cause injury, both to the person being moved and the person helping them make the move. Legislation aims to protect the health and safety of everyone involved in moving and handling activities, through policies, guidelines and risk assessments, and through procedures and agreed ways of working that are written into individual care plans.

The reading and activities in this chapter will help you to:

- Understand anatomy and physiology in relation to moving and positioning individuals
- Understand current legislation and agreed ways of working when moving and positioning individuals
- Be able to minimise risk before moving and positioning individuals
- Be able to prepare individuals before moving and positioning
- Be able to move and position an individual
- Know when to seek advice from and/or involve others when moving and positioning an individual.

**Key term**

Manual involves using human effort, skill, power, energy.

## LO1 Anatomy and physiology in relation to moving and positioning

### 1.1 Anatomy and physiology of the human body in relation to correct moving and positioning of individuals

The musculoskeletal system is the system of muscles, **tendons**, bones, joints and **ligaments**. Its purpose is to move the body and maintain its shape.

**Key terms**

A tendon is a band of tissue that connects a muscle with a bone.
A ligament is a band of tissue that connects bones, typically to support a joint.

There are three types of muscle, cardiac (heart), smooth and skeletal. Each is made up from cells or fibres that have the ability to contract (shorten). Skeletal muscle (also known as striped or striated) is attached to tendons, which attach to bones. When the fibres of a skeletal muscle contract, the muscle shortens, pulling the tendon which pulls on the bone to which it is attached. This results in movement. For example:

- When the biceps muscle contracts, it pulls on the biceps tendon which pulls on the radius, a bone in the forearm. This causes the arm to bend.
- When the triceps muscle contracts, it pulls on the triceps tendon which pulls on the ulna, the other bone in the forearm. This causes the arm to straighten.

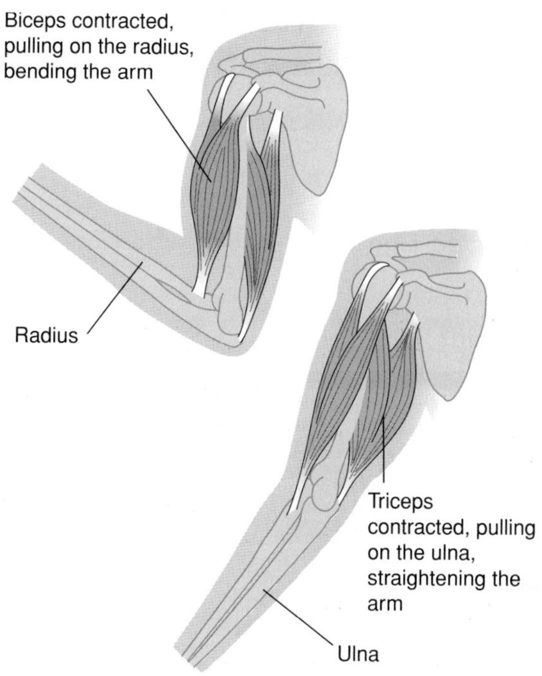


Figure 13.1 The interplay between muscles and bone to create movement

A muscle strain (pulled muscle) happens when muscles and tendons are forced beyond their normal range of movement. It is a very painful condition and can happen during rough manual handling procedures, for example when someone is:

- pulled or jerked, which can tear or over-stretch muscles and tendons
- pushed, forcing muscles and tendons to contract too strongly.

There are two types of bone **tissue**. Cortical or compact tissue forms the dense outer layer of bones and is thickest in places that bear the greatest load. Cancellous or spongy tissue forms the less dense, softer and weaker inner layer of bones, but is also found at the ends of the long bones (the limbs), next to joints and within the vertebrae of the backbone. Spongy bone contains red bone marrow in which blood cells are produced.

## Key term

Tissue is a collection of cells that have the same function.

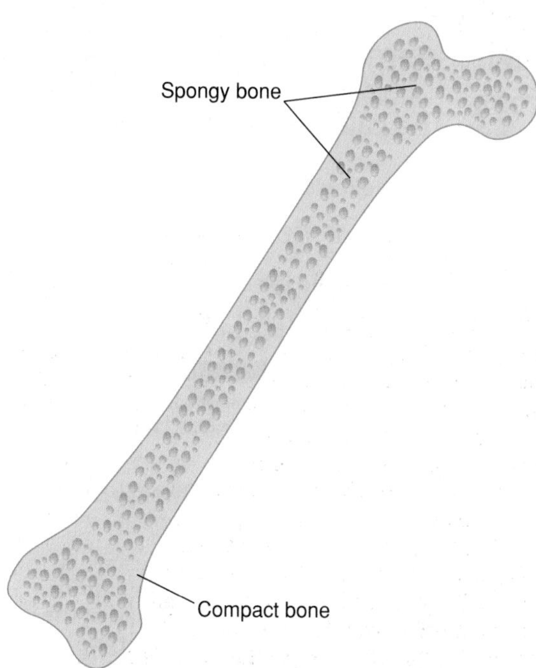


Figure 13.2 Different types of bone

Although it can mend, a **fractured** bone is extremely painful.

1. A simple fracture is the most common type and happens when a bone breaks cleanly. It can be caused by the slightest of pressure, such as a gentle grip or clasp when helping someone move; or by standing for just a very short period, for example when moving from chair to wheelchair.
2. An impacted fracture happens when the ends of two bones are forced into one another, for example when someone puts out their arm to stop themselves falling.
3. A jagged, spiral fracture happens as a result of a sharp sudden twist of a bone, such as when someone is twisted when being repositioned.
4. A compression fracture, where a bone breaks into fragments, can result from being crushed, for example by falling equipment.

## Key term

Fractured means broken.

## Research & investigate 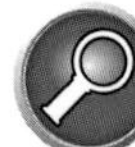

###  1.1 The causes of broken bones

Check out the incidence of broken bones where you work.

- What proportion of these breaks were simple, impacted, jagged or due to compression?
- What caused the breaks?
- How do you think the breaks could have been avoided?

A joint is the connection between two bones. There are three types of joint:

1. Fixed, such as in the skull. There is no movement of bones in a fixed joint.
2. Cartilaginous, in which the bones are firmly joined together by cartilage, for example between the ribs and the vertebrae of the spinal column or back bone. This type of joint allows slight movement only.
3. Synovial, in which the bones are held in place by muscles and ligaments. They allow extensive movement, due to the presence of cartilage and synovial fluid. Cartilage lines the bones forming a smooth, slippery surface, and synovial fluid acts as a lubricant. There are four types of synovial joint (see Table 13.1).

### The spinal column

The spinal column is made up of 24 individual bones called vertebrae, which are stacked on top of each other in a natural curved 'S' shape that provides the body with strength and flexibility. Between the vertebrae are discs or circular pads of cartilage. They have a tough outer layer and a jelly-like centre, allowing them to squeeze or stretch as the vertebrae move, cushioning the vertebrae and acting as shock absorbers.

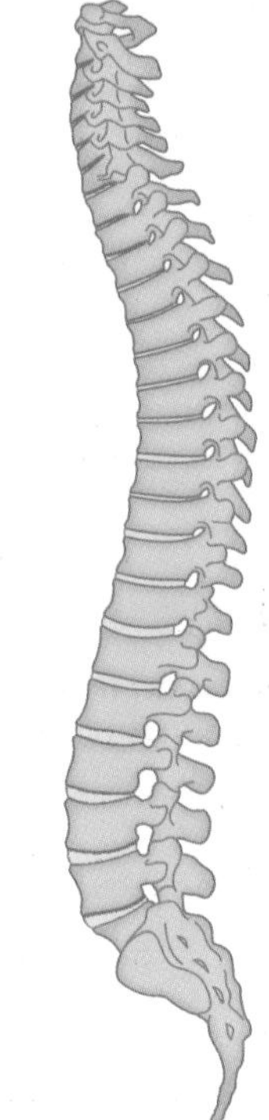

Figure 13.3 The spinal column

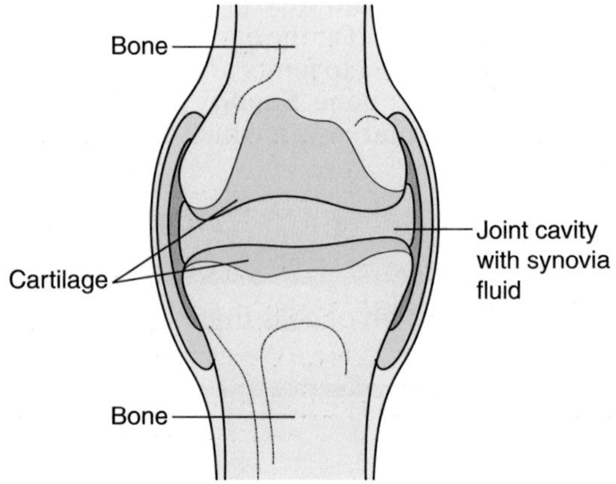


Figure 13.4 A synovial joint

Table 13.1 The four types of synovial joint

| Type of joint | Type of movement | Example of joint |
|---|---|---|
| Ball and socket | Rotation, allowing movement in nearly all directions. | Hip and shoulder. |
| Hinge | Like a door hinge, they allow movement in one direction only. | Jaw, knee and elbow. |
| Gliding | Bones slide over each other. | Wrist and ankle. |
| Pivot | One bone rotates alongside another. | The joint between the atlas and axis vertebrae in the neck, allowing the head to turn from side to side. |

Forcing a joint beyond its normal range of movement can sprain the ligaments holding the bones together. For example, the ligaments on the outside of the ankle can be sprained when the ankle turns over, forcing the sole of the foot to face inward. Sprains also occur when someone is forced into a position, for example when a dragging movement causes twisting or over-stretching of a joint.

## Evidence activity 

### 1.1 Anatomy and physiology of the human body in relation to correct moving and positioning of individuals

This activity enables you to demonstrate your knowledge of anatomy and physiology in relation to moving and positioning the people you support.

Complete the following table to show your understanding of how incorrect moving and positioning can affect the musculoskeletal system and cause injury.

| Moving and positioning technique | Possible effect on the musculoskeletal system. |
|---|---|
| Pulling, jerking. | |
| Pushing. | |
| Gripping, clasping. | |
| Twisting. | |
| Any technique that requires a weakened individual to bear their own weight, for example standing. | |
| Any technique that carries a risk of a fall. | |
| Any technique that uses equipment. | |
| Any activity that prevents the body assuming its natural 'S' shape curve. | |
| Any technique that forces a joint beyond its normal range of movement. | |

## 1.2 The impact of specific conditions on moving and positioning an individual

Many people who use health and social care services need help and support to move and change position. A range of moving and positioning activities is shown in the table below. Organisations that provide support in this way are obliged to have written procedures and agreed ways of working that describe exactly how each manoeuvre must be carried out.

### Time to reflect

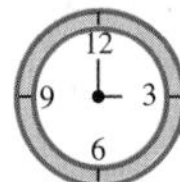

**Your move**

In what ways do you help people to move and reposition?

Why do they need your help?

Do you use the same techniques for everyone you help?

Many people have conditions that affect their mobility and the type of support they need to move and reposition. For this reason procedures must be adapted and agreed ways of working put in place that meet their specific needs.

Specifically tailored moving and repositioning activities must be devised for people who have:

- A history of falls, due, for example, to low BP, vertigo, problems with balance, the side effects of medication, alcohol abuse or low **haemoglobin** levels that bring on fainting.
- Bone and joint conditions, such as rheumatoid arthritis, in which the joints become inflamed and painful; osteoarthritis, in which the cartilage of the joints becomes worn, stiff and painful; and osteoporosis, in which the density of the bones is much reduced, increasing the risk of fracture.
- A physical disability that affects movement and mobility, such as amputation, muscular dystrophy, multiple sclerosis, stroke, Parkinson's Disease, Huntington's Disease, cerebral palsy and epilepsy.
- A sensory impairment, such as impaired sight and hearing, which limit the person's ability to hear how to help in a manoeuvre or see where to move to.

Table 13.2 Moving and positioning activities

| Aim of activity | Objectives of activity |
|---|---|
| Support someone to sit, stand and walk. | • Move backwards and forwards in a chair.<br>• Move from sitting in a chair or on the edge of a bed to standing, and vice versa.<br>• Walk.<br>• Prevent from falling and raise from a fall. |
| Support someone to move in bed. | • Get in and out of bed and turn in bed.<br>• Lie at an angle.<br>• Sit up from lying and onto the edge of the bed.<br>• Slide up and down when lying and sitting.<br>• Maintain the correct posture and appropriate position. |
| Support someone to move laterally (side to side). | • From bed to trolley, and vice versa.<br>• Transfer from bed to chair, and vice versa.<br>• Transfer from chair to chair, commode or toilet, and vice versa. |
| Hoisting. | • Fitting a sling with the person in bed or in a chair.<br>• Fitting a sling with the person in bed or in a chair using glide sheets.<br>• Hoisting from bed to chair, and vice versa.<br>• Hoisting from the floor.<br>• Transferring to the toilet or bath using sling-lifting or a stand aid hoist. |

- A healthcare attachment, such as a **PEG feeding tube** or **catheter**, or who are attached to a storage cylinder of oxygen.
- Reduced **tissue viability**. Reduced tissue viability manifests as skin breakdown and pressure ulcers. Skin breakdown is caused by failure to care for skin that is exposed to moisture from urine, sweat and **exudate**. Pressure ulcers are caused by prolonged pressure of the body on, for example, the bed or chair, and by friction due to pushing and pulling.
- Variations in capability during the day and night, for example, an individual may be able to move themselves during the day but not at all at night.

### Key terms

A catheter is a small tube inserted into the body cavity to, for example, remove fluid or administer medication.
Exudate is fluid that seeps out of injured tissues.
Haemoglobin is the protein in red blood cells that carries the oxygen needed by the body to create energy.
A PEG feeding tube is a tube that is placed through the patient's skin into their stomach as a means of feeding them.
Tissue viability is to do with the ability of the skin to remain intact and healthy.

Specifically tailored moving and repositioning activities must also be devised for people who are:

- Paralysed and unable to move.
- Unconscious. Someone who is **comatose** is unable to understand how to help in manoeuvres.
- Emotionally disturbed, distressed, aggressive or confused or who have diminished understanding, such as a learning difficulty or dementia. Conditions like these can manifest in challenging and unexpected behaviour, which add to the risks of moving and repositioning.

### Key term

Comatose means unable to move voluntarily and unable to understand what is happening.

### Evidence activity

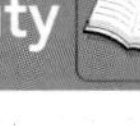

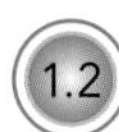

**1.2 The impact of specific conditions on the correct movement and positioning of an individual**

This activity enables you to demonstrate your knowledge of how to move and position people with specific conditions.

Check out your workplace's safe moving and handling procedures for three people with different needs. How do they compare? In what ways are they different? Why are they different?

## LO2 Current legislation and agreed ways of working when moving and positioning individuals

### 2.1 The effect of current legislation and agreed ways of working on working practices related to moving and positioning individuals

The purpose of health and safety legislation (law) is to protect health, safety and well-being. Health and safety policies set out the arrangements that an organisation has for complying with the law. Health and safety procedures and agreed ways of working describe how work activities must be carried out for policies to be implemented and the law obeyed.

## Time to reflect

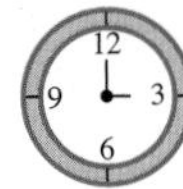

### Laying down the law

- What health and safety law affects the way that you carry out moving and positioning activities?
- What policies does your employer have in place to ensure that you comply with the law when carrying out moving and positioning activities?
- Where are moving and positioning procedures stored in your workplace? When did you last look at them, to make sure that your work practice is accurate?

There are a number of laws that aim to protect everyone involved in moving and repositioning activities. If your job requires you to help someone move or reposition, whether manually or with the help of equipment, you should familiarise yourself with the legislation and your workplace's policies, and ensure that you follow procedures and agreed ways of working to the letter.

The Health and Safety at Work Act 1974 does not specifically cover moving and repositioning activities. However, it does require your employer to:

- write health and safety policies and procedures, including ones that relate to moving and positioning activities, and make you and your colleagues aware of them
- ensure everyone's health, safety and welfare, as far as is reasonably practicable.

In addition it requires you to:

- take reasonable care of yourself and anyone else who may be affected by your activities
- cooperate with your employer in relation to health and safety issues, including those related to moving and repositioning
- not interfere with or misuse anything provided in the interest of health and safety, for example, equipment used for moving and repositioning.

The Manual Handling Operations Regulations 1992 (amended 2002) apply to a wide range of manual moving and repositioning activities, including lifting, lowering, pushing and pulling.

Table 13.3 Responsibilities under the Manual Handling Operations Regulations 1992

| Responsibilities of your employer | Your responsibilities |
|---|---|
| • Avoid hazardous manual handling, so far as is reasonably practicable.<br>• Assess the risk of injury from any hazardous manual handling that can't be avoided.<br>• Reduce the risk of injury from hazardous manual handling, so far as is reasonably practicable. | • Follow safe work practices.<br>• Use equipment that is provided for your safety properly.<br>• Cooperate with your employer on health and safety matters.<br>• Inform your employer if you identify hazardous handling activities.<br>• Take care to ensure that your activities do not put others at risk. |

Getting to Grips with Manual Handling. A Short Guide, HSE, 2006

The Management of Health and Safety at Work Regulations 1999 aim to minimise risks to health and safety through the process of risk assessment. Risk assessment requires your employer to:

- assess the risks associated with moving and repositioning activities
- take sensible measures to tackle them
- ensure that you are competent to carry out moving and repositioning activities, through training and supervision.

The Workplace (Health, Safety and Welfare) Regulations 1992 aim to minimise risks to health and safety associated with working conditions. Your employer must therefore ensure that minimum standards are met with regard to equipment used for moving and repositioning and the environment in which moving and repositioning activities take place, for example the space available, lighting and temperature.

A number of moving and repositioning activities require the use of equipment. The Provision and Use of Work Equipment Regulations (PUWER) 1998 aim to minimise the risks to health and safety associated with the use of equipment. Your employer has a responsibility to ensure that:

- equipment is safe, well maintained and appropriate for the job

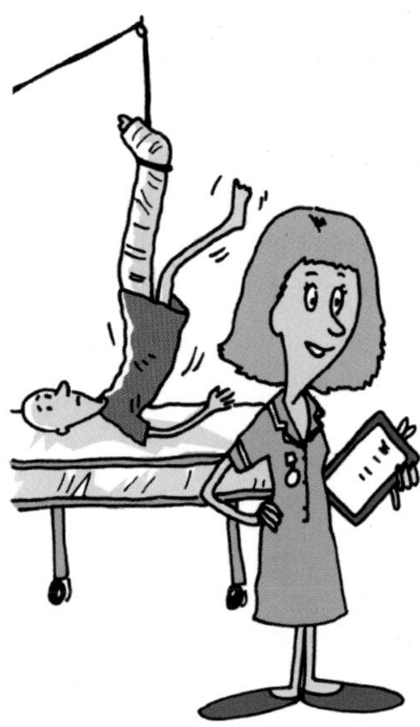

Figure 13.5 Risk assessment

- you use equipment safely and correctly, through training and supervision.

The Lifting Operations and Lifting Equipment Regulations (LOLER) 1998 aim to reduce health and safety risks due to using lifting equipment. Your employer is required to ensure that lifting equipment used for moving and repositioning activities is:

- strong, stable and marked to indicate safe working loads
- safely positioned and installed
- used safely and appropriately, through training and supervision
- maintained and inspected by competent people.

## Research & investigate

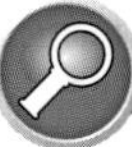

### 2.1 Well equipped?

- What equipment is available at your workplace for carrying out moving and positioning activities?
- What specific activities is it used for?
- How and by whom is it maintained?
- How would you know it was safe to use?

The Personal Protective Equipment at Work Regulations (PPE) 1992 aim to minimise the risks to health and safety associated with cross-infection. Your employer has a responsibility to minimise the risk of cross-infection during moving and repositioning activities by:

- providing you with appropriate PPE
- ensuring that you use and dispose of PPE safely and correctly, through training and supervision.

The Reporting of Injuries, Diseases and Dangerous Occurrence Regulations (RIDDOR) 1995 require that certain work-related injuries, diseases and dangerous occurrences are reported to the Health and Safety Executive (HSE) or local authority. Your employer has a responsibility to train you in how to report injuries and dangerous occurrences associated with moving and repositioning activities.

## Evidence activity

### 2.1 The effect of current legislation and agreed ways of working on working practices related to moving and positioning individuals

This activity enables you to demonstrate your knowledge of how current legislation and agreed ways of working affect working practices related to moving and positioning the people you support.

Think about three different moving and positioning activities in which you participate. For each describe:

- the relevant legislation (law)
- workplace policies that ensure compliance with the law
- your responsibilities in implementing the policies and ensuring best practice.

## 2.2 Health and safety factors to take into account when moving and positioning individuals and using equipment

Moving and repositioning activities, whether manual or with the use of equipment, are health and safety hazards for everyone concerned.

This section looks at the health and safety hazards or risk factors that need to be taken into account when moving and repositioning the people you support.

## The activity

- Musculoskeletal injuries or disorders (MSDs) are the most common occupational illness in the UK. They include back and joint injury, sprains and strains. If the activity requires manual effort, does it involve any of the movements known to cause MSDs? (See Figure 13.6)
- If the activity requires equipment, is it appropriate, safe and well maintained, and do you know how to use it properly? Unless it is safe, well maintained and appropriate for the job, and unless you can use it safely, equipment carries a risk of accident and injury.
- Is the activity appropriate for the person concerned or would an alternative activity meet their needs? You read earlier about conditions that impact on an individual's ability to move and reposition. People with these conditions require specifically tailored support; anything else would put their health and safety at risk.
- Are you trained to carry out the activity and are you confident you can carry it out safely? Never perform any activity for which you haven't been trained and always ask for help if you have any concerns.

## The load

Before attempting to help someone move or reposition, be aware of factors such as their:

- Weight. Would moving them manually put your health at risk? Does the equipment you intend to use indicate that it can carry their weight safely?
- Size. Does their size or shape affect your ability to get hold of them safely and securely?
- Behaviour. Do you anticipate any unexpected movement that would put health and safety at risk?

### Time to reflect

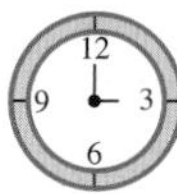

**Been there, got the T-shirt ...**

Have you ever hurt yourself as a result of carrying a heavy, awkward load? How did the experience impact on your ability to carry on as usual? How long were you out of action? What would you say to someone else who appeared to be struggling with an unwieldy, bulky load?

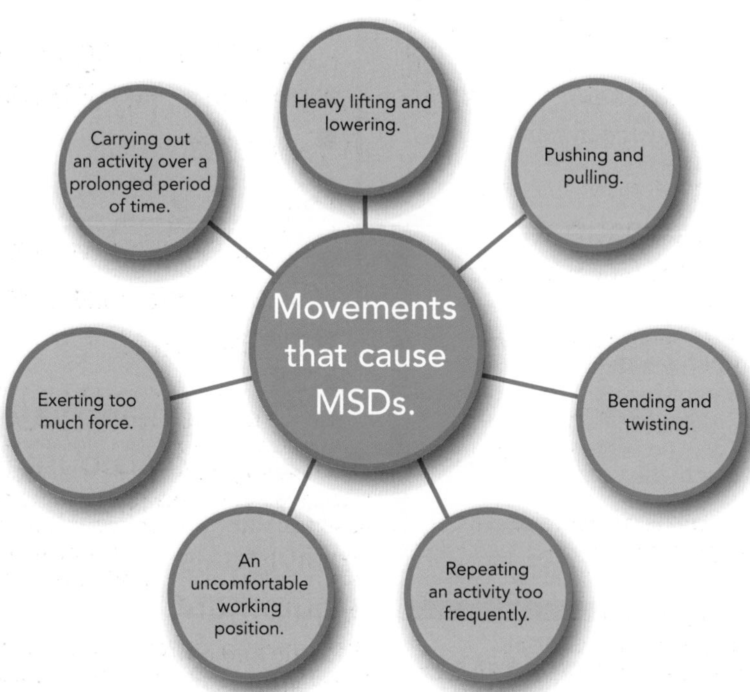


Figure 13.6 Movements that cause musculoskeletal disorders

## The working environment

- Does the environment in which you work constrain your posture, for example, do obstructions or a lack of space restrict your movements or make movement uncomfortable? Postural constraint is a further cause of MSD.
- Is the floor level and free from slip and trip hazards?
- Can you see what you are doing or is the light dazzling or too dim?
- Can you hear or does background noise prevent you from hearing instructions accurately?
- Is there a comfortable working temperature, not too hot and not too cold?
- Is ventilation comfortable, or is it drafty or humid?
- Is the environment clean and fresh-smelling?

### Research & investigate

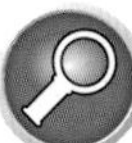

2.2 How safe is your workplace?

Carry out a brief survey of the environment in which you work. On a scale of 1 = excellent and 5 = poor, how does it score with regard to enabling safe moving and positioning? Why have you given it this score? How could you improve things?

## Your capabilities and those of the others in your team

- Are you trained and confident in your ability to do the activity safely?
- Are your clothing and footwear appropriate or do they restrict movement?
- Are you fit and strong enough?
- Do you have a disability that prevents you carrying out certain activities?
- Does your health status affect your ability, for example, are you pregnant or do you have an MSD?
- Are you able to give the activity the time it requires? Or do high job demands, time constraints, fatigue and stress tempt you to cut corners?

## Other factors

- Do you need to take precautions against the risk of cross-infection, for example by using PPE?
- Are you trained and confident in your ability to report and record any accidents and injuries?

### Evidence activity

2.2 Health and safety factors that need to be taken into account when moving and positioning people and using equipment

This activity enables you to demonstrate your knowledge of the health and safety factors that need to be taken into account when moving and positioning people and using equipment.

Think about two people you help to move and position, one of whom requires the use of equipment. For each person, make a list of the health and safety factors you need to consider when helping them move and change position, including those that relate to the equipment.

# LO3 Minimising risks before moving and positioning individuals

## 3.1 Accessing up-to-date copies of risk assessment documentation

Health and safety law relating to moving and positioning requires that every manual or equipment-aided activity is assessed for risks and that steps are taken to eliminate or minimise any risks. The results of risk assessments must be recorded, manually and/or electronically, and everyone involved made aware of the health and safety procedures they contain.

Risk assessment records should be stored in filing cabinets or electronic storage systems in a clearly known and accessible location, for example a staff room or office, so that everyone can keep themselves familiar with their content. Anyone who carries out an activity must follow the procedures described in the risk assessment to the letter.

Risk assessments need to be routinely reviewed and updated to take account of, for example, changes in the law and developments in moving and handling techniques and equipment. Good practice dictates that you keep up to date with the law and the latest moving and handling procedures.

**Practice activity** 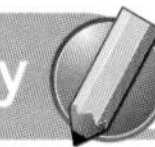

### 3.1 Accessing up-to-date copies of risk assessment documentation

This activity gives you an opportunity to demonstrate that you can access up-to-date copies of risk assessment documentation.

- Where are moving and handling risk assessments stored at your workplace?
- How do you access them?
- Why is it necessary to review them?
- How do you know that the risk assessments you access are up to date?

## 3.2 Preparatory checks using care plans and moving and handling risk assessments

Moving and handling risk assessments record procedures for carrying out activities such as those listed in Table 13.2. Care plans contain information about people's individual abilities and needs, including instructions for moving and handling that are specific to them.

Before helping anybody to move or reposition, check their care plan. This will remind you of any special requirements for the activity and also alert you to whether requirements have changed since you last carried out the activity. If there are no special requirements, check and follow the moving and handling risk assessment for the manoeuvre. Failure to follow procedures laid out in care plans and risk assessments flies in the face of best practice and puts everyone involved at risk.

**Practice activity** 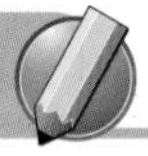

### 3.2 Preparatory checks using care plans and moving and handling risk assessments

This activity gives you an opportunity to demonstrate that you can carry out preparatory checks using a care plan and the moving and handling risk assessment.

Think about three people you help to move and change position.

- What documentation describes the moving and handling activities in which each person needs support?
- Where is this documentation stored?
- Why is it important to follow the procedures described in this documentation?

## 3.3 Identify any immediate risks to the individual

Don't follow procedures blindly. Before you initiate any move, be on the alert for risks that could affect the individual's health and safety.

**Evidence activity** 

### 3.3 Identify any immediate risks to the individual

This activity gives you an opportunity to demonstrate your knowledge of immediate risks to the people you support.

Produce a set of reminder cards to alert your colleagues to risks to people prior to helping them move and reposition. Use the categories 'Activity', 'Load', 'Working environment', 'Workers capabilities' and 'Other factors'.

**Questions to ask yourself prior to carrying out any moving and handling activity**

1. Is the activity still appropriate? Changes in someone's weight, mobility, balance, tendency to fall, sight, hearing and tissue viability can put health and safety at risk. Similarly, changes in their mood, level of dependency, understanding, behaviour and ability to help in the manoeuvre can also affect health and safety.
2. Is the working environment free from obstruction and noise, and is it well lit?
3. Is the equipment that you're going to use appropriate and are you confident and competent in its use?
4. Is there evidence to show that equipment is safe and well maintained?
5. Are you and any others involved in the manoeuvre appropriately trained, fit and healthy, sufficiently strong and appropriately dressed?
6. Is there any possibility of cross-infection? Infection is a major cause of illness and hospitalisation among people living in residential care homes; and healthcare-associated infections (HCAIs) may be serious, even life threatening.

## Actions to take in relation to identified risks

It's very difficult to completely eliminate risks. The aim of risk assessment is to create procedures where risk is reduced 'to the lowest level reasonably practicable.'

Table 13.4 Minimising risks associated with moving and positioning

| Risk factor | Action to take to minimise the risks |
|---|---|
| The activity | Don't carry out any activity unless you've been trained.<br>Don't carry out any activity unless you're sufficiently strong, fit and healthy.<br>If an activity puts great pressure on you, request the support of a team.<br>If a manual activity poses a risk, consider using equipment instead.<br>Don't use equipment unless you've been trained.<br>Use equipment that's appropriate to the activity and the needs of the person concerned.<br>Inspect equipment before use to make sure it's safe and well maintained.<br>Follow procedures within care plans and risk assessments.<br>Report any concerns. |

*Contd.*

| Risk factor | Action to take to minimise the risks |
|---|---|
| The load, ie the person concerned | Prior to the activity, assess the person for changes in their physical and emotional condition that could affect the manoeuvre.<br>Know what can affect their behaviour so you can plan for unexpected movements.<br>Know their weight in order to decide whether you're strong enough to help in the manoeuvre and that the equipment you intend to use can carry them safely.<br>Take their size and shape into account when planning how to grasp or support them.<br>Report any changes in them that could impact on moving and positioning.<br>Report any concerns. |
| Working environment | Don't carry out any activity if there isn't sufficient space for you to move in comfort or use equipment properly.<br>Don't carry out any activity if the light, noise, ventilation and temperature could compromise comfort and safety.<br>Report any concerns. |
| Capabilities | Ensure you are trained in moving and handling, including using equipment.<br>If you work in a team, know your responsibilities and don't let your colleagues down.<br>Ask for supervision to check that you're competent and work safely.<br>Wear appropriate clothing, including PPE if necessary.<br>Stay fit and healthy and let your employer know if you are pregnant or if a manoeuvre causes you pain or discomfort.<br>Report concerns related to high job demands, time constraints, fatigue and stress that you think could interfere with your ability to work safely. |
| Other factors | Follow procedures for working with people who are infected or if you think that you may have an infectious disease.<br>Follow procedures for reporting accidents and injuries related to moving and handling. |

**Evidence activity** 

### 3.4 Actions to take in relation to identified risks

This activity gives you an opportunity to demonstrate your knowledge of what to do in the event that you identify a risk.

Think about three moving and handling manoeuvres that you carry out on a day-to-day basis.

- What risks are associated with each in terms of the activity itself, the load, the working environment, workers' capabilities and other factors, such as risk of infection?
- How would you deal with each risk?

## 3.5 Action to take if an individual's wishes conflict with their care plan in relation to health and safety and their risk assessment

People who use health and social care services have a right to lead their lives independently and to make personal choices about how and when their care is given. For this reason, you should consult with the people you support, to find out how they wish to be cared for and when. Where decisions about care have to be made on someone's behalf, those decisions should take into account any known wishes and beliefs. Providing care and support in ways not agreed by an individual can bring accusations of neglect and abuse.

Conflict can arise when people don't want to be cared for according to their care plan or risk assessment and make decisions that carry an element of risk. For example, they may choose to:

- exercise their independence and move without your help
- not help in a manoeuvre, even though their **active participation** would help and protect you
- not move at all, even though to move is in their best interests.

**Key term**

Active participation means to be an active rather than a passive partner in one's own care and support.

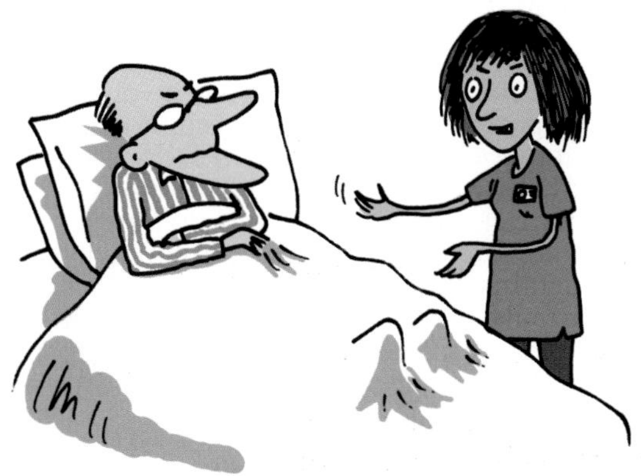

Figure 13.7 In my own time

Although you might think such decisions unwise, everyone has a right to do things that carry an element of risk to themselves, and you have a responsibility to support people in exercising their right to take risks. On the other hand, you also have a responsibility to protect the health and safety of everyone concerned. In the event that someone you support makes a seemingly unwise decision, discuss the safety implications and point out your duty to follow safe procedures and comply with health and safety law. Make every attempt to convince them of the importance of following their care plan or the relevant risk assessment whilst at the same time showing your wish to respect and promote their rights.

If you can't persuade them from making an ill-advised decision, support them according to their wishes and choices and record the incident. If their decision is likely to endanger your health and safety, seek help.

**Evidence activity** 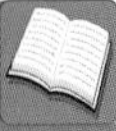

### 3.5 Action to take if an individual's wishes conflict with their care plan in relation to health and safety and their risk assessment

This activity gives you an opportunity to demonstrate your knowledge of what to do in the event that someone's wishes conflict with their care plan in relation to health and safety and their risk assessment.

Check out your workplace's policy for what to do when someone's wishes conflict with the health and safety procedures. Use your findings to produce an information sheet or poster for colleagues who you feel need support in dealing with situations that could become difficult.

## 3.6 Preparing the immediate environment for moving and repositioning activities

### Research & investigate

**3.6 The risks associated with working in a hazardous environment**

With regard to moving and positioning activities, what health and safety hazards are present in your workplace and what risks do they pose?

You read earlier that the Workplace (Health, Safety and Welfare) Regulations 1992 require your employer to minimise risks to health and safety associated with the working environment. Factors within the working environment, which can be someone's own home, that can jeopardise the safety of moving and positioning activities include a lack of space and obstructions, such as general clutter and **fixtures** and **fittings**.

### Key terms

A fixture is any item that is bolted to the floor or walls.
A fitting is any item that is free standing or hung by a nail or hook.

Adequate, accessible space is vital for a normal range of joint and muscle movements. Working in cramped, cluttered conditions uses awkward movements such as twisting, leaning sideways, stooping, overreaching, and turning and balancing on a small area. Awkward movements force the spinal column out of its natural curved 'S' shape, overstretching muscles and joints and causing MSDs, for example:

- **slipped discs**
- joint injury
- sprains and strains.

MSDs are exceedingly debilitating. Apart from long periods of reduced mobility and pain that affect everyday activities and the ability to sleep, they can affect your job prospects.

### Key term

A slipped disc occurs when one of the discs of the spine is ruptured and the jelly-like substance inside leaks out, putting pressure on the spinal cord. It causes intense back pain as well as pain in other areas of the body.

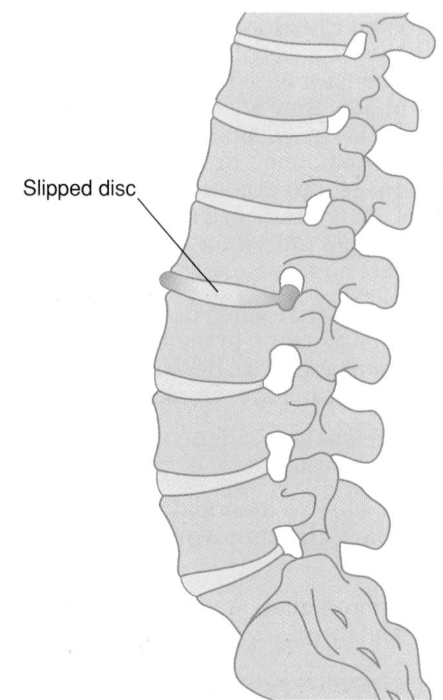


Figure 13.8 A slipped disc

Working in cramped conditions also increases the risk of accidents, for everyone concerned. According to the Health and Safety at Work Act 1974, you have a responsibility to take reasonable care of yourself and anyone else who may be affected by your activities. So before carrying out any moving and positioning activities, make sure that everyone involved has enough space to move freely and comfortably and that there is enough space to use equipment properly. Assess the area for obstructions that could restrict movement, such as furniture, wheelchairs, televisions, shelving, cupboards, even curtains and curtain rails, and deal with them to make the space as tidy and free from clutter as possible. If you are working in a team, coordinate your tasks so that you don't restrict each other.

Other hazards that can jeopardise the safety of moving and handling procedures include:

- slip and trip hazards, for example slippery floors, worn carpets, missing tiles, clutter
- changes in floor level, such as slopes, steps and stairs
- lighting that is uncomfortable and not user-friendly, for example bulbs that provide insufficient light, creating dark areas, and lighting that dazzles or glares
- distracting **ambient** conditions, such as startling or repetitive noise; uncomfortable temperatures, too hot or too cold; high humidity; poor ventilation, including cold drafts; dirt and unpleasant smells.

**Key term**

Ambient means surrounding.

Before carrying out any moving and positioning activities, remove or reduce the risks associated with these hazards 'to the lowest level reasonably practicable'.

## 3.7 Standard precautions for infection prevention and control

Helping someone to move or reposition requires close body contact and, on occasion, contact with blood and body fluids. Standard precautions are the practices adopted by health and social care workers when there is a chance that they may come into contact with blood or body fluids. They are a set of principles designed to minimise exposure to and transmission of a wide variety of **pathogens**.

**Key term**

A pathogen is a disease-producing bacterium, fungi, virus, infestation or prion.

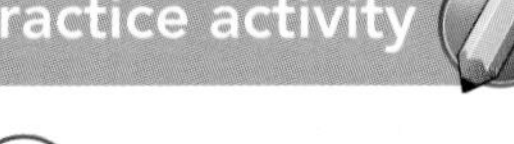

### Prepare the immediate environment ensuring adequate space for the move in agreement with all concerned and that potential hazards are removed

This activity gives you an opportunity to demonstrate that you can ensure the environment is as free from risk as possible.

Complete the following table to show how you ensure that the environment in which you carry out three moving and handling activities is as free from risk as possible.

| Description of moving and handling activity | How I ensure that there is adequate space for the move | Details of other hazards that I remove |
|---|---|---|
| 1. | | |
| 2. | | |
| 3. | | |

Standard precautions.
As it is not always possible to tell who has an infection, always treat blood and body fluids as infected.
Always use good hand hygiene.
Cover any existing cuts or lesions with a waterproof dressing, paying particular attention to hands and forearms.
Wear protective personal clothing.
Use and dispose of sharps appropriately.
Disinfect body fluid spillages correctly.
Dispose of waste carefully and correctly.
Follow infection control procedures where specific precautions are in place,for example, isolation nursing.

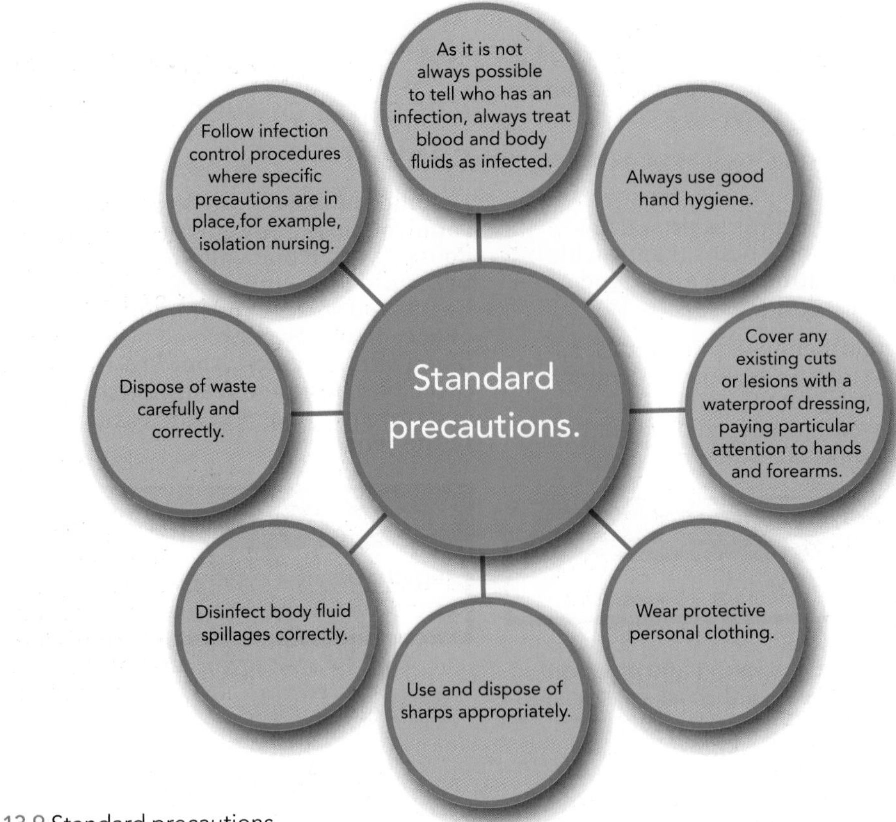

Figure 13.9 Standard precautions

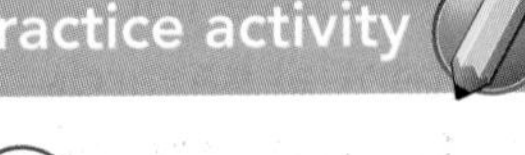


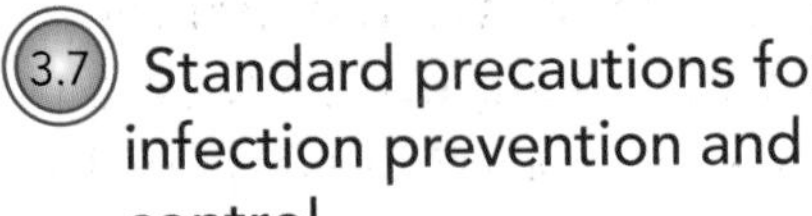


### 3.7 Standard precautions for infection prevention and control

This activity gives you an opportunity to demonstrate that you can apply standard precautions for infection prevention and control.

Think of three moving and handling activities you carry out in which there is a risk of contact with blood or body fluids. For each one, describe the precautions you take to prevent the spread of infection.

# LO4 Preparing individuals before moving and positioning

## 4.1 Communicate effectively with individuals to ensure they understand the details and reasons for the action/activity being undertaken and agree the level of support they require

Unless the people you support understand what is happening to them and why, they can feel a huge loss of independence and dignity and also very frightened. Imagine the feelings associated with having to have, for example, a CT scan or an endoscopy; not knowing why certain things are being done; finding the experience distressing or painful; worrying about how long the procedure will last; and being terrified about the eventual diagnosis. It is essential, therefore, that you reassure the people you support by describing in full any activity you need to carry out and why it needs to be done.

## Time to reflect

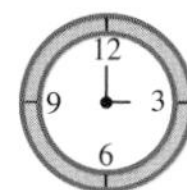

### Do you care?

Does it ever occur to you that the people you support may be frightened, feel they have lost independence and control, or that what they have to undergo takes away their pride and self-respect? If you were in their shoes, how would you like to be treated?

Chapter 1 describes communication techniques that help people understand each other. You need to develop and put effective communication skills into practice to ensure that the people you support understand the details and reasons for your activities with them.

You also need to reach an agreement with them about the level of help and support they require. It's natural that people should want to stay as independent as possible for as long as possible. Taking away someone's independence takes away their control, prevents them from doing what they want to do when they want to do it, and destroys any feelings of self-worth. Reassure the people you work with that you don't intend to 'take over'; that you want to work with them, in a partnership; that you respect what they can do; and that you value their active participation, especially since that makes your job easier and more enjoyable!

Many people find it difficult to admit that they need help and support, especially with everyday activities. Asking for help and support can be embarrassing and challenge their feelings of pride and status. Talk with them about what they can do and what they would like to do. Read between the lines and watch their body language for clues as to where support would be appreciated. It may be as simple as helping them to get up from a chair or clean themselves after using the toilet. It may be that they need help to walk or reposition, because of **vertigo** or pain. Or it may be that movement is tiring, they can't see where they are going, or they are afraid of falling.

## Key term

**Vertigo** is a reeling sensation, a feeling that you are about to fall.

## Time to reflect

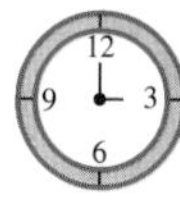

### Can you help?

Think about the people you work with who find it difficult to admit to needing help and support. How do they show their feelings? Are they on the defensive, embarrassed, apologetic? How do you reassure them that it is OK to receive help and support? Why do you think it is important to give this reassurance?

Agreeing the level of support you give maintains independence and dignity. It promotes partnership working and people's right to be cared for in a way that meets their needs and takes account of their choices. The following sections look at how you can give that support, including the use of moving and handling aids and equipment.

## Practice activity

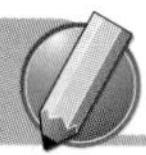

### Communicate effectively with individuals to ensure they understand the details and reasons for the action/activity being undertaken and agree the level of support they require.

This activity gives you an opportunity to demonstrate that you ensure that the people you support understand and agree the details and reasons for your work with them.

Talk to two or three of the people you work with. Ask them for feedback on and how you can improve your ability to:

- communicate to them the details and reasons for your work with them
- agree with them the level of support they need.

They are the experts in their care! Listen to them and act on what they tell you!

## 4.2 Obtaining valid consent for the planned activity

People who use health and social care services have a right to be cared for in a way that meets their needs and takes account of their choices. To impose care on people without respecting their wishes is not only **unethical** it is also illegal.

### Key term

Unethical is behaviour that is neither right, moral nor honourable.

### Time to reflect

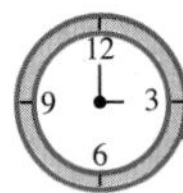

#### 4.2 The right to choose

We all have to conform in one way or another, but life is much more agreeable when we can make choices! How would you feel if your choices were denied, for example if you were told what you could watch on the TV, what to eat, what to wear, and when to get up and go to bed?

Before carrying out a caring activity for a competent adult or child, including helping them to move or reposition, you must obtain their consent. Competence means being able to understand and weigh up the information needed to make a decision. Always assume the people you support are competent unless they demonstrate otherwise. But remember that:

- An unexpected decision or one with which you don't agree does not prove they are incompetent. It might just indicate that they need further information or a simpler explanation.
- They can change their minds and withdraw consent at any time. Always check that consent remains to your caring for them as previously agreed.

### UK country definitions of valid consent

#### England and N Ireland

For consent to be valid, it must be given voluntarily by an appropriately informed person (the person concerned or, where relevant, someone with parental responsibility for a patient under the age of 18) who has the capacity to consent to the **intervention** in question. **Acquiescence** where the person does not know what the intervention entails is not 'consent'.

#### Wales

For consent to be valid, it must be given voluntarily by an appropriately informed person who has the capacity to consent to the intervention in question. The informed person may either be the patient, someone with parental responsibility or a person who has authority under a Power of Attorney. Consent will not be legally valid if the patient has not been given adequate information or where they are under the undue influence of another. Acquiescence where the person does not know what the intervention entails is not 'consent'. Where a patient does not have capacity to give consent, then treatment may be given providing it is given in accordance with the Mental Capacity Act 2005.

#### Scotland

In order for valid consent to treatment to exist, the patient must have been given, and been able to understand, a certain degree of information about the nature, purpose and possible outcomes of the proposed treatment. The case law in Scotland and England broadly suggests that, for the purpose of avoiding civil liability for treatment without consent, a doctor must provide such information as would be provided by a responsible body of medical opinion.

## Key term

An **intervention** is treatment or care provided to improve a situation. **Acquiescence** means consent, agreement.

Some people are competent to make some decisions but not competent to make others. Advocacy services and a variety of different communication methods can help people with learning or communication difficulties to understand any proposed care and treatment. Younger children who fully understand what is involved in a procedure can give consent but when they don't or can't understand, or when they won't give consent, someone with parental responsibility can be asked to do so on their behalf.

Consent must be given voluntarily. Neither you, your colleagues or a person's family and friends are allowed to influence or put pressure on them to consent to care or treatment. In fact, a competent adult is fully entitled to refuse care, even where it would clearly be of benefit. And if an incompetent person indicated in the past, while competent, that they would refuse treatment in certain circumstances (an 'advance refusal'), and those circumstances arise, you must abide by that refusal. However, people can be treated without their consent when:

- the treatment is for a mental disorder and the person is detained under the Mental Health Act 1983
- they are suffering from a notifiable disease (Public Health (Control of Disease) Act 1984).

Consent should be given using a form of communication with which the person is most comfortable, for example it may be spoken, written or be non-verbal, such as British Sign Language or **Makaton**. However, a signature on its own is not sufficient – a consent form must record the decision and discussions that took place in order that the decision could be reached.

## Key term

**Makaton** uses signs and symbols to help people with communication and learning difficulties to communicate.

## Practice activity

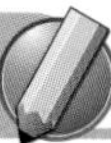

### 4.2 Obtain valid consent for the planned activity

This activity gives you an opportunity to demonstrate that you can obtain valid consent for any moving and handling activity you plan to carry out.

Build on your work for Practice activity 4.1 by checking with the people you support that you do indeed gain their consent for any help and support you plan to give them.

# LO5 Be able to move and position an individual

## 5.1 Follow care plans to ensure that individuals are positioned using agreed techniques and in a way that avoids causing undue pain or discomfort

Moving can be painful and uncomfortable. Bone and joint conditions, strains, sprains and pressure ulcers can make even the slightest movement distressing. Everyone needing help and support to move should be risk assessed to identify techniques that either eliminate the risk of pain and discomfort or reduce it to an absolute minimum. When the person concerned has consented to those techniques they should be written into their care plan and routinely reviewed.

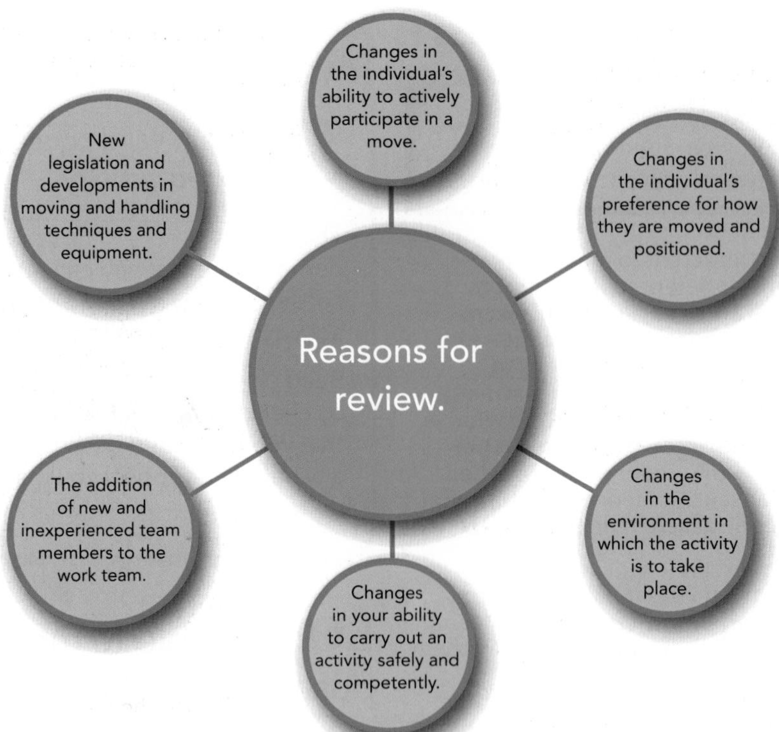


Figure 13.10 Review of moving and handling techniques that are recorded in an individual's care plan

You must follow the instructions within care plans to the letter but remember, only carry out moving and handling activities for which you have been trained and in which you are competent.

## Time to reflect

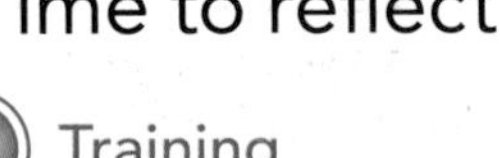

### 5.1 Training

What moving and handling activities have you been trained to carry out?

Do you ever participate in moves for which you have had no formal training?

Imagine that you help someone to move using a technique for which you haven't received training and either they or you get injured. What might be the outcome for you?

Here are Ten Top Tips to ensure that people are moved and positioned using agreed techniques and in a way that will avoid causing undue pain or discomfort.

Before starting the activity:

1. Check the care plan, the moving and handling risk assessment, that equipment is clean, safe and well maintained, and that you have valid consent to carry the activity out.
2. Assess any immediate risks to everyone concerned and get help where you think there is a risk you can't deal with.
3. Tell the person what you need to do, why they are to be moved and handled in a particular way, and help them understand how they can actively participate.
4. Prepare the immediate environment – remove any potential hazards and make sure there is enough space for the move to take place.
5. If appropriate, get help.

Whilst carrying out the activity:

6. Use the correct technique and the correct equipment.
7. Observe the person throughout and if they show any adverse reaction, such as pain and distress, stop and get help.
8. If you run into difficulties, get help.
9. Use appropriate equipment to maintain the person in the required position.

When the activity is finished:

10. Use appropriate documentation to record what you have done, any difficulties you encountered, any pain or discomfort experienced by the person, your suggestions for changes to the activity, and note when the next positioning manoeuvre is due.

## Practice activity 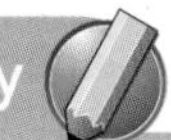

### 5.1 Follow the care plan to ensure that the individual is positioned using the agreed technique and in a way that will avoid causing undue pain or discomfort

This activity gives you an opportunity to demonstrate that you follow care plans to ensure that people are positioned using agreed techniques and in a way that avoids causing undue pain or discomfort.

- Ask your colleagues or a supervisor to observe you as you carry out moving and positioning activities as described in care plans. Act on their feedback to ensure that you use techniques competently and confidently.
- Check with people themselves that the help you give them maintains their comfort. Act on their feedback to ensure you support them in such a way that you avoid causing them any pain or discomfort.

## 5.2 Effective communication with others involved in the manoeuvre

Many moving and positioning activities require teamwork, particularly when the person concerned is heavy or requires a high level of care. Effective team work protects the health and safety of everyone involved.

Ideally team members should be similar in height and strength in order to:

- Avoid awkward movements, such as over-reaching. You read earlier that awkward movements can cause MSDs.
- Ensure that the person's weight is evenly shared. Being overloaded and unbalanced can also cause an MSD.
- Keep the move as smooth and comfortable as possible for everyone concerned.

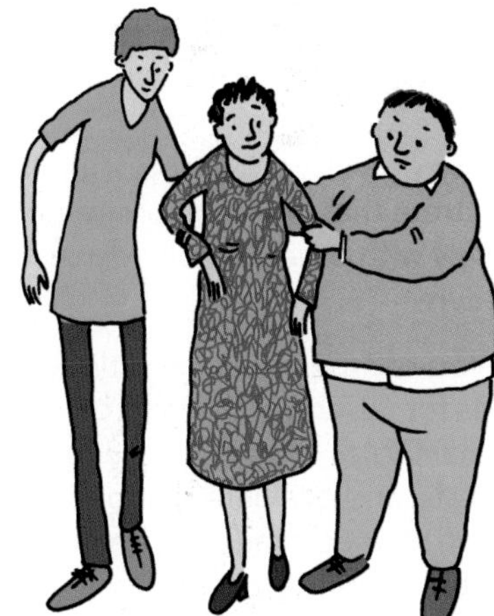

Figure 13.11 Sharing the load?

## Time to reflect 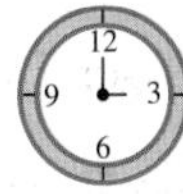

### 5.2 Do as I say, not as I do!

Think about the moving and positioning activities which involve you working with others. How effective are they? What sort of problems have you experienced working in a team? Can you suggest how any problems could be resolved?

An effective team needs a good leader whose experience is worthy of respect and in whom the rest of the team has confidence. Apart from setting a good example by carrying out moving and positioning activities according to agreed techniques, a leader must be able to communicate effectively when:

- ensuring everyone involved, including the person concerned, understands the reason for the manoeuvre and their specific role in enabling it to take place safely
- working with everyone to agree commands, such as 'Ready steady pull'
- issuing commands during the manoeuvre
- evaluating the manoeuvre and how it could be improved.

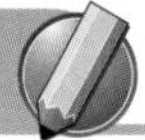

Practice activity

### 5.2 Demonstrate effective communication with any others involved in the manoeuvre

This activity gives you an opportunity to demonstrate that you can communicate effectively with others involved in a manoeuvre.

Keep a log of moving and positioning activities for which you have to give out and explain roles, agree and issue commands, and evaluate manoeuvres. Reflect on your communication skills. Are they effective? Is there room for improvement? What do the others think about your communication skills? Act on their feedback.

## 5.3 Aids and equipment used for moving and positioning

There is a huge number of aids and equipment that can be used to help individuals move, reposition and stay comfortable. They include:

- Mobility scooters and wheelchairs.
- Walking frames, trolleys and sticks.
- Mobile hoists, both manual and electric, that are used to move people from, for example, bed to chair, wheelchair to car.
- Wall and ceiling track hoists, which consist of a rail or track fixed to the wall or ceiling, along which a seat or sling is moved.
- Sling lifts and bath hoists, which are fixed to the floor and have either a sling or a chair seat to lower and raise people into and out of the bath.
- Stand aids, to help a person from sitting to standing and to transfer a short distance.
- Slide sheets, for repositioning a person in bed or moving them from bed to trolley. Their low friction surface prevents pressure ulcers. Some slide sheets have a non-slip area that allows the person to get a heel grip and turn themselves over.
- Monkey poles and bed ladders, to help a person move from lying down to sitting up.
- Inflatable lifting cushions and backrests, to enable people to stand up from a chair and sit up in bed respectively.
- Swivel aids, turntables, turn disks, for transferring people from one sitting or standing position to another.
- Transfer boards for lateral transfer, for example, bed to chair, chair to wheelchair, wheelchair to car.
- Handling belts, for gripping a person prior to a move, often used in conjunction with swivel aids, transfer boards and slide sheets.
- Leg lifters.

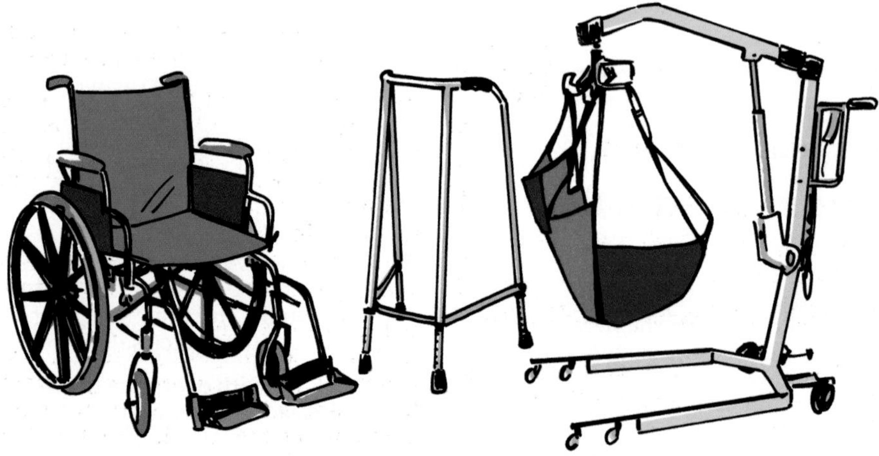

Figure 13.12 Aids and equipment

**Evidence activity** 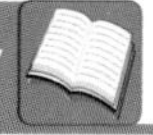

### 5.3 Aids and equipment used for moving and positioning

This activity gives you an opportunity to demonstrate your knowledge about aids and equipment used in moving and positioning activities.

Complete the table below

| Aids and equipment used in moving and positioning activities at my workplace | Function |
|---|---|
| | |
| | |
| | |
| | |

## 5.4 Equipment that maintains the individual in the appropriate position

Because some people are unable to maintain a stable posture, they require frequent repositioning, either unaided or with help. This can be tiring and uncomfortable, disrupt their concentration, affect their quality of life, compromise their dignity and cause pressure ulcers.

**Research & investigate** 

### 5.4 Reposition for repose

What equipment is available at your workplace to help individuals maintain a stable, comfortable posture?

Frequent repositioning can be avoided by using equipment that maintains the appropriate position, for example:

- Support chairs, standing frames and wheeled walkers that have head, arm, knee and foot supports and straps; and chest and hip pads, all of which can be adjusted for comfort and safety.
- Positioning wedges, such as those used to prop someone into position when in bed.
- Orthopaedic supports, braces and immobilising slings.
- Slide sheets that allow movement in one direction only, helping people who tend to slide forwards or to the side to stay upright.

**Evidence activity** 

### 5.4 Equipment for maintaining someone in the appropriate position

This activity gives you an opportunity to demonstrate that you can use equipment to help people maintain an appropriate position.

Make a list of the people you work with who are unable to maintain a stable posture and describe how you help them to do so. Remember to maintain their confidentiality.

## 5.5 Encouraging individuals to actively participate in manoeuvres

You read earlier that active participation involves the people you support being active partners in their care. Active participation is important, for two main reasons:

1. It helps the person stay as independent as possible for as long as possible.
2. It helps protect your health and safety. A problem shared is a problem halved!

Before you carry out a manoeuvre, ask the person how they think they can help and what help they think they would like. Answers will vary on a day-to-day basis, depending on mood, motivation, level of confidence, fear of falling, fear of pain, physical health status and so on. Remind them that you are there to provide support but that you want them to be in control.

Sometimes you may be asked to help in a way that is not within your job scope, in which you haven't been trained, or that you know could risk health and safety. Some moving and handling manoeuvres are so risky that they have been condemned. Be sensitive when explaining why you can't comply with their request, and reach a compromise that will enable you to work within health and safety guidelines whilst at the same time meeting their needs.

**Condemned moving and handling manoeuvres**

Drag lift.

Australian or shoulder lift.

Orthodox or cradle lift.

Any manoeuvres involving the person's hands being placed around the handler's neck or body.

Any manoeuvres involving the lifting of most or the entire body weight of a person without the use of a mechanical lifting aid.

**Evidence activity** 

**5.5 Encouraging active participation in a manoeuvre**

This activity gives you an opportunity to demonstrate that you encourage people to actively participate in moving and positioning manoeuvres.

Think about three moving and positioning activities in which you encourage people to actively participate. In what ways do they help in the move? Why is it useful for them to contribute like this?

## 5.6 Monitoring the individual throughout the activity so that the procedure can be stopped if there is any adverse reaction

You read earlier that it is important to observe people throughout a manoeuvre and that if they show any adverse reaction, to stop and get help. Adverse reactions include:

- distress due to fear, pain, discomfort, a lack of confidence in the handler and anxiety about relying on equipment
- a failure to follow instructions, due to difficulty in hearing or understanding, or a change in the ability or desire to cooperate
- a change in **muscle tone**, unexpected movement, loss of balance
- sprained joints, trapped fingers and limbs, and dislodged healthcare attachments due to poor positioning
- changes in medical status, for example a drop in blood pressure, loss of consciousness, restricted ability to breathe
- fatigue.

Be on the alert for adverse reactions throughout every manoeuvre you perform. If you detect any risks to health and safety, stop what you're doing and get help without delay.

**Key term** 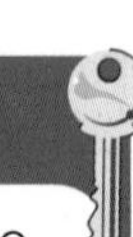

**Muscle tone** is the tension or resistance to movement in a muscle that enables us to keep our bodies in a certain position.

**Evidence activity** 

**5.6 Monitor the individual throughout the activity so that the procedure can be stopped if there is any adverse reaction**

This activity gives you an opportunity to demonstrate that you monitor people when helping them to move or reposition so that you can stop the procedure in the event of an adverse reaction.

Think about three moving and positioning activities that you stopped because of an adverse reaction. What caused the person concerned to react in these ways? What have you learnt from these experiences?

## 5.7 Report and record the activity, including when the next positioning manoeuvre is due

It is extremely important that you follow your workplace's procedures for reporting and recording any moving and positioning manoeuvres you undertake, including accidents, incidents and near misses. Verbal reports should be made to the relevant person; and written records should be made in care plans and on appropriate accident/incident report forms.

## Research & investigate

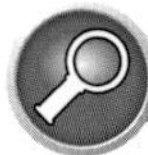

### 5.7 Record keeping

What does your workplace's policy require of you with regard to reporting and recording:

- Moving and handling activities?
- The timing of moving and handling activities?

Report and record any adverse reactions during a manoeuvre. This will trigger a review of the manoeuvre to ensure that the situation does not recur. And use care plans to record details about every manoeuvre that is carried out and when the next is due. Failure to reposition someone, to transfer them when necessary to the toilet or bath, and to generally help them keep moving as much as possible, amounts to neglect. As you read earlier, skin breaks down after a prolonged period of exposure to moisture and pressure ulcers can develop after lengthy periods of sitting or lying in the same position. So it is important that you and your colleagues know when to reposition the people you work with.

Any hazards you identify with the manoeuvre, the person concerned, aids and equipment, and with the working environment must be reported and recorded without delay. Similarly, any accidents, incidents and near misses must be reported and recorded. Unless hazards, accidents, incidents and near misses are reported, their cause can't be investigated and they will continue to put health and safety at risk.

Finally, make sure your colleagues and line manager know about any personal factors such as MSDs, illness or pregnancy that might affect your ability to carry out manoeuvres in the future.

# LO6 Know when to seek advice from and/or involve others when moving and positioning an individual

## 6.1 Seeking advice and/or assistance to move or handle an individual safely

## Time to reflect

### 6.1 Help!

- In what circumstances do you currently get help or advice to carry out moving and handling activities?
- Why might you not seek help?
- What might be the outcome if you carried out an activity for which you didn't feel 100 per cent confident or competent?

If you're pregnant, feel yourself coming down with an infection, have an MSD or are concerned that you're not physically big or strong enough to participate in a particular manoeuvre, get advice from your manager about whether or not you should carry it out.

If you're asked to participate in a manoeuvre in which you haven't been trained, politely refuse but get help. And apply for training! Health and care work depends on people being able to work together – if you can't do a job due to lack of training, you're not much good to anyone!

## Evidence activity

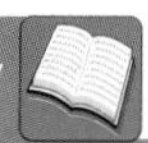

### 5.7 Report and record the activity, noting when the next positioning manoeuvre is due

This activity gives you an opportunity to demonstrate that you know how to report and record moving and positioning activities, including when the next positioning manoeuvre is due.

Produce an information sheet for use in a training session that tells your colleagues how to report and record any moving and positioning activities they undertake and the importance of noting when the next positioning manoeuvre is due.

You may be asked to help in a manoeuvre:

- which isn't included in the care plan
- which isn't within the scope of your job role
- that you know could cause injury.

Get help when you cannot reach a compromise that will enable you to work within health and safety guidelines.

If, despite being trained, you're not confident in being able to carry out a manoeuvre competently, seek advice from an experienced colleague. Ask them to supervise you and help you where necessary until you can demonstrate the required level of competence.

If you have concerns that a manoeuvre is no longer appropriate for someone, because, for example, their health or ability to understand instructions has changed, get help. The manoeuvre may have to be reviewed and adapted.

If you have concerns that any aids or equipment are not sufficiently clean or well-maintained, get help. Don't put health and safety at risk by using unsafe equipment.

**Evidence activity** 

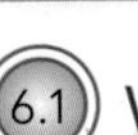

### 6.1 When advice and/or assistance should be sought to move or handle someone safely

This activity gives you an opportunity to demonstrate that you know when to seek advice regarding safe moving or handling.

Make a list of the occasions when, because of fears for safety with regard to moving or handling an individual, you have sought advice or assistance.

## 6.2 Sources of information about moving and positioning individuals

Sources of information about moving and positioning individuals.
Experienced colleagues.
Professionals including back care advisors, H&S and risk assessment staff, moving and handling trainers and assessors, physiotherapists.
The individuals themselves.
Moving and handling risk assessments.
Care plans.
Websites.
Manufacturers instructions for aids and equipment.
Books, Government publications and Guidelines, and specialist journals.
Training courses

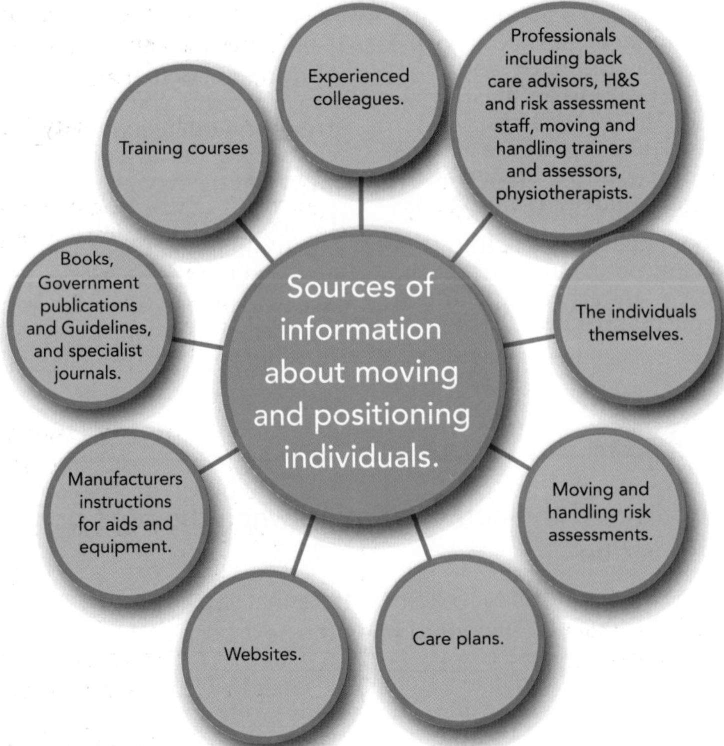

Figure 13.13 Sources of information about moving and positioning individuals

## Evidence activity

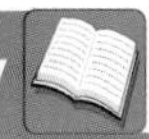

### 6.2 Sources of information that are available about moving and positioning individuals

This activity gives you an opportunity to demonstrate your knowledge of sources of information about moving and positioning the people you support.

Produce a list of sources of information about moving and positioning individuals that can be retained within care plans and risk assessment records.

## Assessment summary

Your reading of this chapter and completion of the activities will have prepared you to demonstrate your learning and understanding of how to move and position individuals in accordance with their plan of care. To achieve the unit, your assessor will require you to:

| Learning Outcomes | Assessment Criteria |
|---|---|
| Learning outcome 1: Understand anatomy and physiology in relation to moving and positioning individuals by: | 1.1 outlining the anatomy and physiology of the human body in relation to the importance of correct moving and positioning of individuals<br>See Evidence activity 1.1 p. 237. |
| | 1.2 describing the impact of specific conditions on the correct movement and positioning of an individual.<br>See Evidence activity 1.2 p. 239. |
| Learning outcome 2: Understand current legislation and agreed ways of working when moving and positioning individuals by: | 2.1 describing how current legislation and agreed ways of working affect working practices related to moving and positioning individuals<br>See Evidence activity 2.1 p. 241. |
| | 2.2 describing what health and safety factors need to be taken into account when moving and positioning individuals and any equipment used to do this.<br>See Evidence activity 2.2 p. 243. |
| Learning outcome 3: Be able to minimise risk before moving and positioning individuals by: | 3.1 accessing up-to-date copies of risk assessment documentation.<br>See Practice activity 3.1 p. 244. |

| Learning Outcomes | Assessment Criteria |
|---|---|
| Learning outcome 3: Be able to minimise risk before moving and positioning individuals by: | 3.2 carrying out preparatory checks using:<br>• the individual's care plan<br>• the moving and handling risk assessment.<br>See Practice activity 3.2 p. 244. |
| | 3.3 identifying any immediate risks to the individual<br>See Evidence activity 3.3 p. 244. |
| | 3.4 describing actions to take in relation to identified risks<br>See Evidence activity 3.4 p. 246. |
| | 3.5 describing what action should be taken if the individual's wishes conflict with their plan of care in relation to health and safety and their risk assessment<br>See Evidence activity 3.5 p. 247. |
| | 3.6 preparing the immediate environment ensuring<br>• adequate space for the move in agreement with all concerned<br>• that potential hazards are removed.<br>See Practice activity 3.6 p. 249. |
| | 3.7 applying standard precautions for infection prevention and control.<br>See Practice activity 3.7 p. 250. |
| Learning outcome 4: Be able to prepare individuals before moving and positioning by: | 4.1 demonstrating effective communication with the individual to ensure that they<br>• understand the details and reasons for the action/activity being undertaken<br>• agree the level of support required<br>See Practice activity 4.1 p. 251. |

| Learning Outcomes | Assessment Criteria |
| --- | --- |
| Learning outcome 4: Be able to prepare individuals before moving and positioning by: | 4.2 obtaining valid consent for the planned activity.<br><br>See Practice activity 4.2 p. 253. |
| Learning outcome 5: Be able to move and position an individual by: | 5.1 following the care plan to ensure that the individual is positioned<br>• using the agreed technique<br>• in a way that will avoid causing undue pain or discomfort<br><br>See Practice activity 5.1 p. 255. |
| | 5.2 demonstrating effective communication with any others involved in the manoeuvre<br><br>See Practice activity 5.2 p. 256. |
| | 5.3 describing the aids and equipment that may be used for moving and positioning<br><br>See Evidence activity 5.3 p. 257. |
| | 5.4 using equipment to maintain the individual in the appropriate position<br><br>See Practice activity 5.4 p. 257. |
| | 5.5 encouraging the individual's active participation in the manoeuvre<br><br>See Practice activity 5.5 p. 258. |
| | 5.6 monitoring the individual throughout the activity so that the procedure can be stopped if there is any adverse reaction<br><br>See Practice activity 5.6 p. 258. |
| | 5.7 demonstrating how to report and record the activity noting when the next positioning manoeuvre is due.<br><br>See Practice activity 5.7 p. 259. |

| Learning Outcomes | Assessment Criteria |
|---|---|
| Learning outcome **6**: Know when to seek advice from and/or involve others when moving and positioning an individual by: | 6.1 describing when advice and/or assistance should be sought to move or handle an individual safely <br>See Evidence activity 6.1 p. 260. |
| | 6.2 describing what sources of information are available about moving and positioning individuals. <br>See Evidence activity 6.2 p. 261. |

Good luck!

## Weblinks

Health and Safety Executive www.hse.gov.uk
Royal College of Nursing www.rcn.org.uk

# GLOSSARY

Acas provides confidential and impartial advice to assist workers in resolving issues in the workplace.

Accessible means easily located, understandable, straightforward and manageable.

An accident is an unforeseen incident that can result in a person being injured.

Active means involved, taking part.

Active participation means to be an active rather than a passive partner in one's own care and support.

Acquiescence means consent, agreement.

Adrenaline is a hormone that stimulates the nervous system, stimulating the heart and breathing, and causes a sense of alertness and excitement.

Allied health professionals are clinical healthcare professionals as distinct from doctors, dentists and nurses, who work in a healthcare team to make the healthcare system function.

Ambient means surrounding.

Ancillary workers in health and social care are staff who do not provide hands-on care.

Apathy means lack of interest, indifference.

Apnoea means a pause in breathing.

Aseptic means free of disease-causing micro-organisms.

Autonomous means independent, not controlled by others.

A barrier hand cream helps reduce the effects of skin contact with a harmful substance.

Braille is a system of writing and printing for blind or visually impaired people. Varied arrangements of raised dots representing letters and numerals are identified by touch.

Bronchi are the large airways that carry air into the lungs.

A carer is someone, who, without payment, provides help and support to a partner, child, relative, friend or neighbour, who could not manage without their help.

A catheter is a plastic tube inserted into the body to drain fluid.

CCTV means Closed Circuit Television.

Citizenship relates to being a citizen of a particular community with the duties, rights and privileges of this status.

Coaching is a method of directing, instructing and training a person or group of people, in order that they achieve some goal or develop specific skills.

Cognitive impairment means difficulty in carrying out cognitive abilities.

Comatose means unable to move voluntarily and unable to understand what is happening.

Common law forms the basis of the legal system.

A communal environment is an environment which is shared by a group of people.

Compensate means to give something, such as money, as payment or reparation for a service or loss.

Competence is to do with having knowledge, understanding and capability.

The complainant is the person making a complaint.

To condone means to ignore, excuse, forgive, make allowances for.

Confabulation means inventing events to fill the gaps in memory.

Confidentiality is keeping a secret within a certain circle of persons.

Conscious means aware, purposely.

Continuing Professional Development is the process by which a workforce can maintain, improve and broaden their knowledge and skills and develop the personal qualities required in their work lives.

The CRB holds information about individuals, such as convictions, cautions, reprimands and warnings.

Critical means examining thoroughly, both the positives and the negatives.

Cross-infection is the spread of pathogens from one person, object, place or part of the body to another.

The Data Protection Act 1998 is legislation for the protection of an individual's information.

Deficiency diseases are caused by a shortage of vitamins or minerals in the diet.

Delict is a concept of civil law in which a wilful wrong or an act of negligence gives rise to a legal obligation between parties, even though there has been no contract between the parties.

Direct payments are local council payments to people who have been assessed as needing help from social services, and who would like to arrange and pay for their own care and support services instead of receiving them directly from the local council.

Discrimination is the acting out of negative prejudices.

Disengage means to detach, withdraw from something.

Disorientation is confusion due to the loss of spatial ability.

Diversity is when many different types of things or people are included in something.

Domiciliary means at home.

Domiciliary care is the provision of care in the individual's own home.

Dyspraxia is a condition which affects ability to perform coordinated movements.

Empathy means identifying with that person's position, in order to understand from their perspective. It is also used to mean understanding and compassion.

Empowering means allowing individuals to have control over their own lives.

An episode of care is one of a series of care tasks in the course of a continuous care activity.

Equality relates to being equal, especially of having the same political, social and economic rights.

The Equality Act 2010 is a legislation framework to protect the rights of individuals and advance equality of opportunity for all.

Evidence-based policies are policies that have been proved to work.

Exudate is fluid that seeps out of injured tissues.

A fitting is any item that is free standing or hung by a nail or hook.

A fixture is any item that is bolted to the floor or walls.

Fractured means broken.

The frontal lobe is the front part of the brain.

A Green Paper is a consultation document issued by the government that contains policy proposals for debate and discussion before a final decision is taken on the best policy option.

Haemoglobin is the protein in red blood cells that carries the oxygen needed by the body to create energy.

A hallucination is seeing and hearing things that don't exist.

Health Protection Units (HPUs) are local centres of the Health Protection Agency (HPA).

A hearing loop provides information on an induction loop system, to assist the hearing impaired by transmitting sound from a sound system, microphone, television or other source, directly to a hearing aid.

Holistic means the 'whole'. In health this tends to mean the whole person and not just physical health.

A holistic approach is one that meets all aspects of an individual's care needs, including physical, intellectual, emotional, social and spiritual.

The HSE is the national independent watchdog for work-related health, safety and illness, working to reduce workplace death and serious injury.

The Human Rights Act 1998 is legislation for the protection of an individual's fundamental rights.

Hypertension means high blood pressure.

Impaired means damaged.

Incidence means occurrence.

Inclusion means to include all.

Inclusive means not excluding any individual or section of society.

An indwelling device is a device that is inserted into body, like a catheter.

Informed means having enough information and knowledge to fully understand.

Integrity means morally-upright, credible, trusting.

Intellectual fitness means being open to new ideas, thinking critically, being creative and curious, and being motivated to learning new things.

Inter-agency working, also known as multi-agency working, means involving two or more agencies.

Interdependence means dependence between two or more people.

Interpersonal skills are the skills we use to interact with others.

An intervention is treatment or care provided to improve a situation.

Isolation nursing is the physical separation of an infected patient from others.

Jargon is the specialist or technical language of a trade or profession.

A label is a 'tag' that we use to describe someone and is usually based on their appearance and behaviour.

Liability is the state of being legally obliged and responsible.

A ligament is a band of tissue that connects bones, typically to support a joint.

List 99 is a list of teachers who are considered unsuitable or banned from working with children in school.

Logistics means the organisation of services, supplies, resources.

Makaton uses signs and symbols to help people with communication and learning difficulties to communicate.

Manual involves using human effort, skill, power, energy.

Media is a means of communication, such as radio, television, newspapers and magazines, that reach or influence people widely.

A mediator is an intermediary third party, which is neutral and helps negotiate agreed outcomes.

Mencap is the leading UK charity for people who have a learning disability and their families.

Mentoring refers to a developmental relationship in which a more experienced person helps someone who has less experience.

Micro-organisms are organisms such as bacteria, parasites and fungi that can only be seen using a microscope.

Mucous membranes are mucous-secreting membranes that line the body cavities and canals that connect with the external air, such as the alimentary canal and respiratory tract.

Muscle tone is the tension or resistance to movement in a muscle that enables us to keep our bodies in a certain position.

Musculoskeletal disorders happen when the musculoskeletal system is injured over time.

The musculoskeletal system is the system of muscles and tendons and ligaments and bones and joints and associated tissues that move the body and maintain its form.

A needle stick injury is a skin puncture by a hypodermic needle or other sharp object.

Neurological disorders are disorders of the brain.

A neurotransmitter is a chemical that transmits messages between nerve cells.

Acting objectively means not being influenced by personal feelings or opinions.

An organic brain disorder is one where a person's behaviour changes because of damage to the brain.

Passive means uninvolved, having things 'done to'.

Paramount means of the upmost importance.

Paraphrasing is rephrasing what you have been told in your own words.

A pathogen is a disease-producing bacterium, fungi, virus, infestation or prion.

A PEG feeding tube is a tube that is placed through the patient's skin into their stomach as a means of feeding them.

A perpetrator is someone who carries out an act of abuse

Perseveration means to use the same words and behaviours over and over again without any specific purpose.

Person-centred planning is a process of life planning for individuals, based around the principles of inclusion and the social model of disability.

Person-centred services aim to improve a person's life by meeting their needs and involving them in the way the services are run.

Pick's Disease is a rare disorder that damages cells in the front part of the brain.

Plaques are insoluble protein deposits that build up around nerve cells.

The PoVA and PoCA schemes were replaced by the Vetting and Barring Scheme in October 2009.

Point of care is the location where care is given.

To be predisposed to a situation means to be inclined to it.

A prejudice is an attitude or way of thinking based on an unfair pre-judgement of a person, rather than on a factual assessment.

Prevalence means the proportion of individuals in a population having a disease.

The Privacy Act 1974 is legislation to protect your privacy.

Prognosis is the prediction of the probable course and outcome of a disease.

Professional registration demonstrates that you have met standards of competence and is a requirement for employment of a number of professionals.

The public sector consists of organisations that are controlled by national and local government.

Reportable injuries are those that need to be reported to the HSE through the RIDDOR reporting system.

A reservoir is an environment in which a micro-organism can live and reproduce.

RIDDOR stands for Reporting of Injuries, Diseases and Dangerous Occurrences Regulations.

The Royal College of Nursing (RCN) represents nurses and nursing, promotes excellence in practice and shapes health policies.

Sector Skills Councils (SSCs) are employer-led organisations that work to boost the skills of their sector workforces.

Self-fulfilling prophecy means a prediction that directly or indirectly causes itself to become true.

Sharps include needles, scalpels, stitch cutters and glass ampoules.

Short term memory (STM) is the ability of the brain to recall recent events.

Single-use equipment is items that can only be used once.

Skin pallor means paleness or rosiness of the skin.

A slipped disc occurs when one of the discs of the spine is ruptured and the jelly-like substance inside leaks out, putting pressure on the spinal cord. It causes intense back pain as well as pain in other areas of the body.

Socio-emotional needs refers to someone's social and emotional needs.

Spatial ability is the ability to understand the way our surroundings are laid out and to be aware of where we are within them.

A spore is a temporary, dormant structure into which a bacterium changes when conditions for its survival become hazardous.

A stakeholder is a person or group having an interest in the success of an activity, enterprise etc.

Standard precautions are based upon a set of principles designed to minimise exposure to and transmission of a wide variety of micro-organisms.

Stigma means shame, disgrace.

Subconscious means not aware, oblivious.

Tangles are insoluble twisted protein fibres that build up inside nerve cells.

A tendon is a band of tissue that connects a muscle with a bone.

Tissue is a collection of cells that have the same function.

Tissue viability is to do with the ability of the skin to remain intact and healthy.

Tort is any wrongdoing for which an action for damages may be brought.

Unethical is behaviour that is neither right, moral nor honourable.

Vertigo is a reeling sensation, a feeling that you are about to fall.

A vesicle is a blister.

Viable means alive and able to reproduce.

The voluntary sector, also known as the third sector, consists of charitable, non-profit-making organisations.

Well-being means in good health, happiness and prosperity.

Western societies are societies in the first or developed world, where medicine is based on science.

Willful means deliberate, intentional.

# INDEX